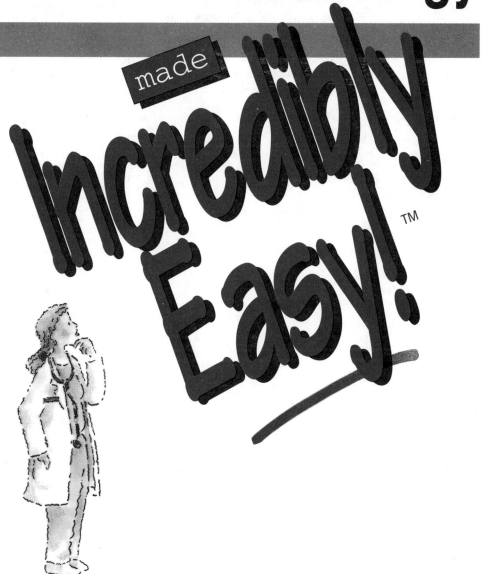

Medical Terminology made Incredibly Easy!™

Springhouse Corporation
Springhouse, Pennsylvania

Staff

Publisher
Judith A. Schilling McCann, RN, MSN

Design Director
John Hubbard

Editorial Director
Michael Shaw

Clinical Manager
Joan M. Robinson, RN, MSN, CCRN

Clinical Editors
Collette Bishop Hendler, RN, CCRN (clinical project manager); Sammie Justesen, RN, BSN; Lori Musolf Neri, RN, MSN, CRNP, CCRN

Senior Associate Editor
Brenna H. Mayer

Editors
Ty Eggenberger, Kevin Haworth, Jacqueline Mills, Stephen Page, Kirk Robinson, Frank Thakuria

Copy Editors
Jaime Stockslager (supervisor), Priscilla DeWitt, Mary T. Durkin, Amy Furman, Kimberly A. J. Johnson, Scotti Kent, Pamela Wingrod

Designers
Arlene Putterman (associate design director), Mary Ludwicki (art director), Joseph John Clark, Lynn Foulk

Illustrators
Bot Roda, Mary Stangl, Bob Neumann, Jean Gardner, Bob Jackson, John Murphy, John Cymerman, Judy Newhouse, Phillip Ashley, Dan Fione

Projects Coordinator
Liz Schaeffer

Electronic Production Services
Diane Paluba (manager), Joyce Rossi Biletz

Manufacturing
Deborah Meiris (director), Patricia K. Dorshaw (manager), Otto Mezei (book production manager)

Editorial and Design Assistants
Tom Hasenmayer, Beverly Lane, Beth Janae Orr, Elfriede Young

Indexer
Ellen Brennan

Printed in the United States of America.

MTIE- D N O
03 02 01 00 10 9 8 7 6 5 4 3 2 1

Library of Congress Cataloging-in-Publication Data

Medical terminology made incredibly easy.
p. ; cm.
Includes index.
1. Medicine—Terminology. 2. Medical sciences—Terminology
[DNLM: 1. Terminology. W 15 M4887 2001]
R123.M394 2001
610'.1'—dc21
00-041974
ISBN 1-58255-041-7 CIP

Contents

Contributors and consultants

Steven R. Abel, PharmD, FASHP
Head of Department of Pharmacy Practice
Purdue University
Indianapolis

Gary J. Arnold, MD, FACS
Associate Professor, College of Nursing
University of Louisiana
Lafayette

Tricia M. Berry, PharmD
Assistant Professor, Department of Pharmacy Practice
Saint Louis College of Pharmacy

Donelle Bussom, RN, MSN, OCN
Medical Affairs Manager
ICON Clinical Research, Inc.
North Wales, Pa.

Susan Christie, PT, BS, ATP
Supervisor, Assistive Technology Center
Bryn Mawr Rehab
Malvern, Pa.

Nancy Cirone, RNC, MSN, CDE
Director of Education
Warminster (Pa.) Hospital

Christine S. Clayton, RN, MS, CNP
Nurse Practitioner, Cardiology Service
Sioux Valley Hospital and University Medical Center
Sioux Falls, S.Dak.

Mary Collins Derivan, RN, MSN, AOCN
Private consultant
Newtown, Pa.

Ellie Z. Franges, MSN, CNRN
Director of Neuroscience Services
Sacred Heart Hospital
Allentown, Pa.

Michelle A. Green, MPS, RHIA, CMA, CTR
Professor
Alfred (N.Y.) State College

Jean Croce Hemphill, RNC, MSN, FNP
Assistant Professor, Department of Family and Community Nursing
East Tennessee State University
Johnson City

Shelton M. Hisley, RNC, PhD, WHNP, ACCE
Assistant Professor, School of Nursing
University of North Carolina
Wilmington

Lucy J. Hood, RN, DNSc
Associate Professor
Saint Luke's College
Kansas City, Mo.

Thomas E. Lafferty, MD
Rheumatology Physician
Ocala (Fla.) Orthopedic Group

Paul J. Mathews, RRT, PhD
Associate Professor
University of Kansas
Kansas City, Mo.

Brady S. Moffett, PharmD
Pharmacy Practice Resident
University of Maryland Medical Center
Baltimore

Debra Shelby, ARNP, RNFA, MSN
Nurse Practitioner
Water's Edge Dermatology
Palm Beach Gardens, Fla.

Kim Siewert, PharmD
Clinical Pharmacist
Cardinal Health System - Ball Memorial Hospital
Muncie, Ind.

Monica R. Walter, RN, MSN, NPC
Nurse Practitioner
Gastrointestinal Specialists, Inc.
Philadelphia

Foreword

Let's start with a quick test. **Dysphagia** is:

A) a type of cheese made from the milk of rare goats.

B) a Greek drama you read in college.

C) the sticking feeling you get in your throat when you have to learn medical terms.

Let's face it. For many people, confronting a long list of medical terminology can create an immediate set of adverse reactions — headache, dizziness, loss of appetite — not to mention dysphagia (difficulty swallowing). If you're involved in health care, you need to have a firm grasp of medical terminology to do your job quickly and efficiently. You want a way to gain that knowledge without reviewing endless lists, memorizing obscure phrases, and forgetting new words as soon as you've learned them. In short, you want to increase your understanding, not your frustration.

That is why the clinical experts at Springhouse created *Medical Terminology Made Incredibly Easy*, a remarkable book that promotes real understanding and retention of the medical terms you need to know — and does it without taking itself too seriously!

The first chapter, "Key concepts of medical terminology," uses an easy-to-read format to build familiarity with medical terminology. Important terms are broken down, along with definitions and examples, providing you with an understanding of *how* medical terms are put together.

Subsequent chapters focus on individual body systems, providing in-depth definitions that help connect words to their meanings. You may find yourself exploring the Greek or Latin origin of a word in order to develop connections between related terms. Alternatively, because many medical terms derive from a person's name, brief biographical sketches place each term in a vivid context. Beautiful illustrations and clear charts also provide visual keys that enhance your learning. In addition, each chapter contains a focus on "real world" uses of words so that your learning is always applicable to actual patient care.

Medical Terminology Made Incredibly Easy also includes a variety of features that promote learning while maintaining a light-hearted, irreverent tone. Checklists at the beginning of each chapter provide a quick review of important terms. Cartoon characters appear regularly to reinforce key points and may even prompt a few chuckles. *Quick quizzes* at the end of each chapter help you assess your progress. Special logos throughout alert you to important information:

Beyond the dictionary further explains a medical term's origins, including interesting side notes to help you remember more easily.

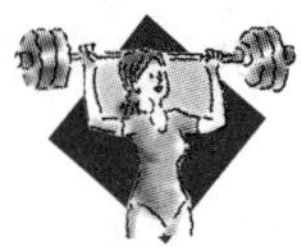

Pump up your pronunciation clearly shows the correct way to pronounce key medical terms. Can you say *Leiomyosarcoma?* LEYE-OH-MY-OH-SAR-KOH-MAH — now you can!

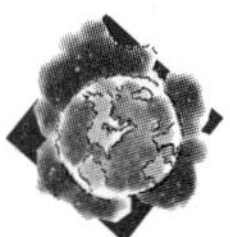

The real world relates medical terminology to commonly used clinical applications and abbreviations you'll encounter in practice.

Health care professionals and students alike will find *Medical Terminology Made Incredibly Easy* an indispensable reference. Students enrolled in a variety of health care disciplines will enjoy learning complex terms in a rewarding way. They'll find that this book serves as an essential complement to the study of anatomy and physiology and pathology. Practicing health care professionals will find their confidence soaring as difficult terms become familiar and discussion about even common terms produces new levels of insight. Enjoy the pleasures of learning medical terminology — without any unpleasant adverse effects.

Cheryl T. Samuels, PhD
Dean and Professor
College of Health Sciences
Old Dominion University
Norfolk, Va.

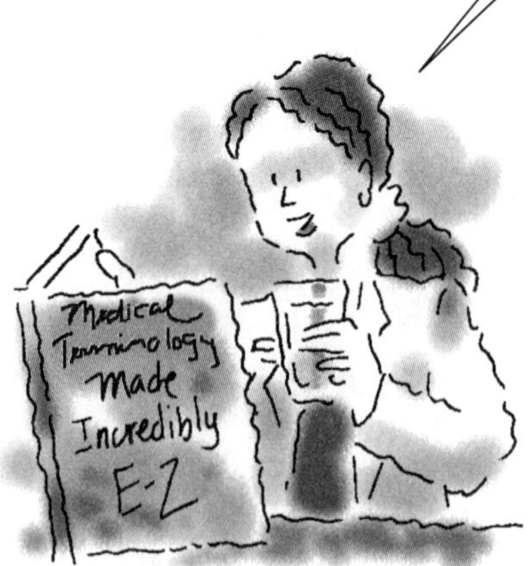
Medical Terminology Made Incredibly Easy (n.): the most intelligent and entertaining way to learn essential medical terms
Medical Terminology Made Incredibly E-Z

Key concepts of medical terminology

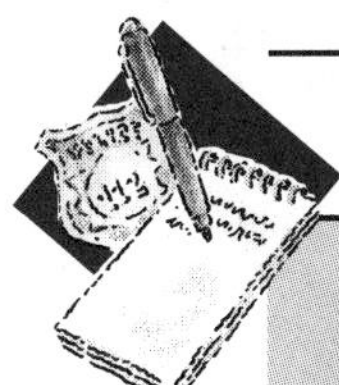

Just the facts

In this chapter, you'll review:

- how to dissect words
- how to quickly find their meaning using roots, prefixes, and suffixes.

Medical terms

Because many medical terms derive from Greek and Latin, learning medical terminology is like learning a new language. Understanding these terms can be easier if you know how to analyze key elements and identify word associations.

Take it apart

Most medical terms are a combination of two or more parts. If you can successfully interpret each part, you can usually grasp the essential meaning of the word. Thus, interpreting the meaning of a medical term requires knowledge of common medical roots, prefixes, and suffixes.

Root it out

A root is the essential component of a word. Many medical roots signify a disease, procedure, or body part. Some roots appear at the beginning of a word, whereas others appear after a prefix, before a suffix, or between a prefix and a suffix. In addition, two or more roots may be combined to form a word (usually with the letter ***-o-***), as in ***cardi-o-pulmonary*** and ***cardi-o-vascular.*** Here are some examples of roots used in different positions:

• a root at the beginning of a word — ***angi***oedema (***angi*** is a root that means *vessel*)
• a root in the middle of a word — en***cephal***ic (***cephal*** is a root that means *head*)
• a root at the end of a word — sclero***derm***a (***derm*** is a root that means *skin*)
• a combination of roots — ***phototherapy*** (***photo*** is a root that means *light;* ***therapy*** is a root that means *treatment*).

In the beginning

A prefix consists of one or more letters attached to the beginning of a root; many prefixes used for medical terms are also applied to standard English vocabulary. To determine the meaning of a prefix in a medical term, consider a familiar word that begins with the same prefix. For example, the prefix ***anti-*** has the same meaning — *against* — in both *antislavery* and *antihistamine,* literally *against slavery* and *against histamine* (the compound that produces allergic reactions).

At last

A suffix is one or more letters attached to the end of a root. When a suffix begins with a consonant, a combining vowel, such as ***o,*** is placed before the suffix. Common suffixing in medical terminology includes adding a ***-y*** to a word to denote a procedure, such as, *gastroscop**y**,* which means *an endoscopic examination of the stomach.* Similarly, adding ***-ly*** to a word denotes an act or process; for example, *splenomega**ly**,* which means *the abnormal enlargement of the spleen.*

If you can understand the building blocks, then you will have the foundation to learn even the most complicated medical terminology.

Break it down; build it up

With a bit of practice, you'll quickly discover how easy it can be to interpret the parts of a medical term and then combine them to identify the term's meaning. For example, in *acrocyanosis,* the root ***acr*** *(extremities)* and the vowel ***o*** are combined with the root ***cyan*** *(blue)* and the suffix ***-osis*** *(condition)* to form a term that means *a condition characterized by blue extremities.* (See *'Dem bones.*)

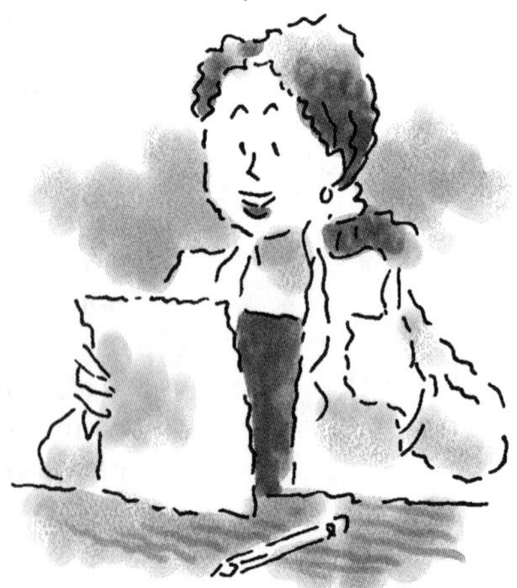

Beyond the dictionary

'Dem bones

A specialist in **osteopathology** studies bone diseases. The root ***oste*** is the Greek word for *bone.* A second root ***patho*** is derived from *pathos,* meaning *disease.* The suffix ***-logy*** is derived from the Greek root ***logia,*** meaning *the study of.* Put these parts together and you have the definition for **osteopathology** — *the study of bone diseases.*

At the root of disease?
A branch of medicine called **osteopathy** maintains that skeletal misalignment impinges on adjacent nerves and blood vessels, causing disease.

Plural words

Plural words in English are usually formed by adding ***s*** or ***es*** to the end of a noun. The rules for forming plurals of many medical terms are different because Greek and Latin have different rules for forming plurals. Generally, words from these two languages form plurals by adding or substituting another vowel or syllable at the end of a word. Examples of plurals of medical terms are:

- *macula* — the plural is *maculae*
- *adenoma* — the plural is *adenomata*
- *glomerulus* — the plural is *glomeruli*
- *pelvis* — the plural is *pelves.*

Pronouncing medical terms

Medical terms can be difficult to pronounce if you've never heard them spoken. In this book, we'll show you how to pronounce words by placing them in all capital letters, with the syllable receiving the greatest stress appearing in tall capitals and the remaining syllables in smaller capitals. For example, in the word cancer, the stress is on the first syllable, so it would appear as follows: CAN-CER.
Here are some additional tips for pronunciation:

- only the ***s*** sound in ***ps*** is pronounced, as in *Pseudomonas*

- only the ***n*** sound in ***pn*** is pronounced, as in *pneumococcal*
- ***g*** and ***c*** assume the soft sounds of ***j*** and ***s***, respectively, when used before ***e***, ***i***, and ***y***; examples are *gene*, *gingivitis*, *cycle*, and *cytology*
- ***g*** and ***c*** have a hard sound in front of other letters, such as *gangrene*, *gastritis*, *cornea*, and *cortex*
- ***ae*** and ***oe*** are pronounced ***ee***, as in *fasciae* and *coelom*
- ***i*** at the end of a word usually denotes a plural and is pronounced ***eye*** or ***ee***
- ***es*** at the end of a word may be pronounced as a separate syllable, as in *nares*, pronounced NAY-REEZ.

Because phonetic spelling isn't used in medicine, it's important to consult a dictionary when in doubt about pronunciation. Also, some terms sound the same but are spelled differently and refer to different things. For example, *ileum* and *ilium* are pronounced alike, but the first term is part of the intestinal tract and the second one is a pelvic bone.

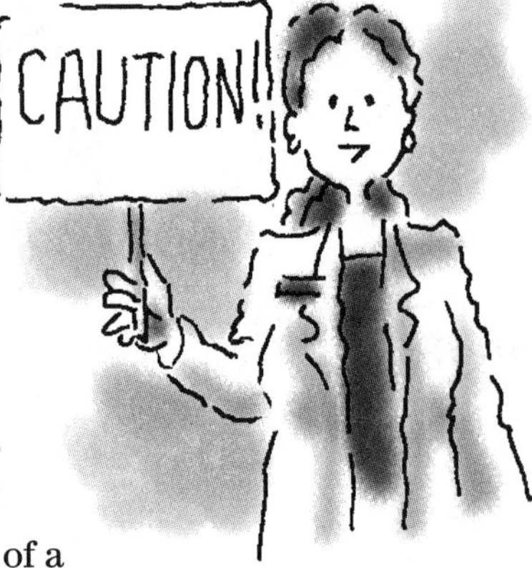
Be careful! Words like **ileum** and **ilium** sound the same but have different meanings.
CAUTION!

Eponyms

Eponyms are medical terms derived from the name of a person, usually a scientist who discovered a body part or disease. Many procedures and tests are also named after the person who invented or perfected them.

Name that condition

Examples of eponyms for medical conditions include:

- **Addison's disease,** a syndrome resulting from insufficient production of hormones from the cortex of the adrenal gland
- **Alzheimer's disease,** a type of irreversible dementia
- **Cushing's syndrome,** a syndrome resulting from the production of excess cortisol from the adrenal cortex
- **Parkinson's disease,** a progressive degeneration of the nervous system that causes weakness, rigidity, and tremors
- **Stokes-Adams syndrome,** a heart condition characterized by sudden loss of consciousness.

Famous body parts

Parts of the body named for their discoverers include:

- **Bartholin's glands,** located in the female perineum

• **Cowper's glands,** located beneath a portion of the male urethra
• **Wernicke's center,** a speech center in the brain.

Featured procedures

Examples of eponyms for medical procedures include:
• **Allen's test,** a test for occlusion of radial or ulnar arteries
• **Belsey Mark IV operation,** a procedure to correct gastroesophageal reflux
• **Heimlich maneuver,** a technique for removing foreign objects from the airway of a choking victim.

What's in a name?

Medical devices such as catheters (tubes passed through body channels) are often named for their inventors; for example:
• the **Foley catheter** is an indwelling urinary catheter
• a **Hickman catheter** is a long-term central venous catheter
• a **Malecot catheter** is a tube used for gastrostomy feedings
• a **Swan-Ganz catheter** is threaded into the pulmonary artery.

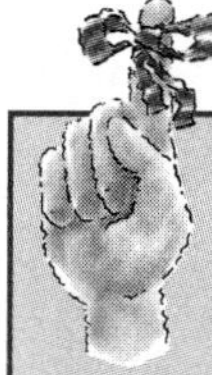

Memory jogger

To remember where a prefix goes and where a suffix goes, you can do two things:

☝ Think of the word *prefix: **Pre-** means before,* so a prefix is a word "fixed" to the word "before" the root. If the prefix comes before, then the suffix comes after.

✌ If that doesn't jazz you, just use the alphabet: ***P*** comes before ***S*** in the alphabet, so a prefix comes before a suffix — and before a root, for that matter, which starts with ***R,*** so now you have ***PRS*** (pretty riveting stuff?).

Word components

Words can be made up of roots, prefixes, and suffixes. (See *Common prefixes, roots, and suffixes*, pages 6 to 13.)

At the root of it all

A root is just what the word implies — where it all starts. A root can be a whole word or part of a word. Roots come from many different languages — such as Greek, Latin, French, and German — and find their way into English.

Perfect prefix

A prefix is a word component or whole word that attaches to the front of a root. A prefix can drastically change the meaning of a word. For example, the prefix ***extra-*** changes the word *ordinary* into *extraordinary.*

(Text continues on page 14.)

Common prefixes, roots, and suffixes

Knowing these common prefixes, roots, and suffixes will help you decipher unfamiliar medical terms.

Word component	Meanings	Examples
Prefixes		
a(n)-	absence, without	anuria (lack of urine output)
ab-	away from	abduct (move away from)
ad-	toward	adduct (move toward)
ambi-	both sides	ambidextrous (using both hands)
ante-	before, forward	anterior (front of the body)
anti-	against	antibody (immune response to an organism)
apo-	away from	apophysis (growth or protuberance)
aut(o)-	self	autoanalysis (self-analysis)
bi-	two	bigeminy (occurring in pairs)
diplo-	double	diplopia (double vision)
dys-	difficult, painful	dysuria (painful urination)
ec-	out of	ectopic (out of place)
end(o)-	inward	endoscope (a device used to examine a body cavity)
eu-	normal, health	euthyroid (normal thyroid function)
ex-	outside	exfoliate (peeling of layers)
hetero-	other, different	heterogeneous (different characteristics)
hyper-	above, beyond	hypernatremia (excess sodium)
infra-	beneath	infra-axillary (below the axilla)
intra-	within, into	intramuscular (into the muscle)
juxta-	near	juxta-articular (near a joint)
macr(o)-	large, long	macromastia (excessive breast size)
mal-	bad, abnormal	malformation (abnormally formed)
mega-	great, large	megacolon (enlarged colon)

Common prefixes, roots, and suffixes *(continued)*

Word component	Meanings	Examples
Prefixes *(continued)*		
meta-	beyond, change	metaphase (second stage of cell division)
micr(o)-	small	microbe (tiny organism)
mono-	one	monochromatic (having only one color)
morph(o)-	shape	morphology (study of the form and structure of organisms)
multi-	many	multifocal (arising from many locations)
olig(o)-	few, little	oliguria (too little urine)
par(a)-	near, beside, accessory to	paracentesis (puncture of a cavity for aspiration of fluid)
peri-	around	pericecal (around the cecum)
pico-	one-trillionth	picornavirus (extremely small RNA virus)
poly-	much, many	polydipsia (excessive thirst)
post-	behind, after	postoperative (after surgery)
pre-	before, in front	preanesthesia (before anesthetic is given)
pro-	favoring, supporting, substituting for, in front of	procoagulant (promotes coagulation)
pseudo-	false	pseudocyst (a cavity resembling a true cyst)
re-	back, contrary	recurrent fever (fever returning after a remission)
retr(o)-	backward	retroauricular (behind the auricle of the ear)
semi-	half	semiflexion (position of a limb midway between extension and flexion)
sub-	under	subclinical (without symptoms)
super-	above	supercilia (the eyebrow)
supra-	above, upon	supraorbital (above the orbit)
tetra-	four	tetralogy (group of four)
trans-	across, through	transdermal (entering through the skin)

(continued)

Common prefixes, roots, and suffixes *(continued)*

Word component	Meanings	Examples
Roots		
abdomin(o)-	abdomen	abdominopelvic (abdomen and pelvis)
acou-	hearing	acoustic (hearing)
acr(o)-	extremity, peak	acrodermatitis (inflammation of skin of the extremities)
aden(o)-	gland	adenocele (cystic tumor in a gland)
adipo-	fat	adipose (fatty)
alb-	white	albumin (protein found in the blood)
andr(o)-	male	androgen (male sex hormone)
angi(o)-	vessel	angiography (X-ray of a vessel)
ankyl-	crooked, fusion	ankylosis (consolidation of a joint)
bili-	bile	biliary (pertaining to bile or the gallbladder)
blast- *or* -blast	embryonic state	blastocyte (embryonic cell)
blephar(o)-	eyelid	blepharitis (inflammation of the eyelid)
brachi(o)-	arm	brachial artery (artery of the upper arm)
brady-	slow	bradycardia (slow heart rhythm)
calc-	heel	calcaneus (heel bone)
carcin(o)-	cancer	carcinoma (malignant growth)
cardi(o)-	heart	cardiac muscle (heart muscle)
caud-	tail	caudal (toward the tail)
cephal(o)-	head	cephalalgia (pain in the head)
cerebr(o)-	cerebrum	cerebral embolism (occlusion of a cerebral vessel by a blood clot)
cervic(i)(o)-	neck	cervical plexus (network of cervical nerves)
chol(e)-	bile	cholecystitis (inflammation of the gallbladder)
chondr(o)-	cartilage	chondritis (inflammation of cartilage)
col(i)(o)-	colon	colitis (inflammation of the colon)

Common prefixes, roots, and suffixes *(continued)*

Word component	Meanings	Examples
Roots *(continued)*		
cost(o)-	rib	costochondral (relating to a rib and its cartilage)
cut-	skin	cutaneous (relating to skin)
cyan(o)-	blue	cyanotic (blue colored)
cyst(i)(o)-	bladder	cystitis (inflammation of the urinary bladder)
cyt(o)-	cell	cytology (study of cells)
derm- *or* -derm	skin	dermatitis (skin inflammation)
dors(i)(o)-	back	dorsiflexion (upward bending of hand or foot)
enter(o)-	intestine	enterocolitis (inflammation of the intestines and colon)
erythr(o)-	red	erythrocytes (red blood cells)
fasci-	bundle	fascia (bundles of muscle fibers)
febri-	fever	febrile (feverish)
fil-	threadlike	filament (fine thread)
galact(o)-	milk	galactose (sugar obtained from milk)
gastro-	stomach	gastritis (inflammation of the stomach)
ger(o)- *or* geront(o)-	aging	gerontology (study of aging)
gest-	carry	gestation (pregnancy)
gloss(o)-	tongue	glossitis (inflammation of the tongue)
glyc(o)- *or* gluc(o)-	sweet	glycogen, glucogen (forms of sugar)
gyn(o)-	woman, particularly female reproductive organs	gynecology (study of women's reproductive organs)
heme(a)(o)- *or* hemato-	blood	hematology (study of blood)
hepat(o)-	liver	hepatitis (inflammation of the liver)
hist(i)(o)-	tissue	histography (process of describing tissue and cells)
hydro-	water, hydrogen	hydrops (excess watery fluid)
hyster-	uterus	hysterectomy (surgical removal of the uterus)

(continued)

Common prefixes, roots, and suffixes *(continued)*

Word component	Meanings	Examples
Roots *(continued)*		
ile(o)-	ileum	ileostomy (surgical opening in the ileum)
ili(o)-	ilium, flank	iliac muscle (muscle that allows thigh movement)
ischi(o)-	hip	ischiopubic (pertaining to the ischium and pubes)
jejun(o)-	jejunum	jejunectomy (excision of the jejunum)
kerat(o)-	horny tissue, cornea	keratectasia (a thin, scarred cornea)
kine(t)(o)-	movement	kinetic (pertaining to motion)
labio-	lips	labiograph (an instrument that records lip movement)
lact(o)-	milk	lactation (secretion of milk by the breasts)
laryng(o)-	larynx	laryngectomy (surgical removal of the larynx)
latero-	side	lateroflexion (flexion to one side)
leuk(o)-	white	leukocytes (white blood cells)
lip(o)-	fat	lipedema (excess fat and fluid in subcutaneous tissue)
lith(o)-	stone	lithocystotomy (surgical removal of bladder stones)
lymph(o)-	lymph	lymphadenia (enlargement of the lymph nodes)
mamm(o)-	breast	mammogram (breast X-ray)
mast(o)-	breast	mastectomy (surgical removal of breast tissue)
melan(o)-	black	melancholia (depression)
meno-	menses	menostaxis (prolonged menstrual period)
ment-	mind	mental illness (psychiatric disorder)
mio-	less, smaller	miosis (excessive contraction of the pupil)
mito-	threadlike	mitochondria (rod-shaped cellular organelle)
my(o)-	muscle	myocele (hernia of muscle)
myc(o)-	fungus	mycology (study of fungi and fungal diseases)
myel(o)-	marrow, spinal cord	myelalgia (pain in the spinal cord)
myx-	mucus	myxoid (resembling mucus)

Common prefixes, roots, and suffixes *(continued)*

Word component	Meanings	Examples
Roots *(continued)*		
nas(o)-	nose	nasolabial (between the nose and lip)
nephr(o)-	kidney	nephritis (kidney inflammation)
ocul(o)-	eye	oculomotor (eye movement)
ophthalm(o)-	eye	ophthalmia (inflammation of the eye)
orchi(o)-	testes	orchitis (inflammation of the testes)
oro-	mouth	oronasal (mouth and nose)
oss- *or* oste(o)-	bone	osteomyelitis (inflammation of bone and muscle)
ot(o)-	ear	otitis (ear inflammation)
ox(y)-	oxygenation	oxyhemoglobin (hemoglobin combined with molecular oxygen)
path(o)-	disease	pathogen (disease-causing organism)
ped(o)-	child	pediatrics (care of children)
pharmaco-	medicine	pharmacotherapy (treatment with medication)
pharyng(o)-	pharynx	pharyngitis (sore throat)
phleb(o)-	vein	phlebitis (inflammation of a vein)
phot(o)-	light	phototherapy (treatment by exposure to light)
plasm(o)-	liquid part of blood	plasminogen (protein found in tissues and body fluids)
pleur(o)-	pleura, rib, side	pleurisy (inflammation of the pleura)
pneum(o)-	lung	pneumonia (inflammation of the lung)
pod(o)-	foot	podiatry (care of the foot)
proct(o)-	rectum	proctectomy (excision of the rectum)
prote(o)-	protein	proteinemia (excess protein in the blood)
psych(o)-	mind	psychiatry (study and treatment of mental disorders)
pulmo(n)-	lung	pulmoaortic (pertaining to the lungs and aorta)
pyel(o)-	kidney	pyelonephrosis (disease of the kidney and renal pelvis)

(continued)

Common prefixes, roots, and suffixes *(continued)*

Word component	Meanings	Examples
Roots *(continued)*		
pyr(o)-	heat	pyrogen (an agent that causes fever)
ren(o)-	kidney	renography (X-ray of the kidney)
rhin(o)-	nose	rhinitis (inflamed mucous membranes of the nose)
rub(r)-	red	bilirubin (bile pigment)
sangui-	blood	sanguineous drainage (bloody drainage)
sarc(o)-	flesh	sarcoma (a highly malignant tumor made of connective tissue cells)
scler(o)-	hard	sclerosis (hardening of tissue)
scolio-	crooked	scoliosis (curvature of the spine)
sensi-	perception, feeling	sensory (pertaining to the senses)
sep-	decay	sepsis (infection in the bloodstream)
soma- *or* somat(o)-	body	somatization (psychiatric condition expressed through physical symptoms)
sten(o)-	narrow	stenosis (narrowing of a body passage)
tachy-	rapid, swift	tachycardia (rapid heart beat)
therm(o)-	heat	thermometer (instrument for measuring temperature)
thorac(o)-	chest	thoracotomy (surgical opening of the chest wall)
thromb(o)-	clot	thrombectomy (excision of a clot from a blood vessel)
toxi(o)-	poison	toxicosis (poisoning)
trache(o)-	trachea	tracheobronchitis (inflammation of the trachea and bronchi)
ur(o)-	urinary, urine	uropoiesis (formation of urine)
vas(o)-	vessel	vasospasm (spasm of a blood vessel)
ven(i)(o)-	vein	venosclerosis (sclerosis or hardening of the veins)
vesic(o)-	bladder	vesicospinal (pertaining to the urinary bladder and spine)

Common prefixes, roots, and suffixes *(continued)*

Word component	Meanings	Examples
Suffixes		
-algia	pain	neuralgia (nerve pain)
-ectomy	surgical removal	splenectomy (removal of the spleen)
-itis	inflammation	colitis (inflammation of the colon)
-lys(i)(o)	breakdown	fibrinolysis (breakdown of a clot)
-oma	tumor	blastoma (cancer composed of embryonic cells)
-osis	condition	fibrosis (formation of fibrous tissue)
-phob	abnormal fear	agoraphobia (fear of open spaces)
-plasia	growth	hypoplasia (incomplete development)
-plasty	surgical repair	angioplasty (surgical repair of blood vessels)
-plegia	paralysis	paraplegia (paralysis of lower body)
-pnea	breathing	apnea (lack of breathing)
-poiesis	production	hematopoiesis (production of blood cells)
-praxia	movement	apraxia (inability to perform purposeful movement)
-rrhea	fluid discharge	diarrhea (frequent soft or liquid bowel movements)
-scope	observe	endoscope (tool for observing the interior of body organs)
-stomy	opening	colostomy (portion of the colon is opened and brought through the abdominal wall)
-taxis	movement	ataxia (uncoordinated movements)
-tomy	incision	thoracotomy (surgical opening of the chest wall)
-tripsy	crushing	lithotripsy (crushing stones in the bladder, kidney, gallbladder, or other organs)
-trophy	growth	hypertrophy (overgrowth)

Sufficient suffix

A suffix is a word unit that attaches to the end of a root. Among other feats, a suffix can change the form of a word from an adjective, for instance, into an adverb. So you could add the suffix ***-ly*** to *extraordinary* to make *extraordinarily* (as in *extraordinarily interesting*).

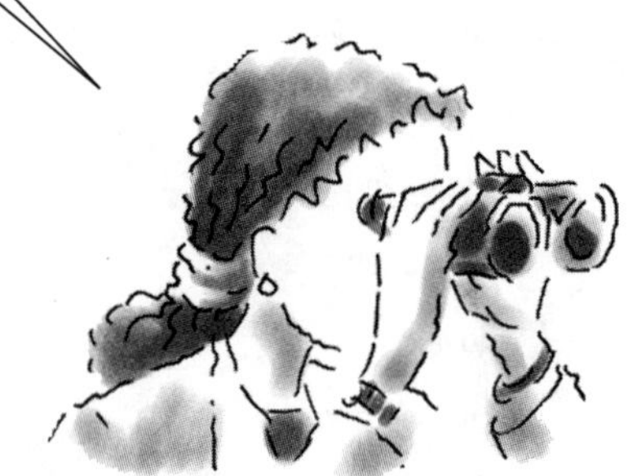

Prefixes and suffixes are important but focus on the root of the word to get the meaning quickly.

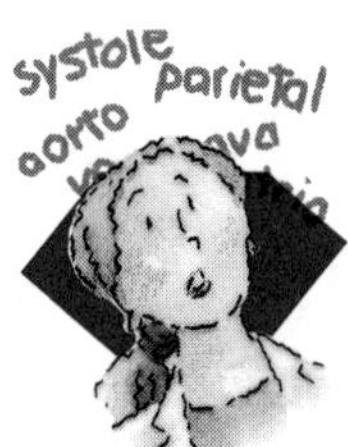

Vocabulary builders

At a crossroads

Completing this crossword puzzle will help build your medical vocabulary. Good luck!

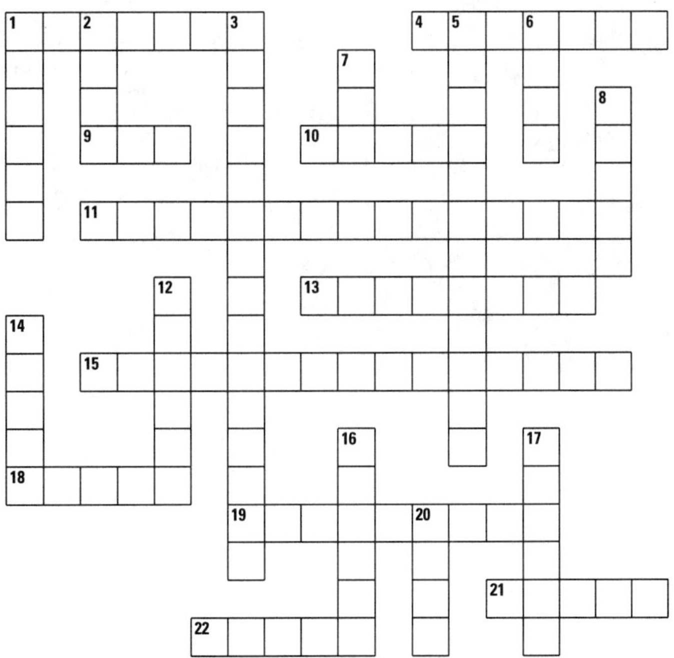

Across

1. Suffix meaning *production*
4. Root for *cancer*
9. Root for *decay*
10. Root for *fat*
11. Suffix in *splenectomy* means this (two words)
13. An eponymic maneuver
15. A speech center in the brain (two words)
18. Root for *male*
19. Root for *eye*
21. Root for *water*
22. Root for *bone*

Down

1. Syllable attached to the beginning of a word
2. Suffix for *inflammation*
3. ***Pro-*** means this (two words)
5. ***Phobia*** is a root meaning this (two words)
6. Second root in *erythrocyte* means this
7. Root of *pediatric*
8. Meaning of root in 7 down
12. Root for *heart*
14. Prefix meaning *upon*
16 Prefix meaning *different*
17. Term derived from a person's name
20. Root for *vessel*

Answers are on page 18.

Match game

Match the following roots and prefixes to the correct answer.

Clues	Choices
1. Super	A. Rapid
2. Tachy	B. Stone
3. Thrombo	C. Above
4. Thermo	D. Large
5. Poly	E. Heat
6. Post	F. After
7. Oxy	G. Clot
8. Mono	H. Oxygen
9. Lith	I. Many
10. Mega	J. One

In medicine, being familiar with roots and prefixes is as essential as being familiar with the human body.

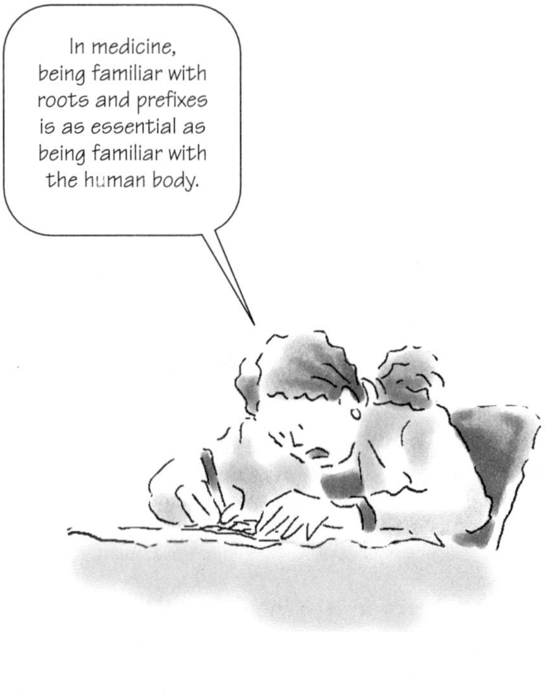

Answers are on page 18.

Scrambled or overeasy

Fill in the answers for the following questions, then unscramble the circled letters to find the answer to the puzzle.

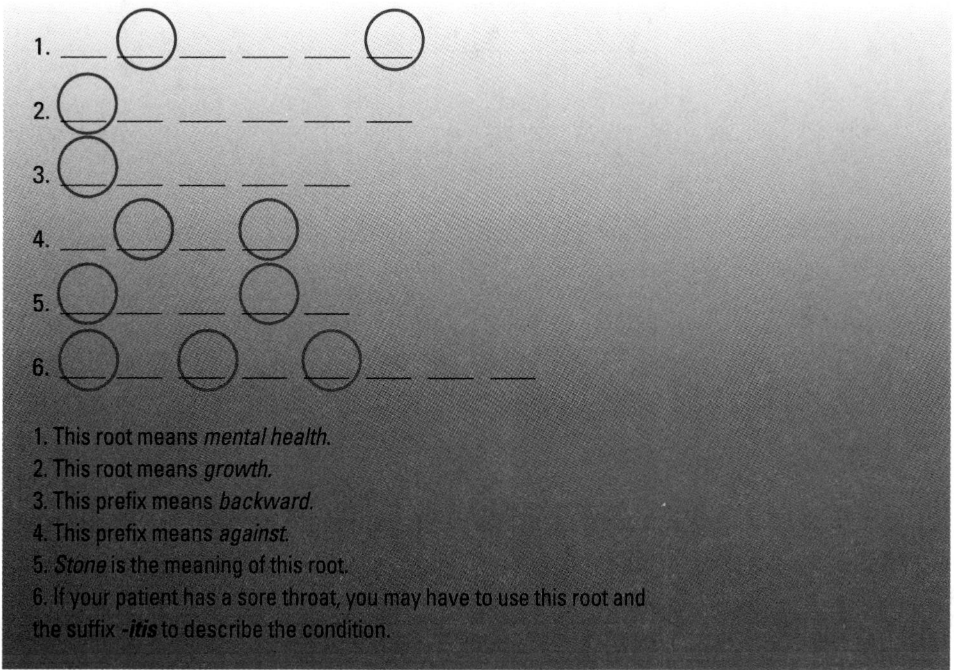

1. This root means *mental health.*
2. This root means *growth.*
3. This prefix means *backward.*
4. This prefix means *against.*
5. *Stone* is the meaning of this root.
6. If your patient has a sore throat, you may have to use this root and the suffix ***-itis*** to describe the condition.

I think we can fix you right up!

Answers are on page 18.

Answers

At a crossroads

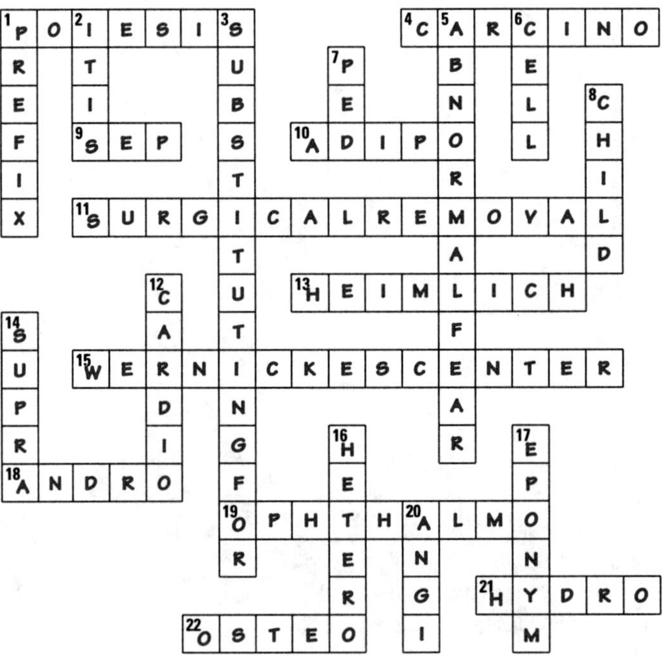

Match game

1. C; 2. A; 3. G; 4. E; 5. I; 6. F; 7. H; 8. J; 9. B; 10. D.

Scrambled or overeasy

1. Psycho; 2. Trophy; 3. Retro; 4. Anti; 5. Litho; 6. Pharyngo.
Answer to puzzle — Rhinoplasty

Body structure

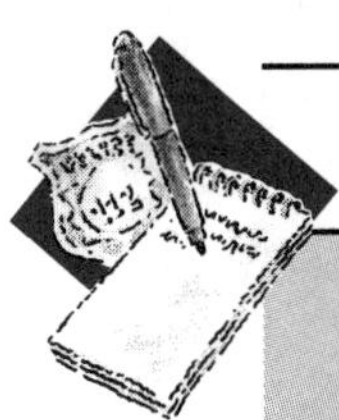

Just the facts

In this chapter, you'll review:

- terminology related to cells, organs, and tissues
- terminology related to the systems of the body
- terminology related to the directions, regions, and positions of the body.

Cells: Nature's building blocks

The cell is the body's basic building block and the smallest living component of an organism. In the late 1600s, British physicist Robert Hooke first observed plant cells with a crude microscope. He decided that the structures reminded him of tiny prison cells—hence the name **cell.** (See *Pronouncing key terms related to the cell*, page 20.)

Specialized units

The human body contains millions of cells grouped into highly specialized units that function together. Large groups of individual cells form tissues, such as muscle, blood, and bone. Tissues in turn form organs, such as the brain, heart, and liver. Organs and tissues are integrated into body systems — such as the central nervous system, cardiovascular system, and digestive system.

Pump up your pronunciation

Pronouncing key terms related to the cell

Below is a list of key terms, along with the correct way to pronounce them.

Adenosine	AH-DEHN-OH-ZEEN
Cytokinesis	SEYE-TOH-KIH-NEE-SISS
Golgi (as in Golgi apparatus)	GOHL-JEE
Meiosis	MEYE-OH-SISS
Mitochondria	MY-TOH-KAWN-DREE-AH
Squamous	SKWAH-MUSS

A peek inside the cell

Cells are composed of many structures, or **organelles,** that each have a specific function. The word **organelles** is from the neo-Latin word ***organella,*** an altered form of ***organum,*** which means *organ.* (See *Just your average cell.*)

Organists

Organelles live in **cytoplasm** — an aqueous mass that is surrounded by the cell membrane. ***Cyto-*** is a Greek prefix that denotes a relationship to a cell. The **cell membrane,** also called the **plasma membrane,** encloses the cytoplasm and forms the outer boundary of each cell.

Nuclear power

The largest organelle is the **nucleus,** a word derived from the Latin word ***nuculeus,*** which means *kernel.* It stores deoxyribonucleic acid (DNA), which carries genetic material and is responsible for cellular reproduction or division.

The typical animal cell is characterized by several additional elements:

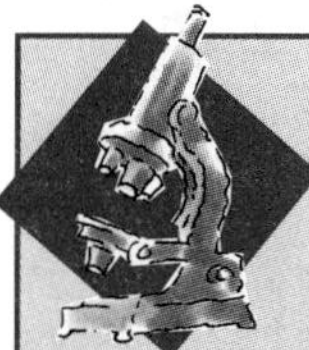

Zoom in

Just your average cell

The illustration here shows cell components and structures. Each part has a function in maintaining the cell's life and homeostasis.

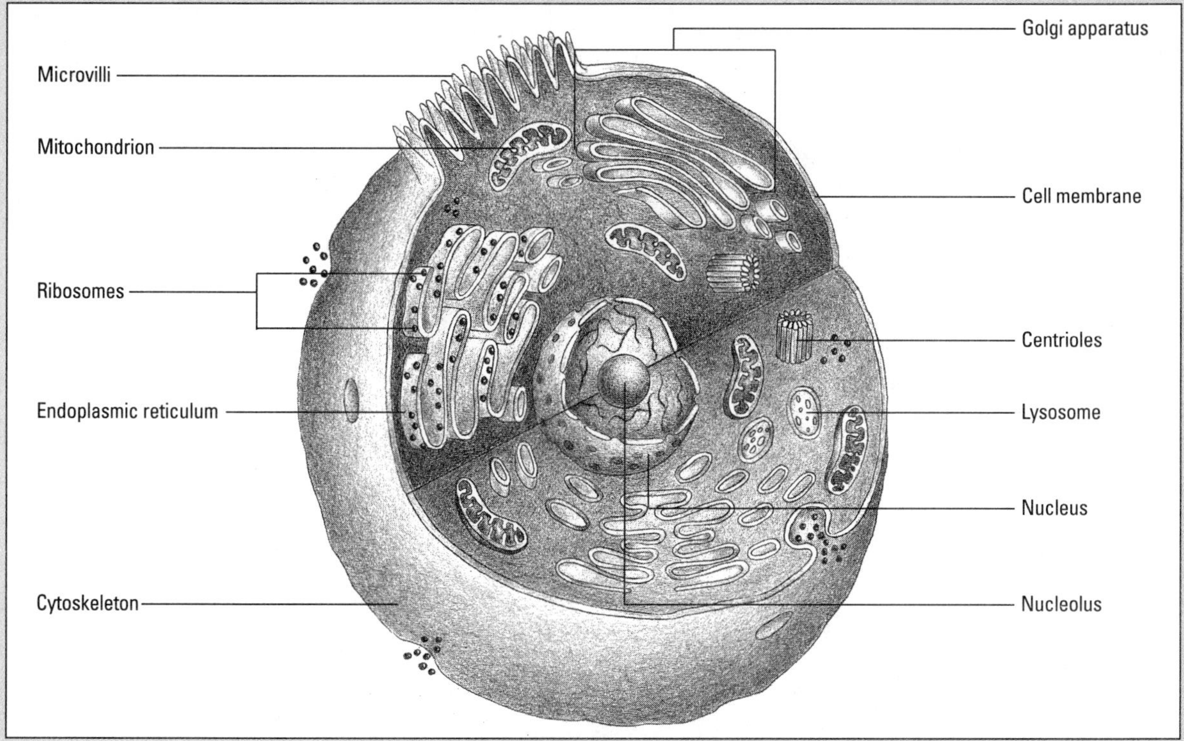

Golgi apparatus
Microvilli
Mitochondrion
Cell membrane
Ribosomes
Centrioles
Endoplasmic reticulum
Lysosome
Nucleus
Cytoskeleton
Nucleolus

- **Adenosine triphosphate,** the energy that fuels cellular activity, is made in the **mitochondria,** the cell's power plant.
- **Ribosomes** and the **endoplasmic reticulum** synthesize proteins and metabolize fat within the cell.
- The **Golgi apparatus** holds enzyme systems that assist in completing the cell's metabolic functions.
- **Lysosomes** contain enzymes that allow cytoplasmic digestion. (See *Why call it a lysosome?*, page 22.)

Cell division and reproduction

Individual cells are subject to wear and tear and must reproduce quickly to replace themselves. Genetic information passes from one generation of cells to the next in an intricate process that is vital to survival. Mistakes here can lead to lethal genetic disorders, cancer, and other conditions.

Making copies

Cells reproduce by splitting into two separate daughter cells through a process called **mitosis,** from the Greek root ***mitos,*** which means *thread,* with the suffix ***-osis,*** which denotes *an action or state.* During mitosis, the nucleus and genetic material divide. The process reaches completion during cell movement, or **cytokinesis;** that is, ***cyto-,*** from the Greek root ***kytos,*** which means *container* or *body,* with the Greek word ***kinesis,*** which means *movement,* when the plasma membrane and cytoplasm divide. (See *Replicate and divide.*)

Getting ready to divide

Before a cell can divide, it must double in mass and content. This begins during the growth phase, or **interphase.** At this phase, **chromatin,** formed of the small, slender rods of the nucleus that give it its glandular appearance, begins to form. Replication and duplication of DNA occur during the four phases of mitosis:

 prophase

 metaphase

 anaphase

 telophase.

Prophase

During **prophase,** the chromosomes coil and shorten and the nuclear membrane dissolves. Each chromosome is made up of a pair of strands, called **chromatids.** Chromatids are connected by a spindle of fibers called a **centromere.**

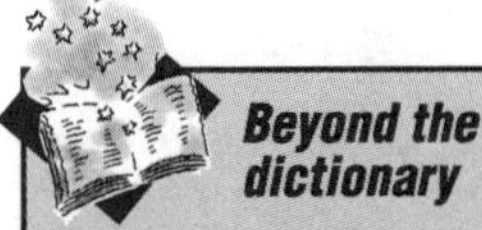

Beyond the dictionary

Why call it a lysosome?

The name **lysosome** comes from the Greek word ***lysis,*** which means *dissolution.* In plain terms, ***lysis*** means *destruction by enzymatic digestion.*

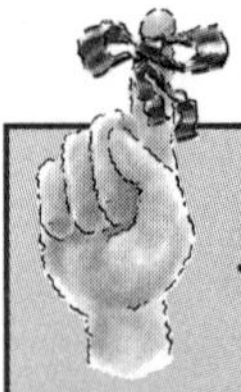

Memory jogger

As a way to remember the processes of mitosis, think of this phrase: "***I p**ulled **m**y **a**ct **t**ogether* (**i**nterphase, **p**rophase, **m**etaphase, **a**naphase, and **t**elophase)."

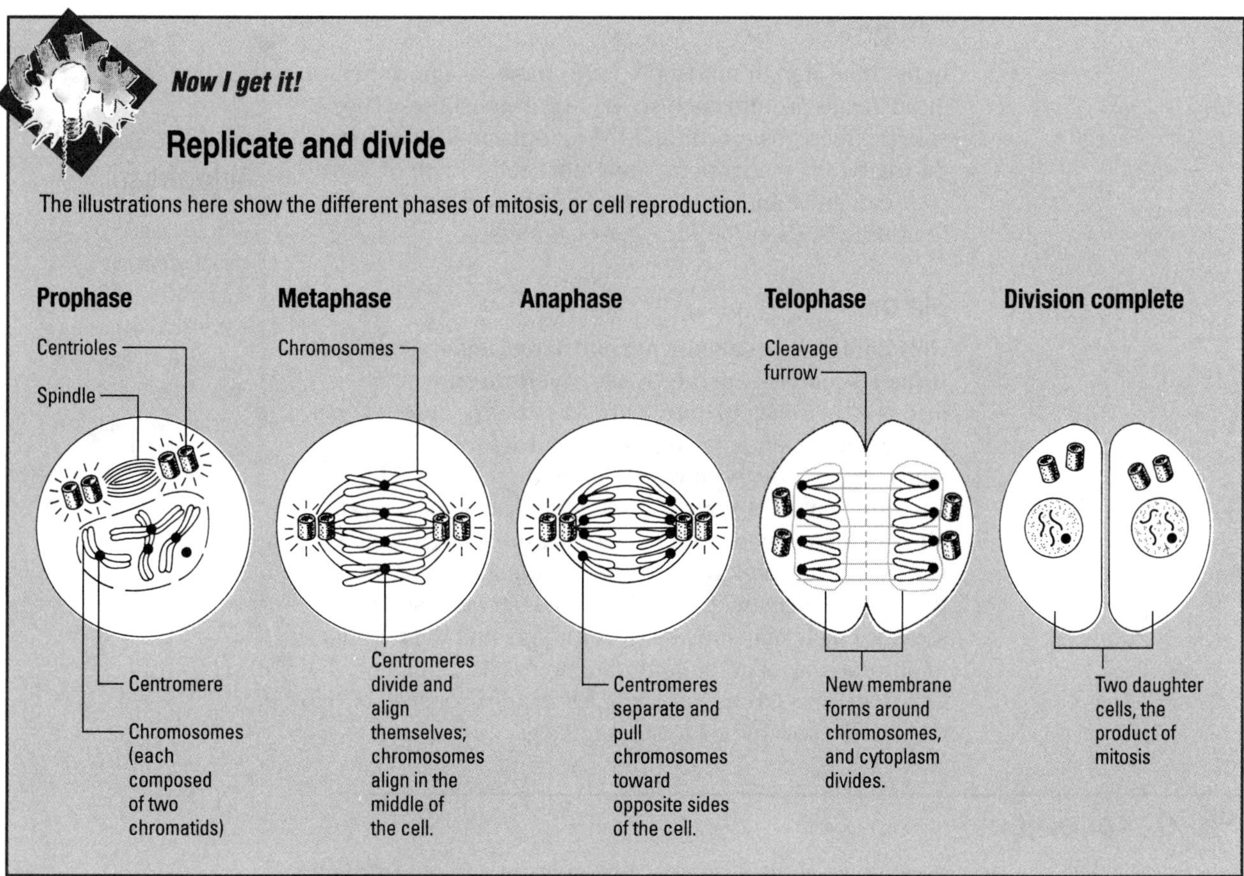
Now I get it!
Replicate and divide
The illustrations here show the different phases of mitosis, or cell reproduction.
Prophase
Centrioles
Spindle
Centromere
Chromosomes (each composed of two chromatids)
Metaphase
Chromosomes
Centromeres divide and align themselves; chromosomes align in the middle of the cell.
Anaphase
Centromeres separate and pull chromosomes toward opposite sides of the cell.
Telophase
Cleavage furrow
New membrane forms around chromosomes, and cytoplasm divides.
Division complete
Two daughter cells, the product of mitosis

Metaphase

During **metaphase,** the centromeres divide, pulling the chromosomes apart. The centromeres then align themselves in the middle of the spindle.

Anaphase

At the onset of **anaphase,** centromeres begin to separate and pull the newly replicated chromosomes toward opposite sides of the cell. The centromere of each chromosome splits to form two new chromosomes, each consisting of a single DNA molecule. By the end of anaphase, 46 chromosomes are present on each side of the cell.

Telophase

In the final step of mitosis — **telophase** — a new membrane forms around each set of 46 chromosomes. The spindle fibers disappear and the cytoplasm divides, producing two new identical "daughter" cells. Each of these cells can grow and develop, perhaps becoming a mother to new cells. (See *Tell me about telophase.*)

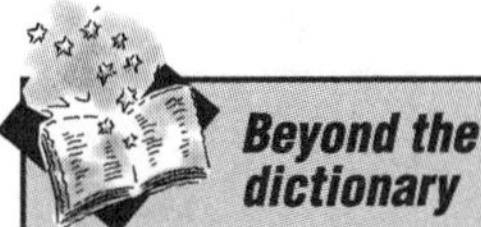

Beyond the dictionary

Tell me about telophase

The prefix ***telo-*** in telophase is derived from the Greek word ***telos,*** which means *an ultimate end.* Telophase marks the end of mitosis, yielding two daughter cells.

Meiosis

Only **gametes** (**ova** and **spermatozoa**) undergo meiosis. **Gamete** comes from the Greek root ***gamet,*** which means either *wife* ***(gamete)*** or *husband* ***(gametes)*** depending on its ending. **Ova** is the plural form of **ovum,** which means *egg*; both words come directly from Latin without change. **Spermatozoa** is the plural form of **spermatozoon,** formed from the Greek ***spermat,*** meaning *seed,* and the Greek root ***zôion,*** meaning *animal.* In this type of cell division, genetic material between similarly structured chromosomes is intermixed, and the number of chromosomes in the four daughter cells diminishes by half. **Meiosis** (Greek, meaning *lessening*) consists of two divisions separated by a resting phase.

Fluid movement

A cell must shuttle various molecules in and out through the plasma membrane and between compartments inside the cell. There are several different ways fluids and **solutes** (dissolved substances) move through membranes at the cellular level.

Going with the flow

In **diffusion,** solutes move from an area of higher concentration to an area of lower concentration. This movement eventually results in an equal distribution of solutes within the two areas. Diffusion is known as **passive transport** because no energy is needed to make it happen. Like fish traveling downstream, solutes involved in diffusion just go with the flow.

Letting fluids through

Osmosis (from the Greek root ***osm,*** meaning *to push,* and the Greek suffix ***-sis,*** which is used to form a noun from a word that was originally a verb) is another passive transport method. Unlike diffusion, osmosis involves the movement of a water (solvent) molecule across the cell membrane from a dilute solution, one with a high concentration of water molecules, to a concentrated one, one with a lower concentration of water.

Osmosis is influenced by the osmotic pressure of a solution. Osmotic pressure reflects the water-attracting property of a solute. It's determined by the number of dissolved particles in a given volume of solution.

Energy required

Unlike passive transport, **active transport** requires energy. Usually, this mechanism moves a substance from an area of lower concentration to an area of higher concentration. Think of this as swimming upstream. When a fish swims upstream it uses energy.

Against the grain

The energy required for a solute to move against a concentration gradient comes from a substance produced within the cell, **adenosine triphosphate,** or **ATP.** Stored in the cell, ATP supplies the energy for solute movement in and out of cells. Some solutes, such as sodium and potassium, use ATP to move in and out of cells in a form of active transport called the **sodium-potassium pump.** Other solutes that require active transport to cross cell membranes include calcium ions, hydrogen ions, amino acids, and certain sugars.

Body tissues: Holding it all together

Tissues are groups of similar cells that perform the same role; each tissue has at least one unique function. Tissues are classified by structure and function and are divided into four types: epithelial, connective, muscle, and nervous.

Epithelial tissue

Epithelial tissue (epithelium) is a continuous cellular sheet that covers the body's surface, lines body cavities, and forms certain glands. It contains at least two types of epithelial cells.

Endothelium and mesothelium

Epithelial tissue with a single layer of squamous cells attached to a basement membrane is called **endothelium.** Such tissue lines the heart, lymphatic vessels, and blood vessels. Tissue that lines the surface of serous membranes, such as the pleura, pericardium, and peritoneum, is called **mesothelium.** Epithelial tissue is classified by the number of cell layers it has and the shape of the cells on its surface.

Recognized by number of cell layers

Depending on the number of cell layers, epithelial tissue may be simple, stratified, or pseudostratified.

Simple epithelial tissue contains one layer of cells.

Stratified epithelial tissue has three or more layers.

Pseudostratified epithelial tissue has only one layer of cells but appears to have more.

The prefix ***pseudo-*** means *false.*

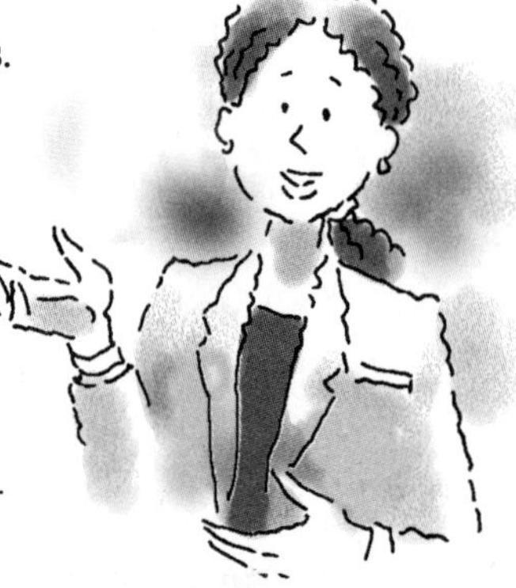

Classified by shape

Based on the shape of its surface cells, epithelial tissue may be squamous, columnar, or cuboidal.

- **Squamous** epithelial tissue has flat surface cells.
- **Columnar** epithelial tissue has tall, cylindrical, prism-shaped surface cells.
- **Cuboidal** epithelial tissue has cube-shaped surface cells.

Connective tissue

Connective tissue includes bone, cartilage, and adipose (fatty) tissue. This tissue binds together and supports body structures. Connective tissue is classified as loose or dense.

Cut loose

Loose connective tissue has large spaces that separate the fibers and cells. It contains much intercellular fluid.

Dense support

Dense connective tissue provides structural support. It has a greater fiber concentration.

Who are you calling fat?

Adipose tissue (fat) is a specialized type of loose connective tissue in which a single fat droplet occupies most of the cell. It cushions internal organs and acts as a reserve supply of energy. (See *Where* adipose *comes from.)*

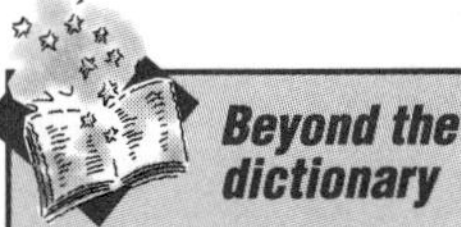

Where *adipose* comes from

Adipose tissue is sometimes referred to as fat. The word **adipose** traces its origins to Greek and Latin. The word ***adiposus*** comes from the combination of the Latin prefix ***adip-*** and the Greek root ***aleipha,*** which means *fat* or *oil.*

Muscle tissue

The three basic types of **muscle tissue** are striated, cardiac, and smooth.

Striated muscle tissue

Striated muscle tissue gets its name from its striped, or striated, appearance. All striated muscle tissue capable of voluntary contraction is called skeletal muscle tissue.

Cardiac and smooth muscle tissue

Cardiac muscle tissue is striated but it contracts involuntarily. **Smooth** muscle tissue lacks the striped pattern of striated tissue; it consists of long, spindle-shaped cells. Its activity is stimulated by the autonomic nervous system and isn't under voluntary control. Smooth muscle tissue lines the wall of many internal organs and other structures, such as the walls of arteries and veins.

Nervous tissue

The main function of **nervous tissue** is communication. Its primary properties are **irritability** (the capacity to react to various physical and chemical agents) and **conductivity** (the ability to transmit the resulting reaction from one point to another). Nervous tissue cells may be neurons or neuroglia.

Neurons consist of three parts: dendrites, the cell body, and axons. Like tiny antennas, **dendrites** receive

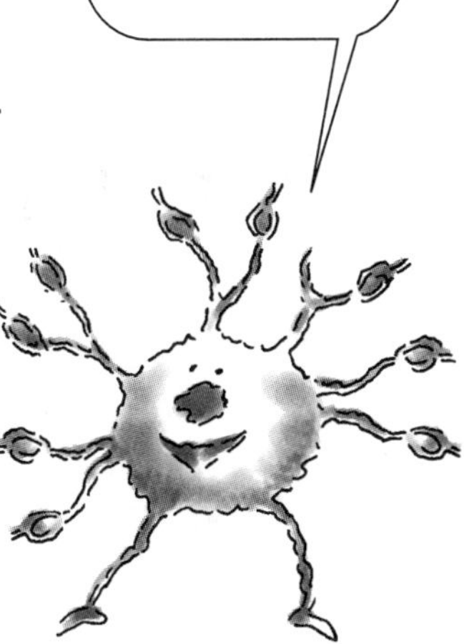

Check out my dendrites. They receive and conduct impulses.

impulses and conduct them into the cell body. **Axons** carry impulses away from the cell body.

Neuroglia form the support structure of nervous tissue, insulating and protecting neurons. They're found only in the central nervous system.

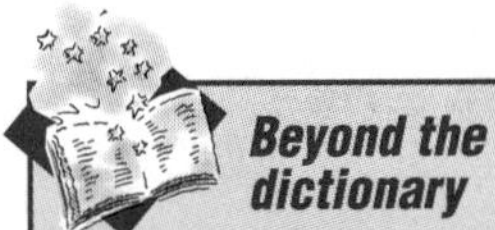

Why call it integumentary?

It's easy to see why **integumentary** is the name for a body system that includes the hair, skin, nails, and sweat glands. The origin of this word is the Latin ***integumentum,*** which means *to cover.*

Organs and systems: The specialists

When a group of tissues handles a more complicated task than any one tissue could perform alone, they're called **organs.**

Organs combine to form **systems,** which perform a more complex function than any one organ can manage on its own. The body depends on these systems in the following ways:

- The **immune system** protects the body from disease and invading organisms.
- The **nervous system** and **special senses** process incoming information and allow the body to respond.
- Reproduction and urine excretion are managed by the **genitourinary system.**
- The **gastrointestinal system** digests and absorbs food and excretes waste products.
- Blood is transported by the **cardiovascular system.**
- The **respiratory system** maintains the exchange of oxygen and carbon dioxide in the lungs and tissues and regulates acid-base balance.
- The **integumentary system,** which includes skin, hair, nails, and sweat glands, protects the body and helps regulate body temperature. (See *Why call it integumentary?*)
- The **muscular system** allows the body to move.
- The **skeletal system** supports the body and gives muscles a place to attach.

Directions, regions, and positions

Determining directions within the body is essential to accurately pinpoint the locations of structures. Terms that describe body planes, cavities, and regions are also useful.

Finding your way around the body

Specific terms define the relationship between body areas and the location of different structures. These terms describe the body in **anatomic position** — standing erect with arms hanging to the side, and palms facing forward:

- **Superior** means *above;* for example, the knees are superior to the ankles.
- **Inferior** means *below;* for example, the feet are inferior to the ankles.
- **Anterior** means *front* or *in front of;* for example, the sternum is an anterior structure. **Ventral** is sometimes used instead of anterior.
- **Posterior** means *back* or *in back of;* for example, the spine is a posterior structure. **Dorsal** may be used instead of posterior.
- **Medial** (midline) means *toward the center.*
- **Lateral** refers to the sides, or *away from the midline.*
- **Proximal** means *nearest to.*
- **Distal** describes a point farthest from point of origin.
- **Superficial** describes a point nearest the body surface.
- **Deep** means *away from the surface.*

Body planes and sections

The body is theoretically divided into three areas called the sagittal, the frontal (coronal), and the transverse planes. (See *Body reference planes*, page 30.)

Sagittal plane

The **sagittal plane** runs lengthwise from front to back and divides the body into right and left sides. A **median sagittal** cut produces two equal halves, each containing an arm and a leg. (Don't try this at home!)

Frontal plane

The **frontal plane** runs lengthwise from side to side, dividing the body into **ventral** and **dorsal** (front and back) sections.

Body reference planes

Body reference planes are used to indicate the locations of body structures. Here are the median sagittal, frontal, and transverse planes, which lie at right angles to one another. The oblique plane, a slanted plane that lies between a horizontal plane and a vertical plane, isn't shown.

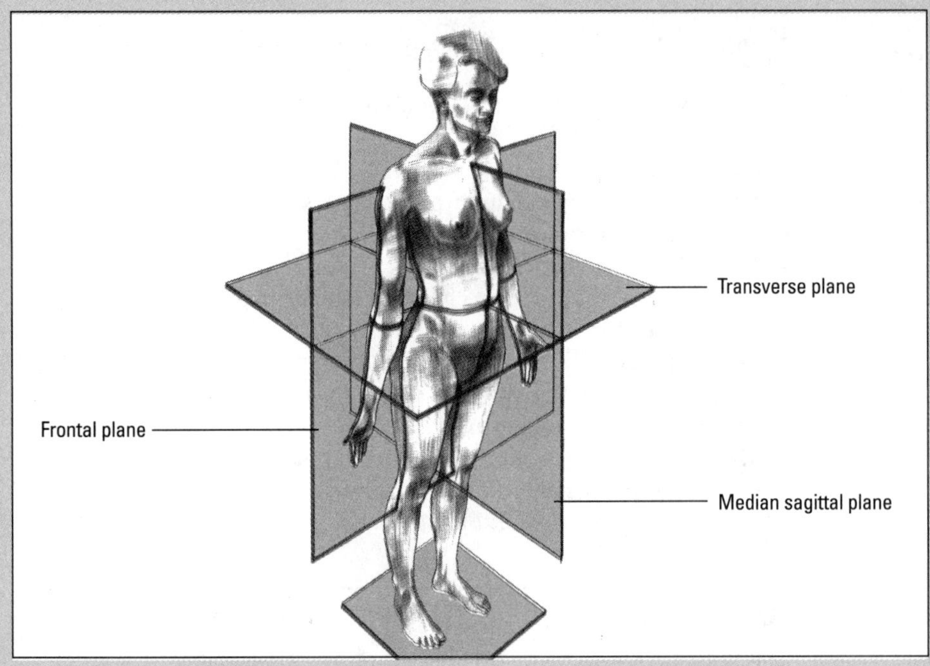

Transverse plane

The **transverse plane,** also called the **horizontal plane,** cuts the body into upper and lower parts. These are known as the **cranial** (head) and the **caudal** (tail) portions.

Body cavities — not the dental kind

A **cavity** is a hollow space within the body that usually houses vital organs. The two major cavities are ventral and dorsal. They're divided into smaller spaces for the internal organs. (See *Locating body cavities.*)

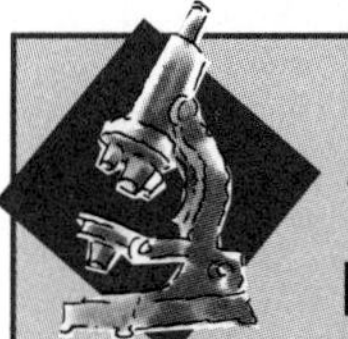

Zoom in

Locating body cavities

The dorsal cavity, in the posterior region of the body, is divided into the cranial and vertebral cavities. The ventral cavity, in the anterior region, is divided into the thoracic and abdominopelvic cavities.

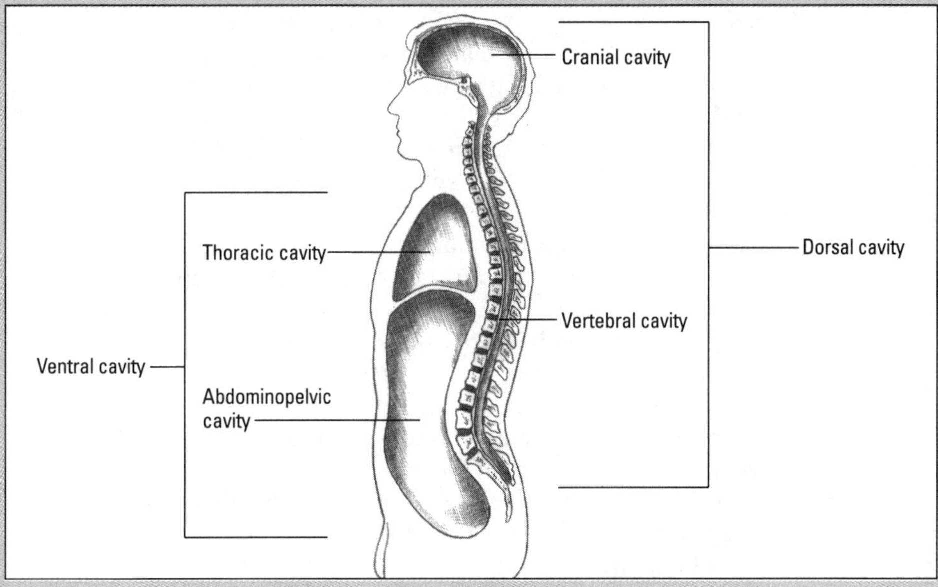

Ventral cavity

The **ventral** cavity contains the **thoracic** (chest) cavity and the **abdominopelvic** cavity. The thoracic cavity is divided into the **mediastinum,** which holds the heart, trachea, and major blood vessels. It also holds the two **pleural** cavities, which enclose the lungs. The **abdominopelvic** cavity has an upper portion, called the **abdominal** cavity and a lower portion called the **pelvic** cavity. The abdominal cavity contains the stomach, intestines, spleen, liver, and other organs. The pelvic cavity contains the bladder, some reproductive organs, and the rectum.

Dorsal cavity

The dorsal cavity includes both the **cranial** and **spinal** cavities. The cranial cavity is relatively small; it houses and protects the brain. The spinal cavity contains the spinal column and spinal cord.

Exploring the abdomen

So many organs and structures lie inside the abdominal and pelvic cavities that special terms are used to pinpoint different areas. Nine regions are identified from right to left and top to bottom:

- The **right hypochondriac region** contains the right side of the liver, the right kidney, and a portion of the diaphragm.
- The **epigastric region** contains the pancreas and portions of the stomach, liver, inferior vena cava, abdominal aorta, and duodenum.
- The **left hypochondriac region** contains a portion of the diaphragm, the spleen, the stomach, the left kidney, and part of the pancreas.
- The **right lumbar region** contains portions of the large intestines and the right kidney.
- The **umbilical region** contains sections of the small and large intestines and a portion of the left kidney.
- The **left lumbar region** contains portions of the small and large intestines and a portion of the left kidney.
- The **right iliac (inguinal) region** includes portions of the small and large intestines.
- The **hypogastric region's** prominent structures include a portion of the sigmoid colon, the urinary bladder and ureters, and portions of the small intestine.
- The **left iliac (inguinal) region** contains portions of the small and large intestines. (See *Anterior view of the abdominal regions.*)

Anterior view of the abdominal regions

The illustration shows the abdominal regions from the front.

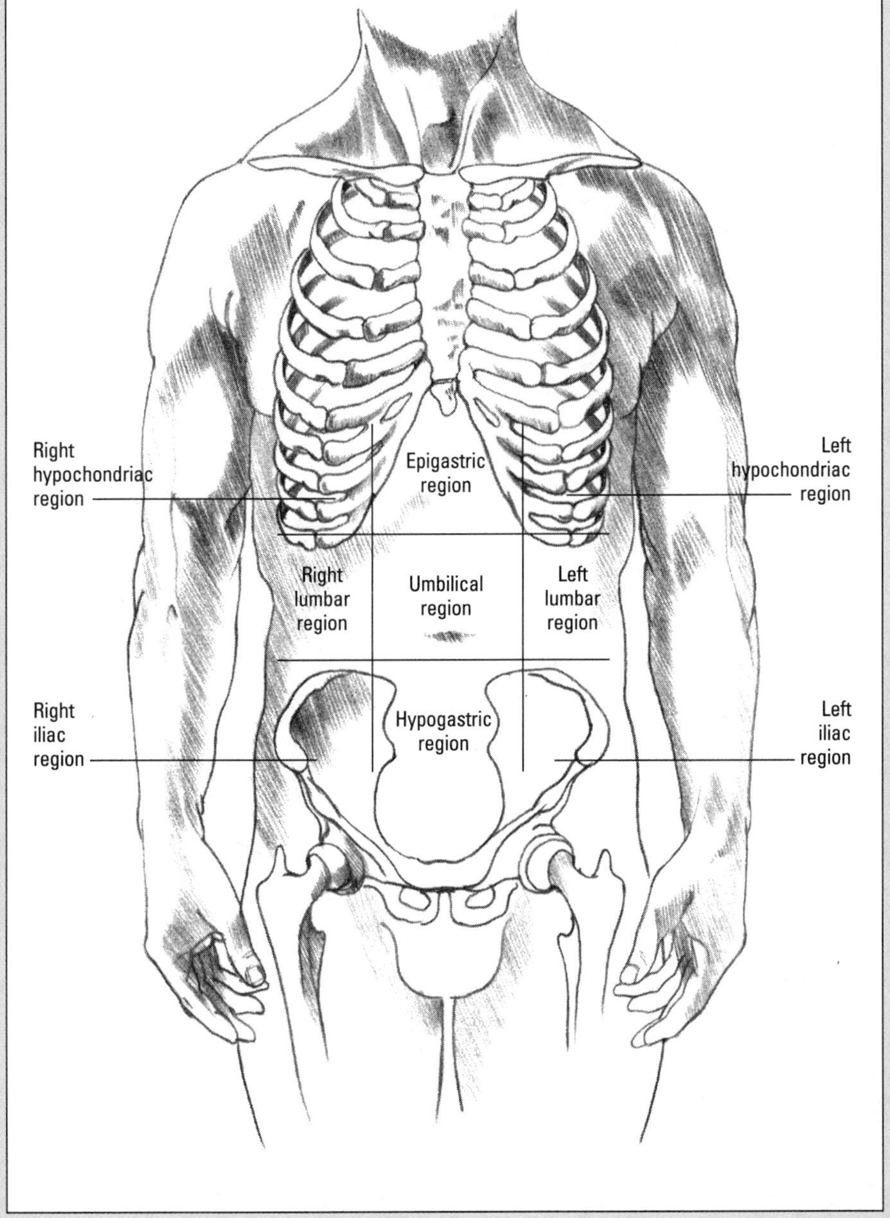

Right hypochondriac region
Epigastric region
Left hypochondriac region
Right lumbar region
Umbilical region
Left lumbar region
Right iliac region
Hypogastric region
Left iliac region

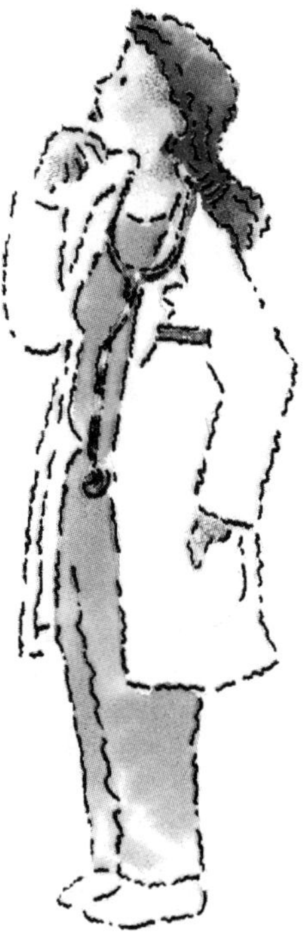

The abdomen has nine distinct regions, divided like a tic-tac-toe board.

Positions

Patients may be placed in several positions for examination, testing, and treatment. These positions are described by many terms. The most frequently used include:

- **Fowler's** — head of bed raised, knees slightly flexed
- **lateral recumbent,** or **Sims'** — lying on the left side with the right thigh and knee drawn up
- **lithotomy** — lying on the back with the hips and knees flexed and the thighs abducted and externally rotated
- **supine** — lying flat on the back
- **prone** — lying face down
- **Trendelenburg's** — lying flat with the head lower than the body or legs
- **reverse Trendelenburg's** — lying flat with the head higher than the body or legs.

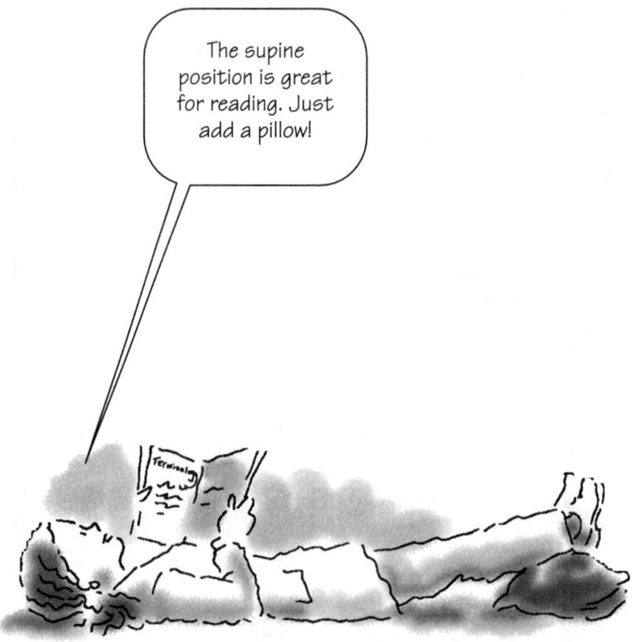
The supine position is great for reading. Just add a pillow!

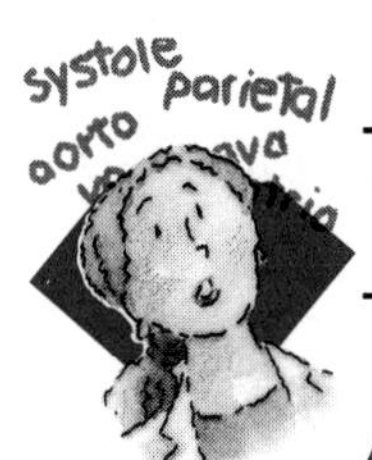

Vocabulary builders

At a crossroads

Completing this crossword puzzle will help build your medical vocabulary. Good luck!

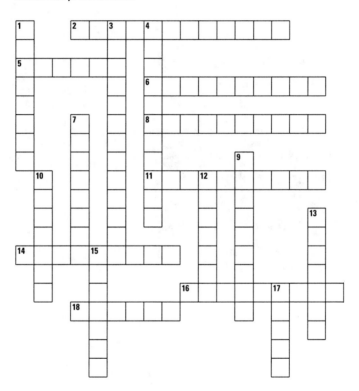

Across

2. Site of adenosine triphosphate production
5. Only type of cell that undergoes meiosis
6. Name for the structures of a cell
8. Growth phase of mitosis
11. Type of epithelial tissue that has three or more layers
14. Support structure of nervous tissue
16. The final step of mitosis
18. Eponym for a position in which the head of the bed is raised and the patient's knees are slightly flexed

Down

1. One of three body reference planes
3. Eponym for a position in which the patient's head is lower than his body or legs
4. Cell movement
7. Word that means *in front of*
9. When solutes move from an area of higher concentration to an area of lower concentration
10. Largest organelle
12. Type of tissue in which a fat droplet occupies most of the cell
13. Process of cell division from the Greek word for *thread*
15. Passive transport method whose root comes from the Greek for *to push*
17. Physicist to first coin the term *cell*

Answers are on page 38.

Match game

Tissues are groups of similar cells that perform the same role. Each tissue also has at least one unique function. Match the clue to the correct type of tissue.

Clues

1. Tissue that lines the surface of serous membranes, such as the pleura, pericardium, and peritoneum
2. Epithelial tissue that has only one layer of cells but appears to have more
3. Tissue that has cube-shaped surface cells
4. Tissue that has large spaces that separate the fibers and cells and contains a lot of intercellular fluid
5. Tissue with a striped appearance
6. Nervous tissue that consists of three parts: dendrites, cell body, and axons

Choices

A. Loose connective
B. Mesothelium
C. Neurons
D. Pseudostratified
E. Cuboidal
F. Striated muscle

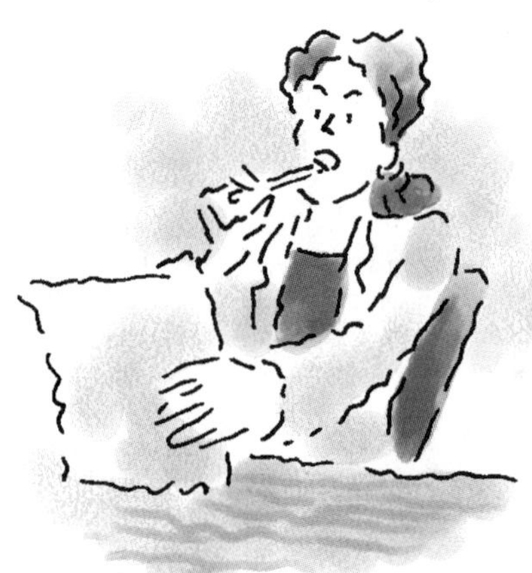

Knowing the different tissue types brings you one step closer to mastering anatomy.

Answers are on page 38.

Scrambled or overeasy

Mr. Cell is hungry but has lost the organelle responsible for digesting foreign material. Fill in the blanks, then unscramble the circled letters to find the organelle that will help Mr. Cell fulfill his craving.

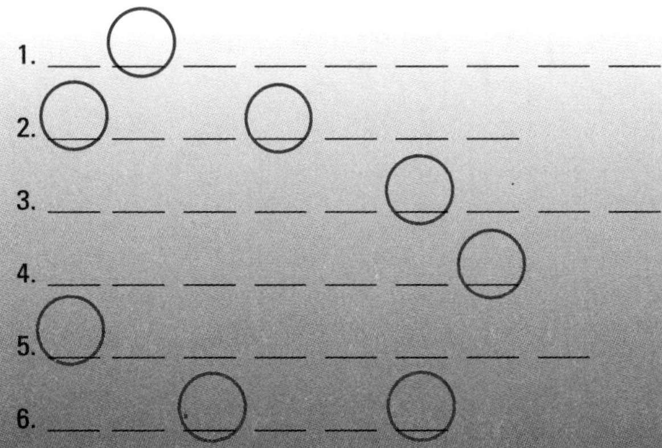

1. This is an aqueous mass that is surrounded by the cell membrane.
2. Only gametes (ova and spermatozoa) undergo this type of reproduction.
3. Particles or solutes move from an area of higher concentration to an area of lower concentration in this type of movement.
4. The cavity that houses and protects the brain.
5. This plane runs lengthwise front to back and divides the body into right and left sides.
6. This prefix means *false.*

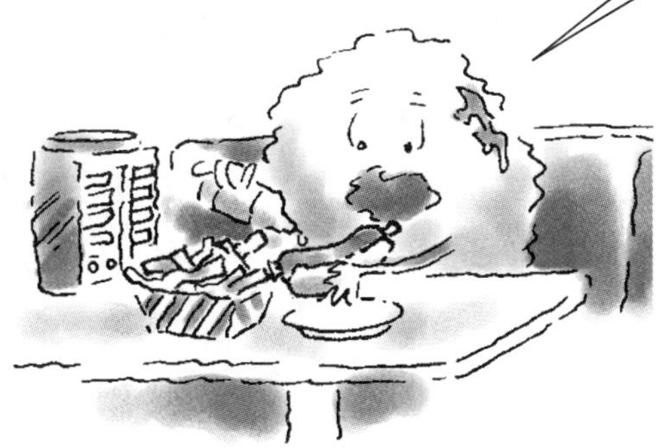

I'm hungry...and I need something other than a knife and fork!

Answers are on page 38.

Answers

At a crossroads

1 S			2 M	I	3 T	O	4 C	H	O	N	D	R	I	A			
A					R		Y										
5 G	A	M	E	T	E		T										
I					N		6 O	R	G	A	N	E	L	L	E	S	
T					D		K										
T			7 A		E		8 I	N	T	E	R	P	H	A	S	E	
A			N		L		N										
L			T		E		E					9 D					
	10 N		E		N		11 S	T	R	12 A	T	I	F	I	E	D	
	U		R		B		I			D		F					
	C		I		U		S			I		F				13 M	
	L		O		R					P		U				I	
14 N	E	U	R	15 O	G	L	I	A		O		S				T	
	U			S						S		I				O	
	S			M					16 T	E	L	O	P	17 H	A	S	E
			18 F	O	W	L	E	R				N		O		I	
				S										O		S	
				I										K			
				S										E			

Match game

1. B; 2. D; 3. E; 4. A; 5. F; 6. C.

Scrambled or overeasy

1. Cytoplasm; 2. Meiosis; 3. Diffusion; 4. Cranial; 5. Sagittal; 6. Pseudo.
Answer to puzzle — Lysosome

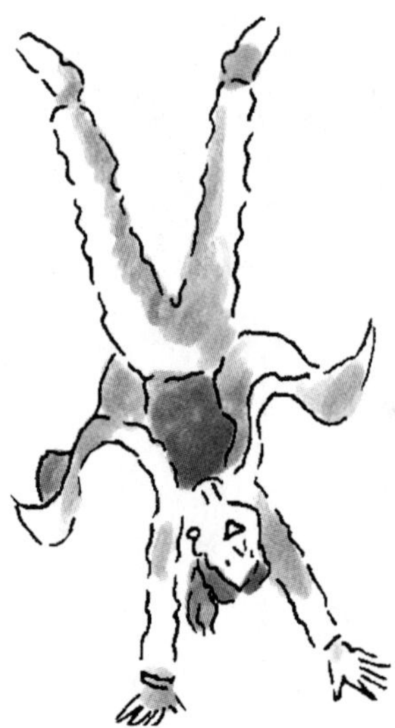

3

Skeletal system

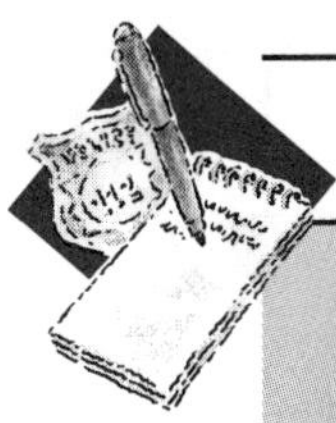

Just the facts

In this chapter, you'll review:

- terminology related to the anatomy of the skeletal system
- terminology that will help you describe your patient's signs and symptoms
- tests that help diagnose skeletal system disorders
- skeletal disorders and their treatments.

Anatomy of a skeleton

The 206 bones of the skeletal system carry out six important anatomic and physiologic functions:

- They protect internal tissues and organs; for example, the 33 vertebrae surround and protect the spinal cord.
- They stabilize and support the body.
- They provide surfaces for muscle, ligament, and tendon attachment.
- They move through lever action when contracted.
- They produce red blood cells in the bone marrow (a process called **hematopoiesis,** from the Greek ***haima,*** or blood, and ***poiesis,*** meaning *making* or *forming*).
- They store mineral salts, for example, approximately 99% of the body's calcium. (See *Pronouncing key skeletal terms*, page 40.)

Bones 'r us — in two parts

The skeleton is divided into two parts: the **axial** (from the Latin ***axis,*** meaning *axle* or *wheel*) and **appendicu-**

Pump up your pronunciation

Pronouncing key skeletal terms

Below is a list of key terms, along with the correct way to pronounce them.

Acetabulum	AS-EH-TAB-YUH-LUHM
Arthrocentesis	AHR-THROW-SEHN-TEE-SISS
Arthrodesis	AHR-THROW-DEE-SISS
Astragalus	AHS-STRAHG-AH-LUSS
Calcaneus	KAHL-KAY-NEE-USS
Canaliculi	KAHN-AH-LIHK-YOO-LEYE
Cartilaginous	KAHR-TIH-LAJ-IH-NUSS
Coccyx	KOCK-SIHKS
Hematopoiesis	HEE-MAT-OH-POY-EE-SISS
Hyaline	HIGH-AH-LEEN
Kyphosis	KEYE-FOH-SISS
Lambdoidal	LAM-DOY-DUHL
Malleolus	MAH-LEE-OH-LUSS
Medullary	MEHD-YOO-LAHR-EE
Occipital	OHK-SIHP-IH-TAHL
Periosteum	PEHR-EE-OSS-TEE-UHM

lar (from the Latin ***appendare,*** meaning to *add* or *append*). The **axial skeleton** forms the body's vertical axis and contains 74 bones in the head and torso; it also includes 6 bones of the middle ear, for a total of 80 bones.

The **appendicular skeleton** contains 126 bones and includes the body's **appendages,** or upper and lower extremities. (See *The body's bones.*)

The body's bones

The human skeleton contains 206 bones; 80 form the axial skeleton and 126 form the appendicular skeleton. The illustrations below show some of the major bones and bone groups.

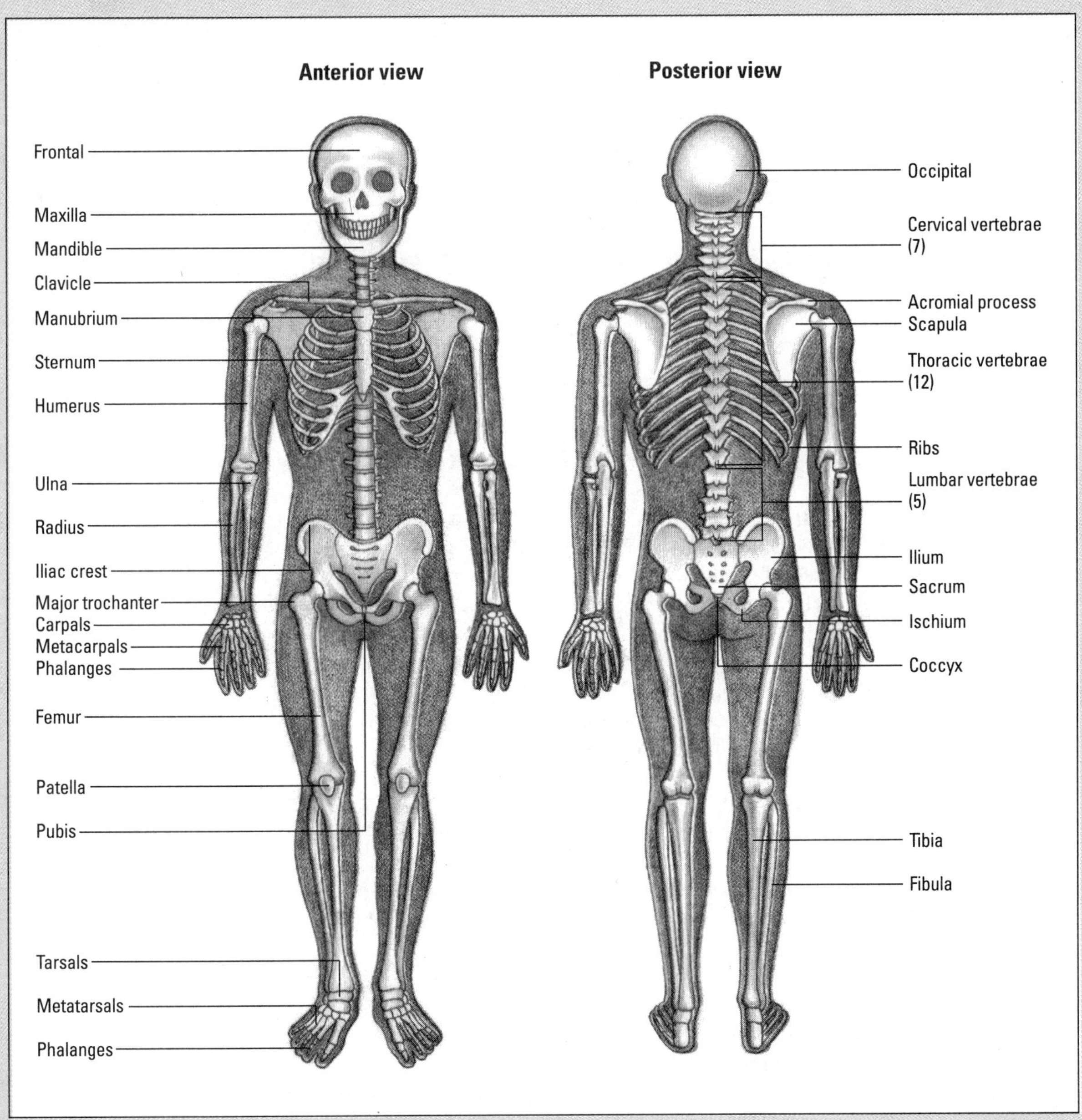

The axial skeleton

The axial skeleton forms the long axis of the body and includes bones of the skull, vertebral column, and rib cage.

The skull

The **skull** contains 28 irregular bones in two major areas: the brain case, or **cranium** (from the Greek ***kranion,*** meaning *upper part of the head*) and the **face.** Eight bones form the cranium, 14 bones make up the face, and the inner ears contain 6 **ossicles** (from the Latin ***ossiculum,*** meaning *bone*), or 3 small bones in each ear. The jaw bone, or **mandible** (from the Latin ***mandibula,*** meaning *jaw*) is the only movable bone in the skull. (See *Bones of the skull.*)

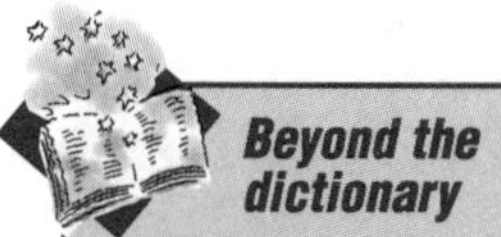

Fontanel is a little fountain

Fontanel, also spelled **fontanelle,** derives from French and means *little fountain.* It can also refer to any membrane-covered area between two bones.

Getting it together

Sutures are immobile joints that hold the skull bones together. The **coronal suture** unites the frontal bone and the two parietal bones. In infants, this suture isn't closed, leaving a diamond-shaped area (called the **anterior fontanel**), which is covered only by a membrane. This soft spot closes between ages 10 and 18 months. At the back of the head of infants, the **posterior fontanel** closes by age 2 months. (See *Fontanel is a little fountain.*)

A real airhead

Sinuses are air-filled spaces within the skull that lessen the bone weight, moisten incoming air, and act as resonating chambers for the voice.

Up front

The sinuses, the forehead, and the area directly behind it are part of the **frontal bone.** This bone also forms the **orbits** (eye sockets) and the front part of the cranial floor. The coronal suture separates the frontal bone from the parietal bones.

Take it from the top

The main part of the skull consists of a number of bones sutured together:

• The **coronal suture** connects the frontal bone with the parietal bones.

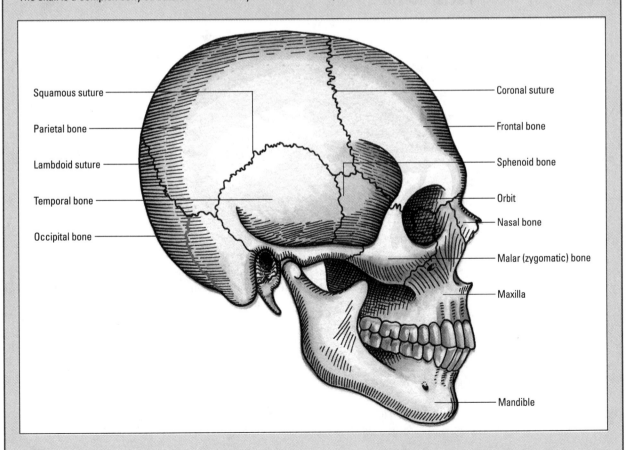

- Two **parietal bones** crown the head, forming the roof and the upper part of each side of the skull.
- The **squamous suture** connects the parietal bones with the temporal bones.
- **Temporal bones** form the lower part of the sides of the skull and part of its floor. They contain structures of the middle and inner ear and the **mastoid sinuses**.
- The **lambdoid suture** connects the parietal bones to the occipital bone.

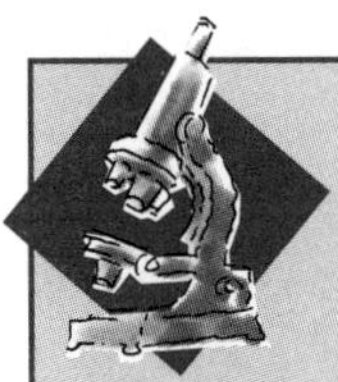

Zoom in

Bones of the skull

The skull is a complex bony structure. It's formed by two sets of bones, the cranial bones and the facial bones.

Squamous suture
Parietal bone
Lambdoid suture
Temporal bone
Occipital bone
Coronal suture
Frontal bone
Sphenoid bone
Orbit
Nasal bone
Malar (zygomatic) bone
Maxilla
Mandible

• The **occipital bone** forms the rear portion and the base of the skull and forms a movable joint with the first cervical vertebra.
• A large opening in the base called the **foramen magnum** (that is, *large hole*) allows the spinal cord to pass from the skull into the spine.

A bat in the belfry

The **sphenoid bone** looks like a bat with outstretched wings and legs extended to the back. Located in the cranial floor, this bone is an anchor for the frontal, parietal, occipital, and ethmoid bones. It also supports part of the eye sockets and forms the lateral walls of the skull. The **sphenoid sinuses** are large air-filled spaces within the sphenoid bone.

Facial bones

The bones of the face include:
• two **maxillary bones** that form the upper jaw, nose, orbits, and roof of the mouth as well as the **maxillary sinuses**
• the cheekbones, called **zygomatic** or **malar bones,** that attach to chewing muscles
• two **nasal bones** that form the upper part of the bridge of the nose (**cartilage** forms the lower part)
• the **mandible** that forms the lower jaw.

The spinal column

The flexible spinal column contains 24 **vertebrae** (plural of **vertebra**), the **sacrum**, and the **coccyx.** (See *Some thorny words of the spine.*)

Joints between the vertebrae allow forward, backward, and sideways movement. The spinal column supports the head while suspending the ribs and organs in front. It also anchors the pelvic girdle and provides attachment points for many important muscles. The spinal column contains:
• seven **cervical** (neck) vertebrae, which support the skull and rotate
• twelve **thoracic** (chest) vertebrae, which attach to the ribs
• five **lumbar** (lower back) vertebrae, which support the small of the back

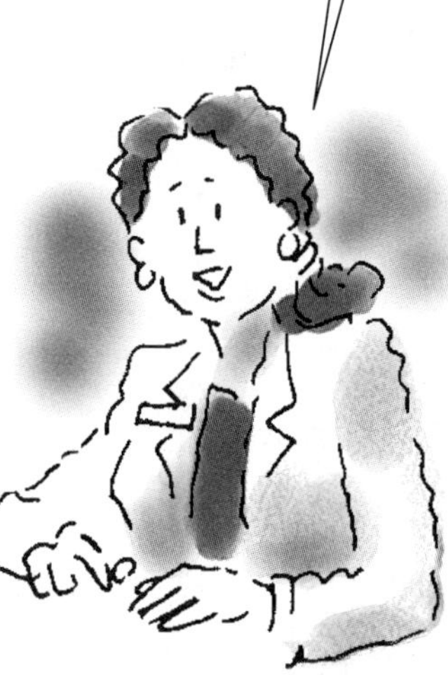
Joints between the vertebrae allow forward, backward, and sideways movement. Not all at once, though!

Beyond the dictionary

Some thorny words of the spine

Spine comes from the Latin word ***spina,*** which means *thorn,* and is related to **spike** as well. Latin writers likened the thorn to the prickly bones in animals and fish and, thus the word also became the designation for the vertebral column.

Vertebra and spondylo
Also from Latin, **vertebra** derives from a verb meaning *to turn.* Therefore, it formerly designated any joint—not just those of the spine. A Greek word, ***spondylos,*** means the same as **vertebra.** It shows up in words like **spondylitis,** which is an inflammation of the vertebra.

Sacrum and coccyx bringing up the rear
The **sacrum** was formerly know as the **os sacrum,** literally the *holy bone,* so called because it was thought to be a particularly choice bit and so was offered to the gods in sacrifice. The **coccyx** derives its name from the Greek word for the cuckoo, ***kokkyx.*** The Greek anatomist Galen thought this triangular bone resembled the shape of the bird's bill.

• the **sacrum,** a single bone that results from the fusion of five vertebrae and attaches to the pelvic girdle
• the **coccyx,** or tailbone, which is located at the bottom tip of the spinal column and is a single bone formed from the fusion of four or five vertebrae.

The spinal column is curved to increase its strength and make balance possible in an upright position. The vertebrae are cushioned by intervertebral disks composed of cartilage. (See *The spinal column,* page 46.)

Sternum

Located in the center of the chest, the **sternum** is a flat, sword-shaped bone that is attached to the **clavicles** (collar bones) and the innermost part of the first seven pairs of ribs.

Living in a cage

The sternum, ribs, and thoracic vertebrae form a protective enclosure around the vital organs. Known as the

Zoom in

The spinal column

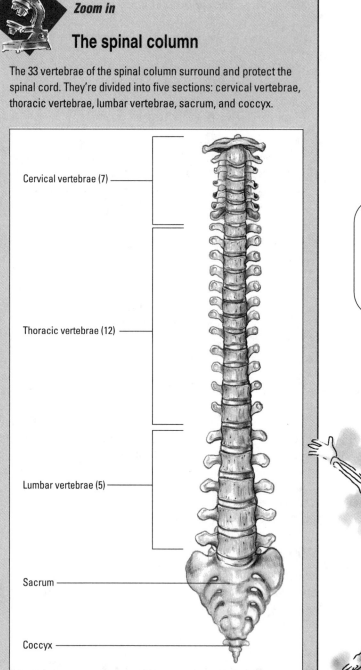

The 33 vertebrae of the spinal column surround and protect the spinal cord. They're divided into five sections: cervical vertebrae, thoracic vertebrae, lumbar vertebrae, sacrum, and coccyx.

Cervical vertebrae (7)

Thoracic vertebrae (12)

Lumbar vertebrae (5)

Sacrum

Coccyx

Yep. I have 33 of these — and they're all perfect specimens, if I do say so myself.

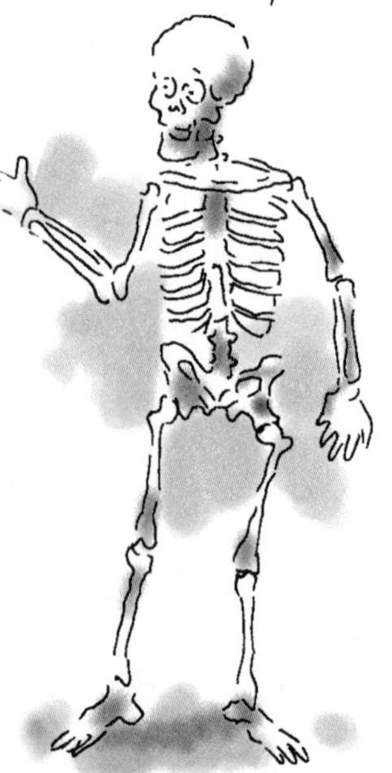

thoracic cage, or **thorax,** this flexible structure protects the heart and lungs and allows the lungs to expand during respiration.

Ribs

The flat, curved bones attached to the thoracic portion of the spinal column are called ribs.

Ribs — true or false?

The term **costal** refers to ribs. The first seven ribs are attached to the sternum by **costal cartilage;** they're called **true ribs.** The remaining five ribs are called **false ribs,** because they aren't attached directly to the sternum. All ribs are independently attached to the spinal column.

Appendicular skeleton

The appendicular skeleton includes the upper and lower extremities.

The upper extremities

The **clavicles,** or collarbones, are two flat bones attached to the sternum on their anterior side and to the scapulae (shoulder blades) laterally. This forms the **sternoclavicular joint.** The **scapulae** are a pair of large, triangular bones that are located at the back of the thorax. These bones, plus the clavicles, form the shoulder girdles.

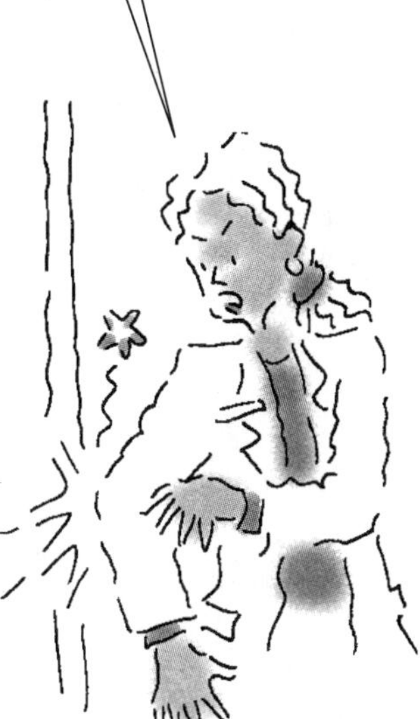
The ulna and the radius articulate with the humerus to form the elbow joint.

Armed and dangerous

The **humerus,** or upper arm bone, is a long bone with a shaft and two bulbous ends. The two long bones of the lower arm are the **ulna,** located on the little finger side of the humerus, and the **radius,** on the thumb side. These bones articulate with the humerus to form the elbow joint. The **wrists** are composed of eight small, irregular **carpal** bones aligned in two rows. Ligaments bind the carpals together.

A handful of terms

The bones of the hand are comprised of metacarpal bones and phalanges. (See *Bones of the hand,* page 48.)

The way these bones come together enables movement of the hand:

Zoom in

Bones of the hand

A view of the right hand, illustrating the positions of the carpals, metacarpals, and phalanges.

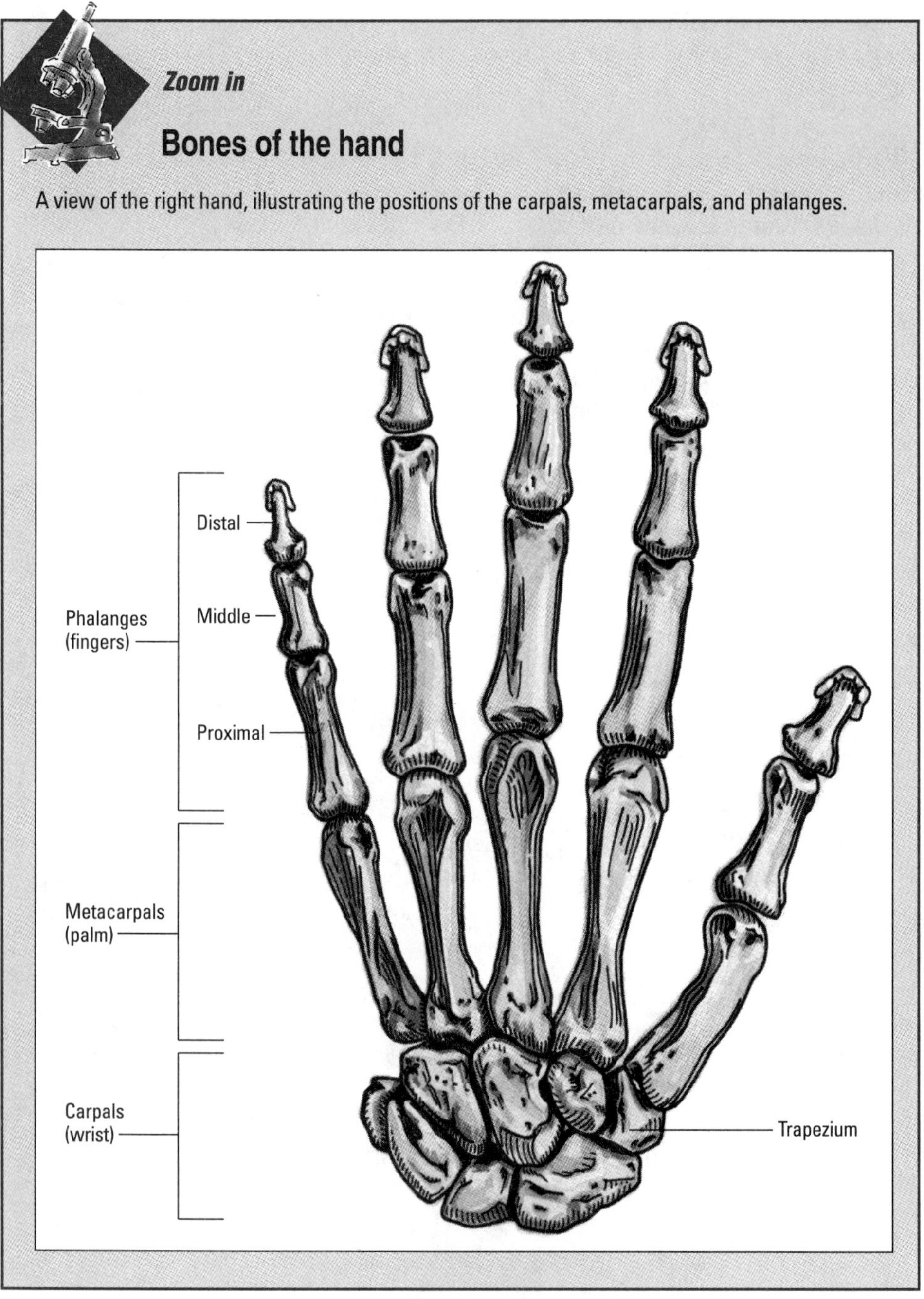

- Five small long **metacarpal** bones attach to the carpals and form the palm of the hand.

• **Phalanges,** or finger bones, are miniature long bones. Each finger has three phalanges, while the thumb has two. (See *A phalanx of phalanges.*)
• The thumb **metacarpal** has a freely movable joint, allowing a wide range of movement between the thumb metacarpal and the **trapezium,** the carpal at the base of the thumb.

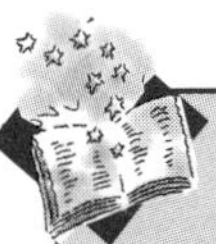

Beyond the dictionary

A phalanx of phalanges

Phalanges is the plural of the Greek word ***phalange,*** or ***phalanx.*** The latter is a term applied to Greek and then Roman army troop formations noted for their closely joined and unified maneuvers.

Lower extremities

The lower extremities contain bones of the hip, thigh, leg, ankle, and foot.

Girdle words

Three pairs of bones fuse during childhood to form the **pelvic girdle,** the broadest bone in the body. This bone supports the trunk, protects the abdominal organs within its basin, and attaches the lower extremities to the body. The three pairs of fused bones include the **ilium,** which is the largest and uppermost of the three; the **ischium,** the lower and strongest set of bones; and the **pubis,** a pair of anterior bones that meet at the **symphysis pubis** — a cartilaginous joint.

Give 'em a leg up

The two **femurs,** or upper leg bones, are the longest and heaviest bones in the body. They connect at the proximal end with the hip, articulating with the **acetabulum,** or hip socket. The femurs connect with the **tibia** at the distal end. The kneecap, or **patella,** is a small, flat bone that protects the knee joint and overlaps the distal end of the femur and the proximal end of the tibia.

The word **patella,** for kneecap, is a Roman word that means *a small, flat dish* — just what the kneecap looks like. Ow!

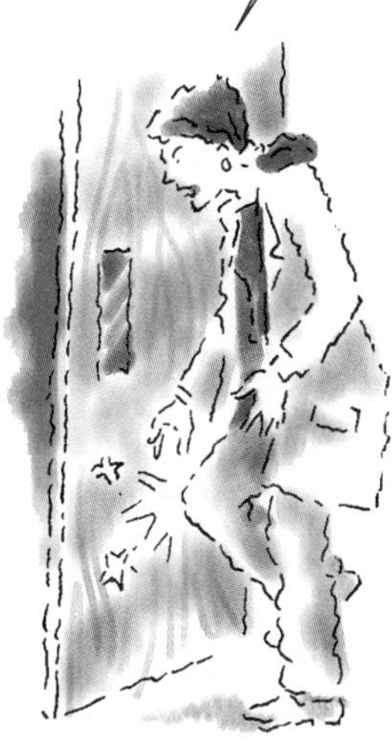

Below the knee

The **tibia,** sometimes called the shinbone, is the largest and strongest of the lower leg bones. It articulates with the femur at the proximal end, and meets the fibula and the talus at the distal end. The **fibula** connects with the tibia at its proximal and distal ends. The fibula's distal end also articulates with the talus. The articulation of the fibula, tibia, and talus bones creates the bony prominence on the outside of the ankle, called the **lateral malleolus.**

Now, fleetly, to the foot

The foot bones form a strong, stable arch with lengthwise and crosswise support. Strong ligaments and tendons of the leg muscles help the foot bones maintain their arched position:

- Seven short **tarsal bones** structurally resemble the wrist, and they articulate with the tibia and fibula.
- The **talus bone** (astragalus) forms part of the ankle joint.
- The heel is called the **calcaneus** and is the largest tarsal bone.
- The **scaphoid bone** is also called the **navicular** because of its boat shape.
- The **cuneiforms** are three wedge-shaped bones forming the arch of the foot.
- Five **metatarsal bones** form the foot and articulate with the tarsal bone and the phalanges.
- The fourteen **phalanges** (toes) are similar to fingers, with three bones in each toe except the great toe, which, like the thumb, contains only two bones.

Anatomy of bones

Bones are classified according to their shape: long, short, flat, or irregular:

- **Long bones** are the main bones of the limbs, except the patella, and those of the wrists and ankles.
- **Short bones** are the bones of the wrists and ankles.
- **Flat bones** include the sternum, scapulae, and cranium, among others.
- **Irregular bones** include the vertebrae and hip bones.

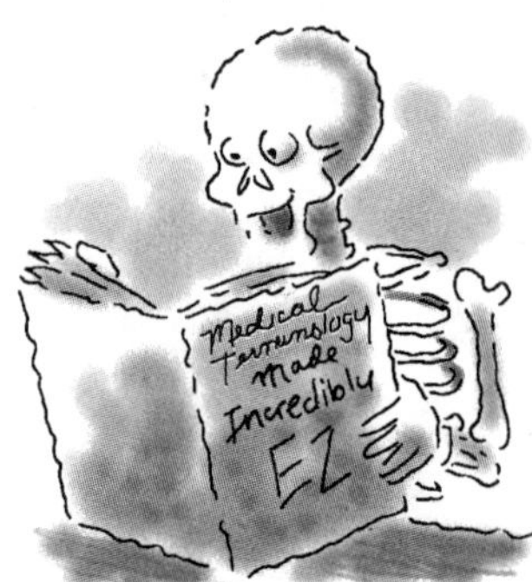
Words will never hurt me. But let's keep sticks and stones out of it!
Medical Terminology Made Incredibly EZ

Hard or soft

All bones consist of two types of bone material: an outer layer of dense, smooth **compact bone** and an inner layer of spongy, **cancellous** (porous) bone. Compact bone is found especially in the shaft of long bones and in the outer layers of short, flat, and irregular bones. Cancellous bone fills the central regions of the epiphyses (the end of a long bone where bone formation takes place) and the inner portions of short, flat, and irregular bones.

Long bones

Long bones contain a number of visible, common structures:

- **Epiphyses** (singular: **epiphysis**): The bulbous ends of long bones that provide a large surface for muscle attachment and give stability to joints.
- **Articular cartilage:** A thin layer of hyaline cartilage that covers and cushions the **articular** (joint) surfaces of the epiphyses.
- **Periosteum:** A dense membrane that covers the shafts of long bones; it consists of two layers — a fibrous outer layer and a bone-forming inner layer.
- **Medullary cavity:** A cavity filled with bone marrow.
- **Endosteum:** A thin membrane that lines the medullary cavity and contains **osteoblasts** (bone-producing cells).

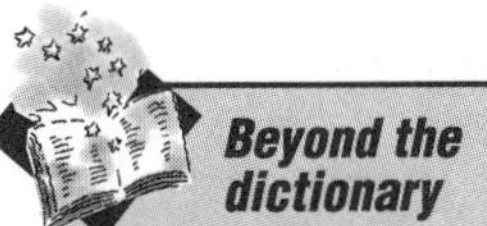

Haversian systems

The **haversian systems** were named in honor of the 17th century British doctor and anatomist Clopton Havers, who discovered them.

Feeding the long bones

Within the compact bone are **haversian systems**. (See *Haversian systems.*)

These systems are made up of the following structures:

- **lamellae** — thin layers of ground substance
- **lacunae** — small hollow spaces
- **canaliculi** — small canals
- **haversian canals** — minute canals that contain blood and lymph vessels, nerves, and sometimes marrow.

Blood reaches bone by arterioles in haversian canals; by vessels in Volkmann's canals, which connect one haversian canal to another and to the outer bone; and by vessels in the bone ends and within the marrow. (See *Two views of a long bone*, page 52.)

To marrow, and to marrow, and to marrow...

In a child's body, nearly all the bones contain **red bone marrow.** In an adult, red bone marrow is found in the femur, ribs, vertebrae, and the ends of the humerus in the upper arm. Red bone marrow performs **hematopoiesis,** making new red blood cells for the body.

Bone growth and resorption

Bones grow both in length and in thickness. At the epiphyses (ends), they grow longer, and at the diaphyses (shafts), they grow in diameter through the activity of os-

Zoom in

Two views of a long bone

Here is a look at the long bone from interior and cross-section views.

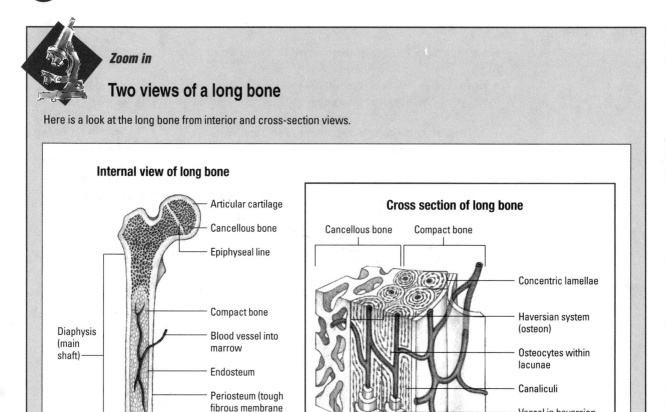

Internal view of long bone

Articular cartilage
Cancellous bone
Epiphyseal line
Compact bone
Blood vessel into marrow
Endosteum
Periosteum (tough fibrous membrane sheath)
Diaphysis (main shaft)
Epiphysis

Cross section of long bone

Cancellous bone
Compact bone
Concentric lamellae
Haversian system (osteon)
Osteocytes within lacunae
Canaliculi
Vessel in haversian canal
Volkmann's canal
Trabeculae

teoblasts in the periosteum. A hormone secreted by the anterior lobe of the pituitary gland controls bone growth. (See *Bone up on* osteo- *and* oss-.)

As osteoblasts add new tissue to the outside of a bone, large phagocytic cells called **osteoclasts** eat away bony tissue in the medullary cavity to keep the bone from becoming too thick. A healthy bone is constantly broken down, reabsorbed, and repaired long after it stops growing in size. During adulthood, bone formation, or **ossifi-**

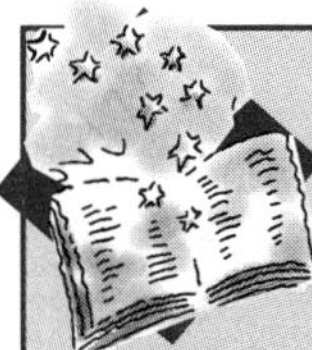

Beyond the dictionary

Bone up on *osteo-* and *oss-*

Osteon, Greek for *bone,* provides a key word-forming root for medical terms relating to bones, ***oste-*** or ***osteo-*. Osteoblast** is a compound of ***osteo-*** and ***-blast,*** another common medical root derived from a Greek word that means a *bud* or a *shoot of a developing organism;* an **osteoblast** is thus *a cell that buds forth new bone tissue.* The Greek word ***clast,*** on the other hand, means *to break* or *fragment.* Therefore, an **osteoclast** is *a cell that breaks down bone.*

The Romans had a name for it

Another very common root for forming words is the Latin word ***os,*** or ***oss-,*** also meaning *bone.* This root is contained in words like **ossify,** meaning *to change* or *become bone,* and **ossification,** *the process of becoming bone.*

cation, and bone **resorption** balance one another so that each bone remains a constant size. During childhood and adolescence, ossification is faster than resorption and bones grow larger.

Cartilage

Cartilage is a dense connective tissue that consists of fibers embedded in a strong, gel-like substance. Unlike rigid bone, cartilage has the flexibility of firm plastic.

Cartilage supports and shapes various structures, such as the auditory canal and the intervertebral disks. It also cushions and absorbs shock. Cartilage has no blood or nerve supply.

Types of cartilage

Cartilage may be fibrous, hyaline, or elastic:

- **Fibrous cartilage** forms at the symphysis pubis and the intervertebral disks.
- **Hyaline cartilage** covers articular bone surfaces (where one or more bones meet at a joint), connects the ribs and sternum, and appears in the trachea, bronchi, and nasal septum.
- **Elastic cartilage** is located in the auditory canal, external ear, and epiglottis.

How bones move

Bones are rigid structures and can't bend without damage, so individual bones move at joint sites, or **articulations.** Every bone in the body except the hyoid bone, which anchors the tongue, is connected to another bone by flexible connective tissue.

Classifying joints

Joints can be classified by the type of movement they allow and by their structure.

How does it move?

The three classes of joints identified by the range of movement they allow are:

- **synarthrosis** — immovable
- **amphiarthrosis** — slightly movable
- **diarthrosis** — freely movable.

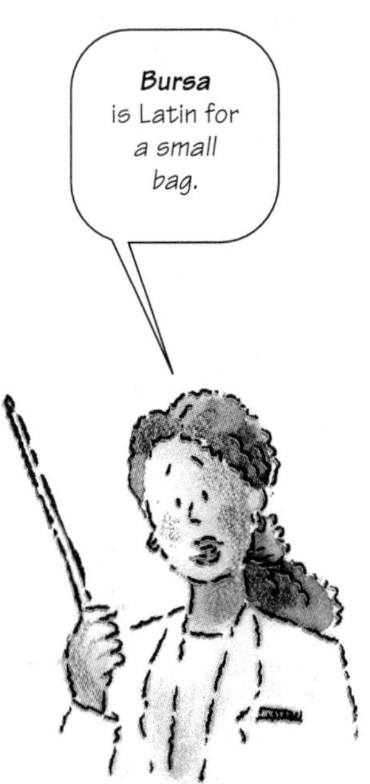
Bursa is Latin for a small bag.

What is it made of?

By structure, a joint may be classified as fibrous, cartilaginous, or synovial. In **fibrous joints,** the articular surfaces of the two bones are bound closely by fibrous connective tissue and little movement is possible. The cranial sutures are examples of fibrous joints.

In **cartilaginous joints,** cartilage connects one bone to another; these joints allow slight movement. An example is the symphysis pubis (the junction of the pelvic bones).

Body surfaces in the **synovial joints** are covered by articular cartilage and joined by **ligaments** (dense, strong, flexible bands of fibrous connective tissue that bind bones to other bones) lined with synovial membrane. Freely movable, synovial joints include most joints of the arms and legs. Synovial joints also include an **articular capsule** — a saclike envelope, whose outer layer is lined with a vascular synovial membrane. This membrane contains synovial fluid — a viscid fluid, produced by the synovial membrane that lubricates the joint.

Small **bursae** (singular: **bursa**) are synovial fluid sacs located at friction points of all types of joints as well as between tendons, ligaments, and bones. Bursae cushion these structures and decrease stress on adjacent ones.

Synovial subdivisions — joints to live in

Based on their structure and the type of movement, synovial joints fall into various subdivisions:

- **Gliding joints,** such as the wrists and ankles, allow adjacent bone surfaces to move against one another.
- **Hinge joints,** such as the elbows and knees, permit movement in only one direction.
- **Pivot joints,** also called **rotary joints,** allow a movable bone to pivot around a stationary bone. The neck and elbows contain pivot joints.
- **Condylar,** or **knuckle joints,** contain an oval head of one bone that fits into a shallow depression in a second bone. The union between the radius (arm bone) and the carpal bones of the hand is an example of a condylar joint.
- **Saddle joints** resemble condylar joints but allow greater freedom of movement. The only saddle joints in the body are the carpometacarpal joints of the thumb.
- **Ball-and-socket joints** get their name from the way their bones connect — the spherical head of one bone fits into a socket of another bone. The hip and shoulder joints are the only ball-and-socket joints in the body.

Saddle joints resemble condylar joints but allow greater freedom of movement. The only saddle joints in the body are the carpometacarpal joints of the thumb.

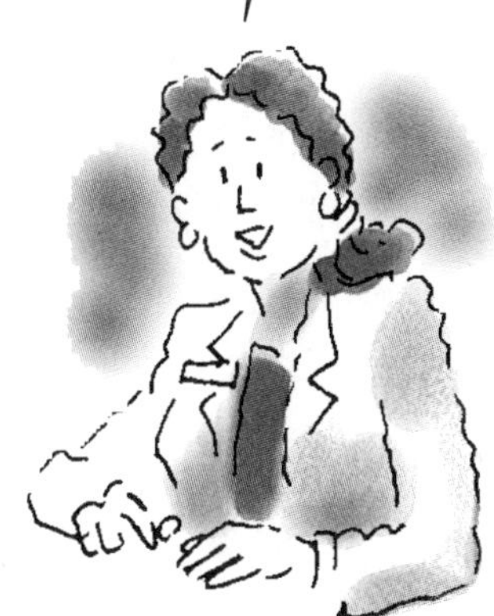

Physical examination terms

Tests to determine bone and joint diseases or injuries include blood tests, aspiration tests, and radiologic tests.

Blood tests

Several blood tests help determine bone and joint disorders:

- **Alkaline phosphatase (ALP)** is an enzyme produced by several organs, including the bones, liver, and intestines. Because blood concentrations of ALP rise with increased activity of bone cells, high ALP levels help diagnose bone disorders.
- **Erythrocyte sedimentation rate (ESR)** is the rate at which red blood cells settle in a tube of unclotted blood. An elevated ESR indicates inflammation.
- **Rheumatoid factor** is a blood test used to distinguish rheumatoid arthritis from other disorders.

• **Serum calcium** measures the amount of calcium in the blood. Abnormally high levels are present with Paget's disease of the bone.

Aspiration tests

Aspiration tests use fluid withdrawn by a suction device, usually a needle:

• In **arthrocentesis,** a joint space is punctured with a needle to aspirate synovial fluid for analysis or to remove accumulated fluid. (See *Arthrocentesis.*)

• In **bone marrow aspiration,** a needle is forced through the outer cortex of a flat bone — such as the sternum or iliac crest — and bone marrow is aspirated for analysis.

• In **lumbar puncture,** a needle is inserted into the subarachnoid space surrounding the spinal cord to remove a sample of cerebrospinal fluid.

Beyond the dictionary

Arthrocentesis

Arthrocentesis becomes a simple compound word when its components are understood. ***Arthro-*** comes from the Greek word ***arthron,*** which means *joint,* and ***-centesis*** derives from the Greek word ***kentesis,*** which means *puncture.* So **arthrocentesis** must be *a joint puncture.*

Radiologic tests

• **Bone X-ray,** the simplest radiologic procedure, is used to examine a bone for disease or fracture.

• A **computerized tomography (CT) scan** uses X-rays directed at multiple angles; subsequent analysis by a computer provides a total picture of the bone. (See *Cat's tale.*)

• **Arthrography** employs contrast dye to observe the interior of a joint, such as the knee, shoulder, ankle, or elbow. Dye is injected into the joint space, and a CT scan records images of the joint.

• **Bone densitometry** is a noninvasive technique that uses X-rays to measure bone mineral density and identify the risk of osteoporosis. The results are analyzed by computer to determine bone mineral status.

• A **bone scan** helps detect bony metastasis, benign disease, fractures, avascular necrosis, and infection. After I.V. administration of a radioactive material, a counter detects the gamma rays, indicating areas of increased uptake, indicating an abnormality.

• **Myelography** is a radiographic examination of the spinal column following administration of a contrast material.

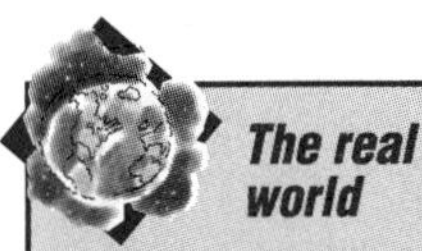

Cat's tale

You may also hear a **CT scan** referred to as a **CAT scan,** which is short for *computerized axial tomography.*

Procedures

• **Arthroscopy** is also used to observe the interior of a joint — most often the knee. A fiberoptic viewing tube is inserted directly into the joint, allowing a doctor to examine its interior.
• A **bone marrow biopsy** removes a piece of bone containing intact marrow.
• **Magnetic resonance imaging** uses an electromagnetic field and radio waves to transfer visual images of soft tissue, such as tendons, to a computer screen.

It's easy when you break it apart: ***arthr-*** is the root for *joint;* ***-algia*** is the suffix for *pain.*

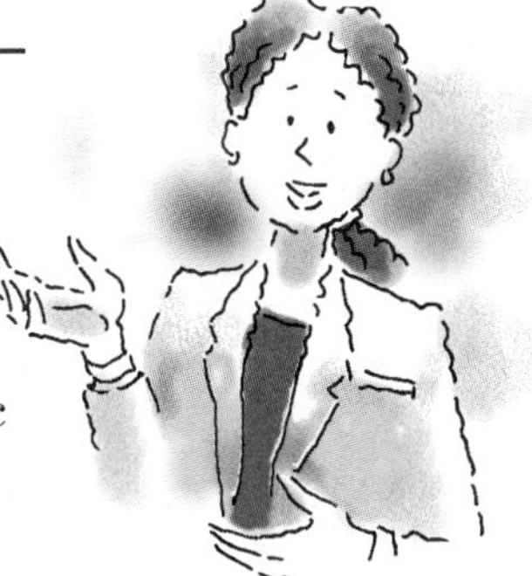

Additional terms

Here are some other terms you should bone up on:
• **arthralgia** — pain in a joint
• **arthredema** — joint swelling
• **arthropyosis** — pus formation in a joint cavity
• **bursitis** — inflammation of a bursa, the fluid-filled sac that prevents friction within a joint
• **chondralgia** — pain originating in the cartilage
• **chondritis** — inflammation of the cartilage
• **chondromalacia** — softening of the cartilage
• **coxitis** — inflammation of the hip joint
• **epiphysitis** — inflammation of the epiphysis of a bone
• **hemarthrosis** — bleeding into a joint
• **hydrarthrosis** — accumulation of watery fluid in a joint
• **kyphosis** — the Greek word for *hunchback*, an outward curvature of the thoracic spine
• **lordosis** — inward curvature of the lumbar spine; also known as sway back
• **lumbago** — pain in the lower back (lumbar) region
• **ostealgia** — bone pain
• **osteitis** — inflammation of bone
• **osteochondritis** — inflammation of bone and cartilage
• **osteolysis** — degeneration of bone from calcium loss.

Disorders of the skeletal system

Disorders of the skeletal system include fractures, dislocations, herniations, cancer, and other diseases.

Fractures and other injuries

Fracture, a traumatic injury or break in the bone tissue, is most commonly seen in the long bones of the arms and legs. Fractures can be caused by direct injury or can occur spontaneously when bone is weakened by disease; the latter is called a pathologic fracture. **Closed** (simple) **fracture** is seen when the broken bone doesn't protrude through the skin. **Open** (compound) **fracture** occurs when the bone breaks through the skin, causing tissue damage.

Fracture features

Fractures can be classified according to the bone fragment position or by the fracture line:

- **Colles' fracture** — a fracture of the radius at the lower end of the wrist in which the bone fragment is displaced posteriorly.
- **Linear fracture** — a fracture that runs along the length of a bone without displacing the bone fragment.
- **Comminuted fracture** — a bone is broken into two or more fragments.
- **Greenstick fracture** — the fracture is incomplete, but there is bowing in the bone.
- **Transverse fracture** — the fracture line extends across the bone.

Bone away from home

Dislocation, displacement of a bone from its normal position within the joint, can occur at birth called a **congenital dislocation,** or may be caused by a disease or trauma. With a dislocation, joint tissue is torn and stretched, possibly rupturing blood vessels. **Subluxation,** partial dislocation that separates the joint's movable surfaces, occurs most commonly in the shoulder, hip, and knee.

Don't play with this disk

Herniated disk, a ruptured area in the cartilage that cushions the intervertebral disks of the spinal column, is a painful condition. Cartilage balloons out from the disk and puts pressure on the nerve roots. Herniation can happen suddenly with lifting or twisting or may result from degenerative joint disease and other chronic conditions.

Diseases

Some of the most common diseases of the skeletal system and terms to describe skeletal disorders are presented here:

- **Ankylosing spondylitis** is a chronic, progressive inflammatory disease that sometimes causes the spine to **fuse.** It involves ligaments and tendons, not synovial membranes as in rheumatoid arthritis.
- **Osteoarthritis,** also known as **degenerative joint disease,** affects the joints of the hand, knee, hip, and vertebrae. It's a major cause of disability.
- **Osteomalacia** is softening of the bones; it's the adult form of rickets.
- **Osteomyelitis** is a generalized infection of bone and bone marrow, most commonly caused by staphylococci that travel to the bone as a result of trauma or surgery.
- **Osteoporosis** is a disorder in which bone mass is reduced and fractures may occur after minimal trauma.
- **Rickets** is a condition of abnormal bone growth in children caused by insufficient vitamin D, calcium, and phosphorus.
- **Rheumatoid arthritis** is a chronic autoimmune disorder that affects the synovial membranes. Painful inflammation of the joints may lead to crippling deformities and affect many organ systems.
- **Scurvy** is a condition caused by lack of vitamin C in the diet, which results in abnormal bones and teeth.

Beyond the dictionary

Word for bone tumor

A word for bone tumor begins with the common root ***osteo-***, meaning *bone.* ***Chondr-*** is a root meaning *cartilage*, and ***-oma*** is a suffix meaning *tumor.* **Osteochondroma** thus is *a tumor of the bone and cartilage.*

Bone tumors

Bone tumors can be **benign** (noncancerous) or **malignant** (cancerous).

Osteochondroma is a common tumor that causes projections (spurs) at the end of long bones. (See *Word for bone tumor.*)

Osteosarcoma is a fast-growing malignant tumor of skeletal tissue with a high fatality rate. Common sites of involvement are the tibia, femur, and humerus, but this tumor commonly metastasizes to the lungs.

Chondrosarcoma is a large, slow-growing malignant tumor that affects the hyaline cartilage. It occurs most often in the femur, spine, pelvis, ribs, or scapula.

Treatments

Noninvasive treatment for bone and joint injuries include:

- a **splint,** which is a removable appliance that immobilizes, restrains, and supports the injured area
- a **cast,** which is a rigid dressing that is placed around an injured body part to support, immobilize, and protect it and promote healing
- a **closed reduction,** which is a manual alignment of a fracture and may precede the application of a cast
- **traction,** which uses a system of weights and pulleys to immobilize and relieve pressure on a fractured bone.

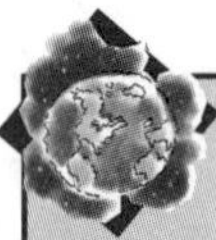

The real world

Let's reduce that reduction

In the real world, you may hear people refer to open reduction with internal fixation as an "ORIF."

Bones, bones — a fixation on bones

Some fractures require **internal fixation** devices, such as pins, plates, screws, wires, and surgical cement to stabilize the bone fragments. An **open reduction with internal fixation** is a surgical procedure that allows the surgeon to directly align the fractured bone and apply internal fixation devices. (See *Let's reduce that reduction.*)

Back off!

These terms relate to invasive treatment of joints and bones:

- **Arthrectomy** is the excision of a joint.
- **Arthrodesis** uses a bone graft typically from the patient's iliac crest to fuse joint surfaces; **spondylosyndesis** is this procedure applied to the vertebrae. (See *Spondylosyndesis.*)
- **Arthroplasty** surgically reconstructs a joint.
- **Bone marrow transplant** involves I.V. administration of marrow aspirated from the donor's bones to a recipient.
- In **chemonucleolysis,** a drug is injected into a herniated disk that dissolves the **nucleus pulposus,** the pulpy, semifluid center of the disk.
- **Costectomy** is the surgical removal of a rib.
- **Diskectomy** removes an intervertebral disk.
- **Hip replacement** replaces a diseased hip joint with a **prosthesis** (artificial substitute for a missing body part).
- **Laminectomy** removes bony arches of vertebrae.
- **Laminotomy** divides the lamina of a vertebra.
- **Ostectomy** is the surgical excision of bone.
- **Osteotomy** is cutting of bone.
- A **sternotomy** cuts through the sternum.

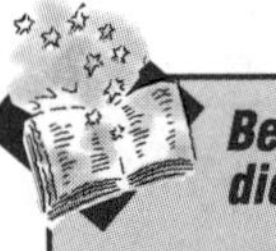

Beyond the dictionary

Spondylosyndesis

Spondylo- comes from the Greek word ***spondylos,*** which means *vertebra;* ***syndesis*** is the Greek word that means *binding together.* Therefore, **spondylosyndesis** is *binding together of the spine,* or *spinal fusion.*

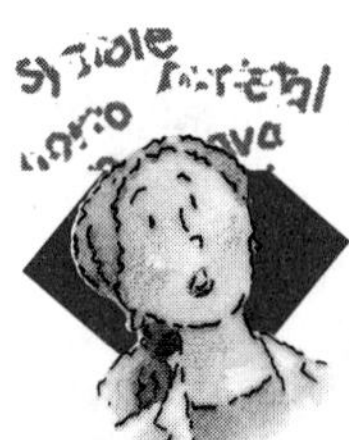

Vocabulary builders

At a crossroads

Completing this crossword puzzle will help build your medical vocabulary. Good luck!

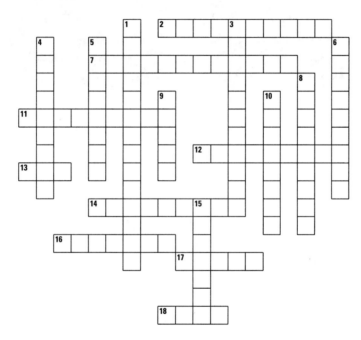

Across

2. Bone's membrane
7. Another name for a joint
11. Dense connective tissue
12. Collarbones
13. Color of marrow that makes blood cells
14. Ends of a long bone
16. Mineral found in bones
17. Bag of synovial fluid
18. Rigid dressing on an extremity

Down

1. Degenerative joint disease
3. Immature bone cells
4. Fingers and toes
5. Jaw bone
6. Main shaft of a long bone
8. Bone cavity
9. Upper leg bone
10. Two bones at top of the head
15. Immovable joints

Answers are on page 64.

Finish line

The root ***osteo-***, meaning *bone*, forms many words related to bone disorders and diseases. Complete the sentences below by filling in the blanks with the appropriate word that begins with ***osteo-***.

1. Osteo______________ is a disorder in which bone mass is reduced.
2. A generalized infection of the bone marrow is called osteo______________.
3. A term used to describe the cutting of a bone is osteo______________.
4. A cell that destroys bone tissue is an osteo______________.
5. Osteo____________ is a common tumor that causes spurs at the end of long bones.

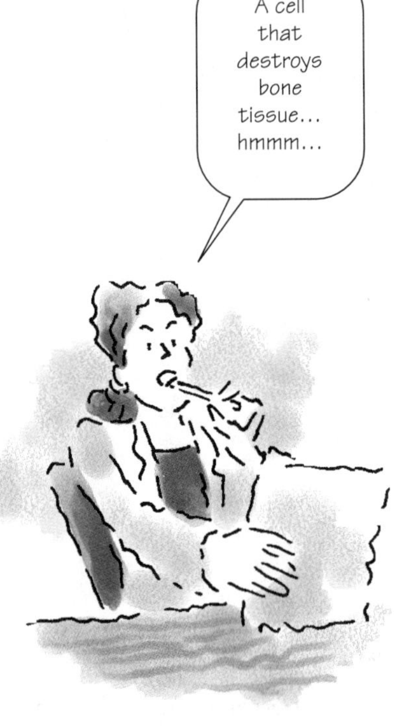

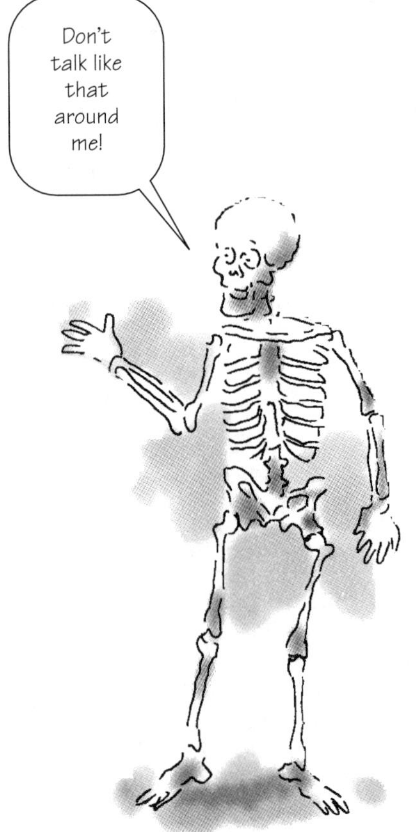

Answers are on page 64.

Scrambled or overeasy

Fill in the blanks with the appropriate word. Unscramble the letters in the circles to answer the puzzle.

1. This is the suture that connects the frontal bone with the parietal bones.
2. This is the cartilage that attaches the sternum to the ribs.
3. The lower arm bone on the thumb side is called this.
4. This is the type of joint in the wrists and ankles.
5. This is the term for displacement of a bone from its normal position.
6. This is the term for joint swelling.
This joint really makes my bones move.

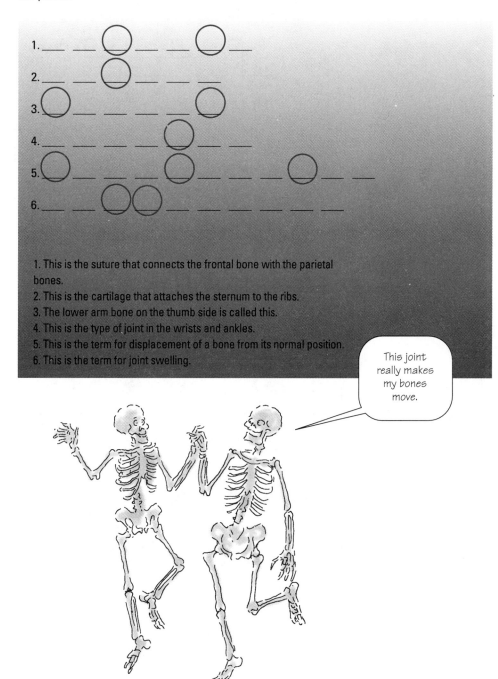

Answers are on page 64.

Answers

At a crossroads

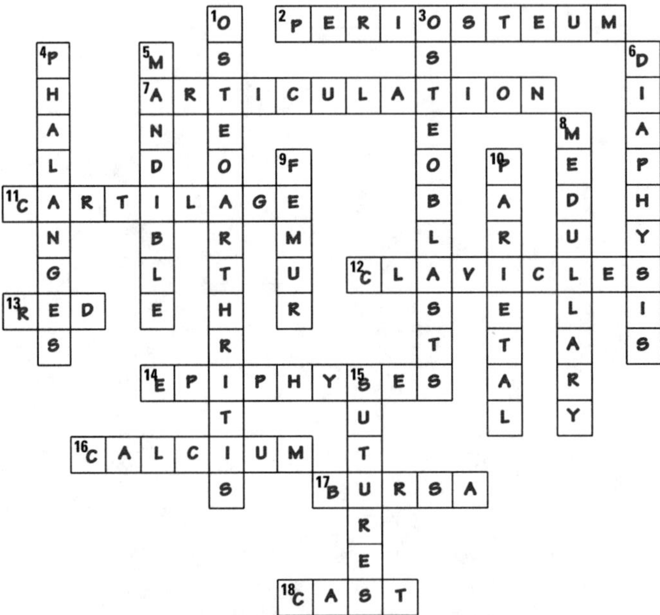

Finish line

1. Porosis; 2. Myelitis; 3. Tomy; 4. Clast; 5. Chondroma.

Scrambled or overeasy

1. Coronal; 2. Costal; 3. Radius; 4. Gliding; 5. Dislocation; 6. Arthredema.
Answer to puzzle — Diarthrosis

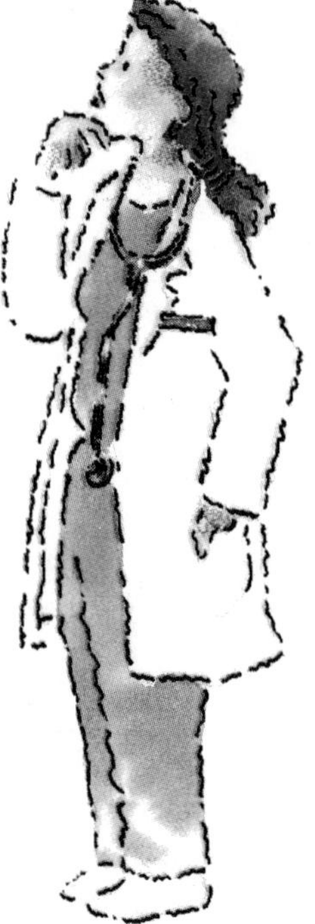

Skeletal system is done — only 11 more systems to go!

Muscular system

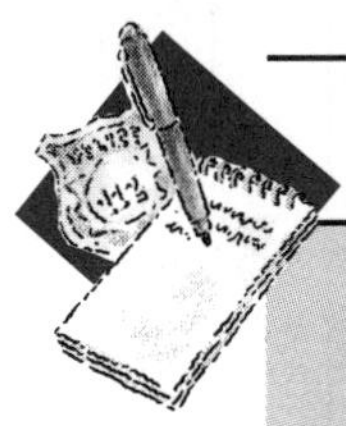

Just the facts

In this chapter, you'll review:

- terminology related to the structure and function of the muscular system
- terminology needed for physical examination of the muscular system
- tests that help diagnose muscular disorders
- disorders of the muscular system and their treatments.

Muscle structure and function

A key to learning terminology related to the muscular system is knowing the medical prefix for muscle, ***my(o),*** from the Greek word for muscle, ***mys.*** Combined with other words, this prefix forms such terms as **myology** (the study of muscles), **myocardium** (heart muscle), and **myositis** (inflammation of voluntary muscle tissues). (See *A close look at myocardium* and *Pronouncing key muscular system terms*, page 66.)

More than just heavy lifting

Muscles have three functions:

 support the body

 permit movement

 produce body heat.

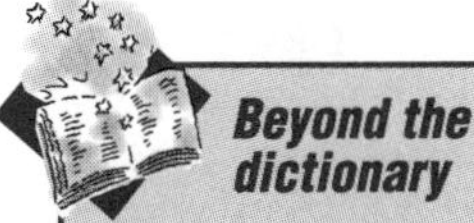

A close look at myocardium

The Greek word for *muscle* is ***myo,*** and ***cardiac*** is the Greek word for *heart.* Therefore, **myocardium** means *heart muscle.*

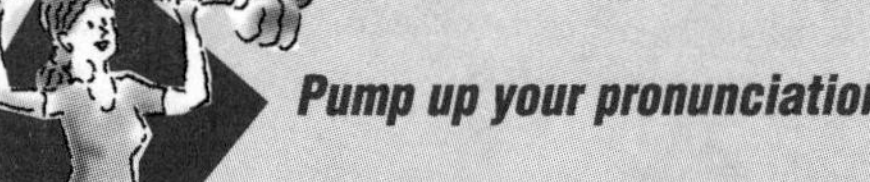

Pump up your pronunciation

Pronouncing key muscular system terms

Below is a list of key terms, along with the correct way to pronounce them.

Term	Pronunciation
Aspartate aminotransferase	AHSS-PAHR-TATE AH-MEE-NOH-TRANS-FUR-AYZ
Buccinator	BUCK-SIH-NAY-TOR
Creatine kinase	CREE-AH-TIHN KEYE-NAYZ
Epimysium	EPP-IH-MIHZ-EE-UHM
Gastrocnemius	GASS-TROH-NEE-MEE-UHS
Leiomyosarcoma	LEYE-OH-MEYE-OH-SAHR-COH-MAH
Myasthenia gravis	MEYE-AHS-THEE-NEE-AH GRAH-VIHS
Myokinesimeter	MEYE-OH-KIHN-NEES-IH-MEE-TUHR
Myositis purulenta	MEYE-OH-SEYE-TIHS PYOO-ROO-LEHN-TAH
Sarcolemma	SAHR-COH-LEHM-AH
Torticollis	TOOR-TIH-KAWL-IHS
Trapezius	TRAH-PEE-ZEE-UHS

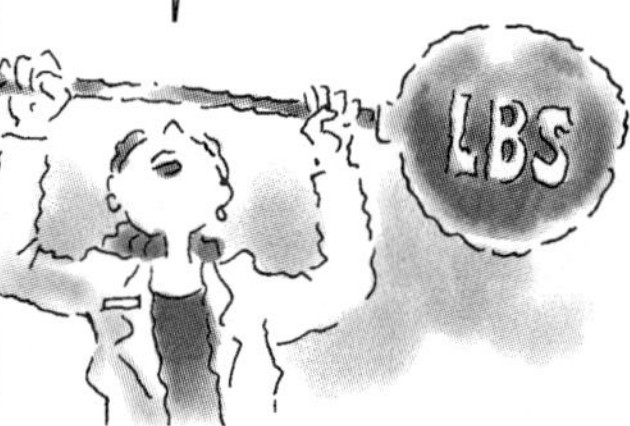

Our bodies have about 600 muscles — not all of them are as easy to identify as my biceps brachii!
500
LBS

They're also an integral part of internal organs, such as the heart, lungs, uterus, and intestines.

Tissue issue

The three major types of muscle in the human body are classified by the tissue they contain:

- **Skeletal** muscles are **voluntary** (controlled by will) muscles that attach to the skeleton and consist of **striated** (in thin bands) tissue. They move body parts and the body as a whole, maintain posture, and implement voluntary and reflex movements. Skeletal muscles also generate body heat. (See *A close look at skeletal muscles.*)
- **Visceral** muscles are **involuntary** (not controlled by will) muscles that contain smooth muscle tissue. They're found in such organs as the stomach and intestines. (See *Gut reaction.*)

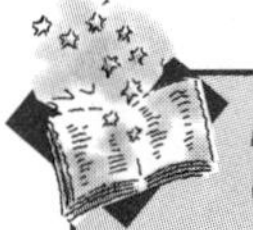

Beyond the dictionary

Gut reaction

The word **visceral** is derived from the Latin ***viscera,*** meaning *internal organs.* **Visceral** also means *intensely emotional* or *instinctive.* Think of a "gut reaction."

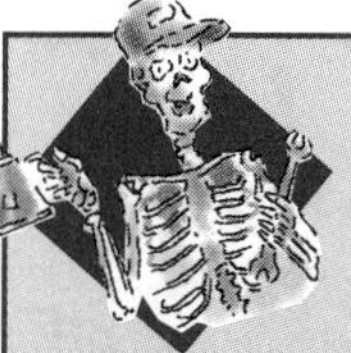

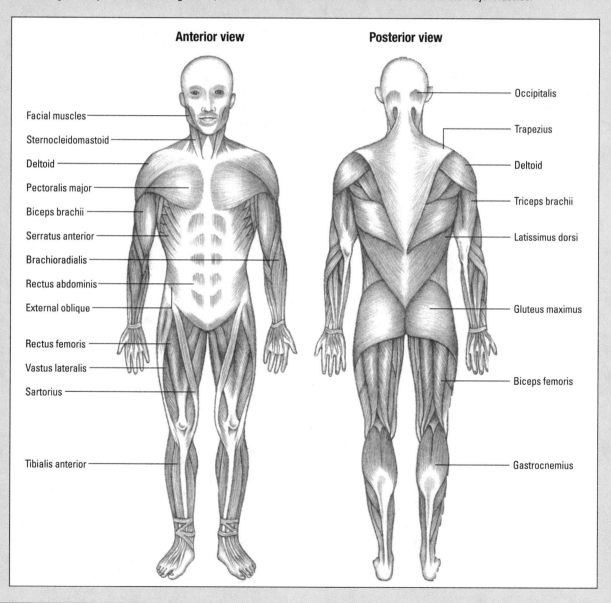

Body shop

A close look at skeletal muscles

Each muscle is classified by the movement it permits. For example, flexors permit the bending of joints, or flexion; abductors permit shortening so that joints can be straightened, or abducted. The illustration below shows some of the major muscles.

Anterior view

Facial muscles
Sternocleidomastoid
Deltoid
Pectoralis major
Biceps brachii
Serratus anterior
Brachioradialis
Rectus abdominis
External oblique
Rectus femoris
Vastus lateralis
Sartorius
Tibialis anterior

Posterior view

Occipitalis
Trapezius
Deltoid
Triceps brachii
Latissimus dorsi
Gluteus maximus
Biceps femoris
Gastrocnemius

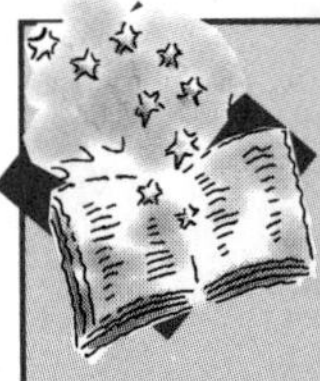

Beyond the dictionary

Origins of sarcolemma and sarcoplasm

A muscle fiber's plasma is called **sarcolemma membrane,** and its cytoplasm is called **sarcoplasm.** In Latin, ***sarco*** means *flesh.* Both **sarcolemma** and **sarcoplasm** share this Latin root.

- **Cardiac** muscle is made up of involuntary, striated tissue. It's controlled by the autonomic nervous system and specialized **neuromuscular** (meaning both nerve and muscle) tissue located within the right atrium.

The muscles' makeup

Muscle tissue cells perform specialized activities and vary greatly in size and length. Because they're usually long and slender with a threadlike shape, muscle cells are called **fibers.**

Connective tissue holds muscle fibers together. Bundles of muscle fibers are enclosed by a fibrous membrane sheath called **fascia.**

Although muscle cells have the same parts as other cells, several of their structures have special names. A muscle fiber's plasma membrane is called a **sarcolemma** and the cytoplasm is called **sarcoplasm.** (See *Origins of sarcolemma and sarcoplasm.*)

The word **ligament** comes from the Latin ***ligare,*** which means *to tie or bind.* That is exactly what ligaments do to your bones.

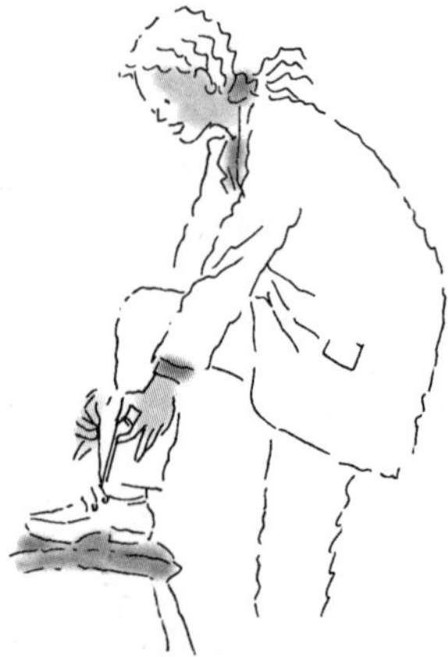

Muscles and bones — holding it together

Tendons are bands of fibrous connective tissue that attach muscles to the **periosteum,** a fibrous membrane that covers the bone. Tendons enable bones to move when skeletal muscles contract, creating energy through the release of the enzyme **adenosine triphosphate** from the cells.

Ligaments are dense, strong, flexible bands of fibrous connective tissue that bind bones to other bones. Ligaments in the skeletal muscle system connect the **articular** (relating to a joint) ends of bones. They provide stability and can either limit movement or make movement easier. Deeper inside the body, ligaments support the organs.

Most skeletal muscles are attached to bones either directly or indirectly. In a direct attachment, the **epimysium** (fibrous sheath around a muscle) of the muscle fuses to the **periosteum** of the bone. In an indirect attachment, the fascia extends past the muscle as a tendon or **aponeurosis** (deeply set fascia), which in turn attaches to the bone. In the human body, indirect attachments outnumber direct attachments.

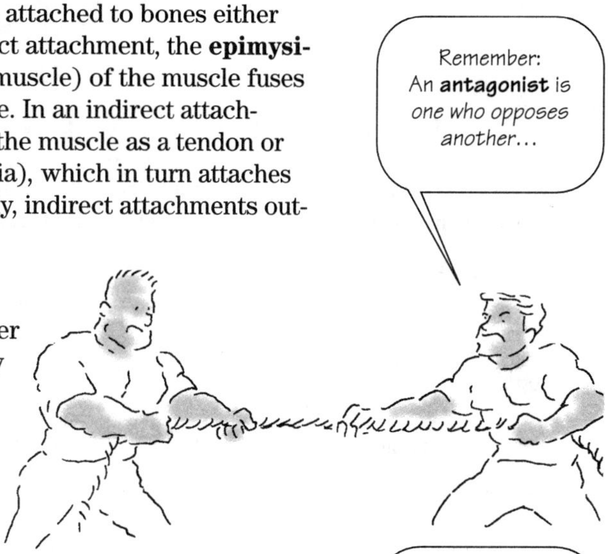

Remember: An **antagonist** is *one who opposes another...*

Putting it in motion

Muscles depend on one another for movement; a muscle rarely acts on its own. **Prime movers** are muscles that actively produce a movement. **Antagonists** are muscles that oppose the prime movers and relax as the prime movers contract. **Synergists** contract along with the prime movers and help execute the movement or provide stability.

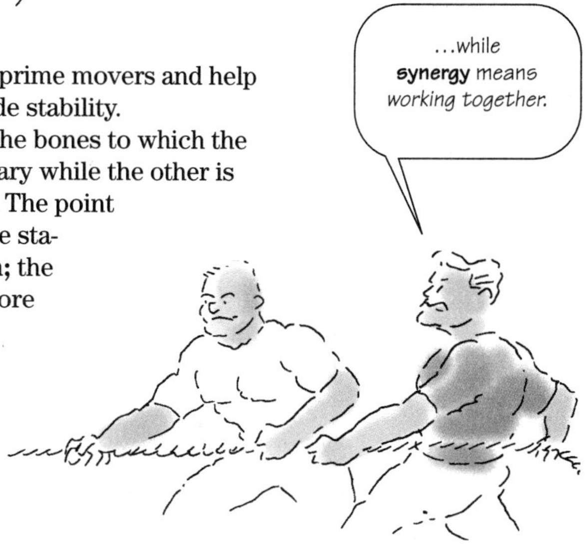

...while **synergy** means *working together.*

During contraction, one of the bones to which the muscle is attached stays stationary while the other is pulled in the opposite direction. The point where the muscle attaches to the stationary bone is called the **origin;** the point where it attaches to the more moveable bone, the **insertion.** The origin usually lies on the **proximal** (nearest to) end of the bone and the insertion site on the **distal** (farthest away) end.

Key muscles

The name of a skeletal muscle may come from its location, action, size, shape, attachment points, number of divisions, or direction of fibers. (See *Muscle structure,* page 70.)

Scalp muscles

The top of the head contains no muscles but has a broad, flat tendon called the **epicranial aponeurosis** that con-

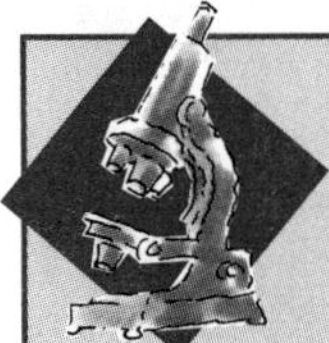

Zoom in

Muscle structure

Each muscle contains cell groups called muscle fibers that extend the length of the muscle. A sheath of connective tissues — called the **perimysium** — binds the fibers into a bundle, or **fasciculus.**

A strong sheath

A stronger sheath, the **epimysium,** binds the fasciculi together to form the fleshy part of the muscle. Beyond the muscle, the epimysium becomes a tendon.

Fine fibers

Each muscle fiber is surrounded by a plasma membrane called the **sarcolemma.** Within the **sarcoplasm** (or cytoplasm) of the muscle fiber lie tiny myofibrils. Arranged lengthwise, myofibrils contain still finer fibers, called thick fibers and thin fibers.

Myosin
Actin
Myofibril
Sarcoplasm
Perimysium
Endomysium
Sarcolemma
Bone
Epimysium
Nuclei
Tendon
Motor neuron
Nerve ending
Fasciculus

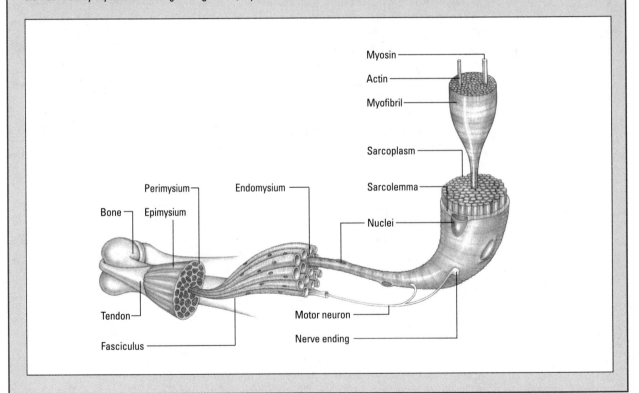

nects to three nearby muscle groups. (See *Dissecting epicranial aponeurosis.*)

• The **occipitofrontal group** houses both the **occipitalis** muscle, which pulls the scalp backward, and the **frontalis** muscle, which pulls it forward. Raising the eyebrows and wrinkling the forehead use the frontalis muscle.

- The **temporoparietal group** includes the **temporalis** muscle, which tightens the scalp and moves the ears forward.
- The **auricular group** contains three muscles (the **anterior, superior,** and **posterior**), which move the ear forward, upward, and backward.

Beyond the dictionary

Dissecting epicranial aponeurosis

Epicranial aponeurosis looks intimidating until you break it down. In Greek, ***epi*** means *upon,* ***kranion*** means *skull,* ***apo*** means *away,* and ***neuron*** means *tendon.* Epicranial aponeurosis is a fibrous membrane that covers the **cranium,** or skull, between the occipital and frontal muscles of the scalp.

Facial muscles

Facial expressions, such as a smile, frown, and a look of surprise, depend on specialized muscles.

Blow, muscle, blow

The **buccinator** muscle, also called the **trumpeter** muscle, compresses the cheeks for smiling or blowing (***bucca*** means *cheek* in Latin). The **corrugator supercilii** draws the eyebrows together in a frown (***corrugatus*** means *wrinkled,* as in a corrugated box). When the eyes widen in surprise, the **orbicularis oculi** (***orbit*** means *around* and ***ocul*** means *eye*) moves the eyelids.

Chew on this

The **masseters** are the chewing muscles (***masticate*** means *chew*), and the **pterygoids** open and close the mouth. The prefix ***pteryx-*** means *wing* and describes the shape of these muscles. (See *Saying pterygoid isn't p-terribly difficult.*)

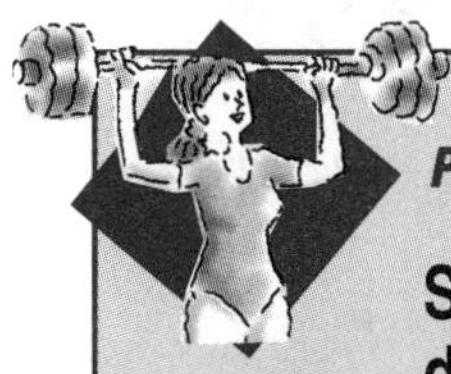

Pump up your pronunciation

Saying pterygoid isn't p-terribly difficult

English doesn't have a sound for the consonant cluster ***pt*** at the beginning of a word. **Pterygoid** is derived from the Greek word for *wing,* ***pteryx.*** When ***pt*** is pronounced in English, the ***p*** is simply silent, as it is when you say the name of the "winged" dinosaur, the pterodactyl. Therefore, pterygoid is pronounced TEHR-IH-GOYD.

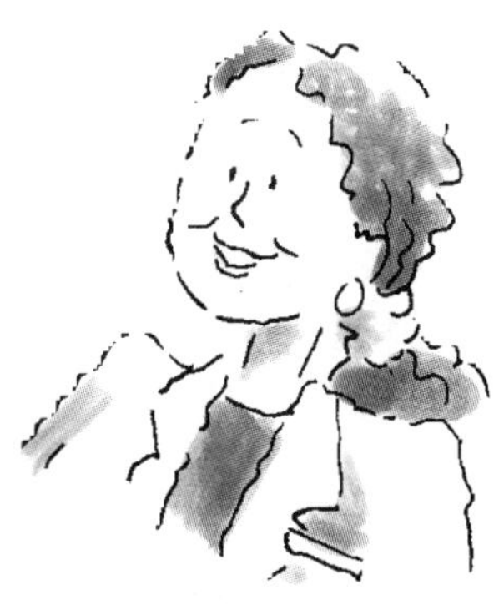

When you see my cheeks (or **buccae,** in Latin) go up in a smile, you know I'm using my buccinator muscles!

Neck and shoulder muscles

Sternocleidomastoid muscles are paired muscles on either side of the neck that allow the head to move. This name combines the muscles' origins in the **sternum** and **clavicle** with their insertion point in the **mastoid process** of the temporal bone.

There's no shrugging this muscle off

The **trapezius** muscle on the back of the neck raises and lowers (shrugging) the shoulders. Arms can be crossed when the **pectoralis major** muscle adducts and flexes the upper arm.

Thorax muscles

The **diaphragm,** a dome-shaped muscle located in the chest, flattens during inspiration to increase the size and volume of the thoracic cavity. This allows air to enter the lungs.

Remember that **abduct** means to draw away and **adduct** means to "add" it to the main plane of the body.

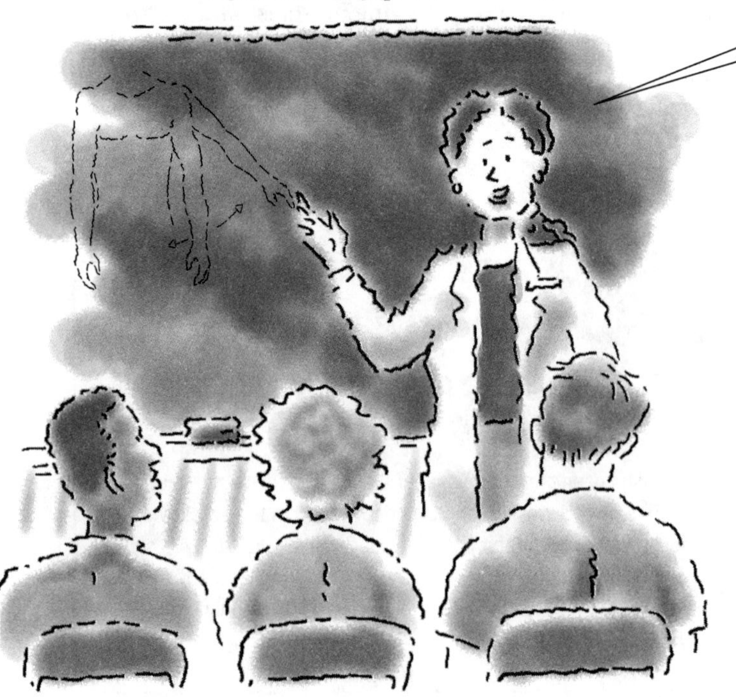

Now for a little ribbing

The **external intercostal** (***costa*** means *rib* in Latin) muscles lift the ribs during breathing and the **internal intercostals** lower them. The use of these muscles is most noticeable when a person is out of breath.

Abdominal muscles

Muscles in the abdominal cavity form three layers, the **external oblique** (the outermost), the **internal oblique** (the middle), and the **transversus abdominus** (the innermost), with fibers running in different directions.

A muscular girdle

The three layers form a strong "girdle" of muscle that protects and supports the internal organs. These muscles contract during childbirth, defecation, coughing, and sneezing. The **rectus abdominis** muscle runs down the midline of the abdomen and helps flex the spinal column as well as support the abdomen.

Arm and hand muscles

Several important muscles contribute to the movement of the arms and hands:

- **triceps brachii,** which extends the lower arm
- **brachialis,** which flexes the lower arm
- **biceps brachii,** which flexes the lower arm and **supinates** (turns upward) it along with the hand
- **pronator teres,** which flexes and **pronates** (rotates the forearm so that the palm of the hand faces downward) the lower arm.

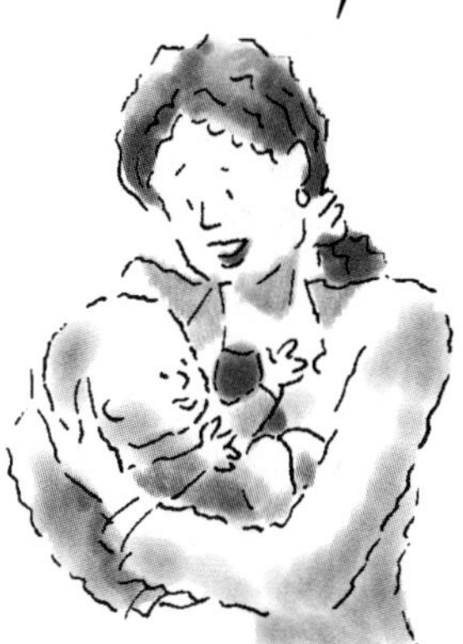

The prefix ***brachi-*** comes from the Latin word that means *arm,* ***brachium,*** from which we also get the word **embrace!**

It's all in the wrist

Many small muscles work together to flex and extend the wrists, hands, and fingers. Here are a few examples:

- **Flexor** muscles bend the fingers.
- **Lumbrical** muscles allow fine movements of the hand.
- The **flexor carpiradalis** and the **flexor carpiulnaris** both flex and adduct the wrist joint.

Pelvic floor muscles

A muscular "floor" called the **perineum** supports the pelvic organs and protects the diamond shaped pelvic opening. The perineum occupies the space between the

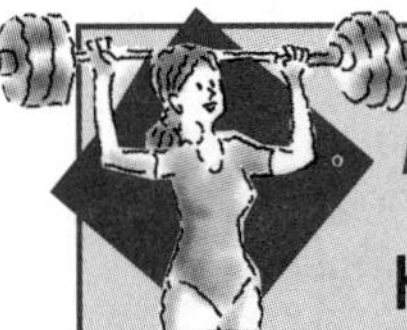

Pump up your pronunciation

How do I say coccygeus?

Coccygeus is pronounced COCK-SIHJ-EE-UHS. It's derived from ***coccyx***, the Greek name for the *cuckoo*, whose bill was thought to have a similar shape to the small bone (henceforth termed the **coccyx**) at the base of the spinal cord in the human body.

anus and vagina in females and the anus and scrotum in males.

The **levator ani** muscle and the **coccygeus** muscle support the pelvic organs and contribute to childbirth and defecation. The **sphincter ani** muscle keeps the anus closed. (See *How do I say coccygeus?*)

Thigh and upper leg muscles

Three groups of muscles affect movement in the thigh and upper leg area.

The first group includes those that cross the front of the hip:

- The **internal obturator** laterally rotates the thigh and extends and abducts the thigh when it's flexed.
- The **external obturator,** along with both the **superior** and **inferior gemellus,** laterally rotates the thigh as well.
- The **piriformis** laterally abducts, rotates, and extends the thigh.
- The **quadratus femoris** flexes and extends the leg in addition to laterally rotating the thigh.

Bringing up the rear

The second group consists of the **gluteals** (from the Greek word ***gloutos,*** which means *buttocks*). The **gluteus minimus** and **medius** abduct and rotate the thigh while the **gluteus maximus** extends and rotates the thigh.

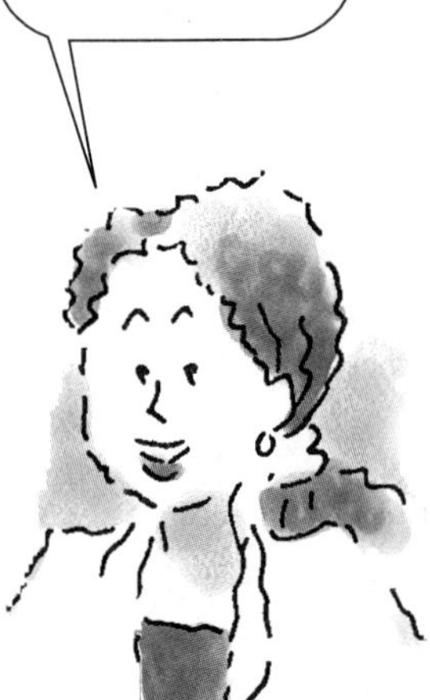

Don't let all this muscle talk wear you out. Remember, the more you learn, the easier it gets!

Adduction is the function

The third group, the **adductors,** includes the powerful **longus, brevis,** and **magnus** muscles, which draw back

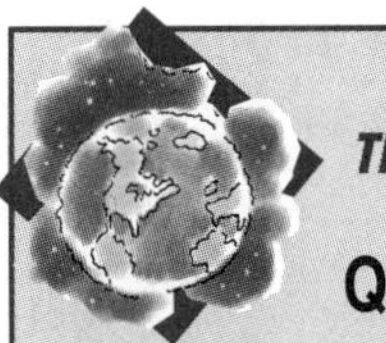

The real world

Quads

While working out in the gym, you often hear the word **quads** applied to the thigh muscles as a whole. In medical terminology, it's important to know the four muscles that make up the **quadriceps femoris** — the **rectus femoris, vastus lateralis, vastus medialis,** and **vastus intermedius.**

the thigh after abduction. The **gracilis** flexes and adducts the leg as well as adducting the thigh.

Lower leg muscles

Two groups of muscles move the lower leg. The first, the **quadriceps femoris,** includes the **vastus lateralis, medialis,** and **intermedius** — all of which work to extend the leg — and the **rectus femoris,** which flexes the thigh and extends the leg. (See *Quads.*)

The second group of muscles passes behind the thigh, and their tendons form the **hamstrings,** from which the group takes its name. The **semimembranosus** and **semitendinosus** extend the thigh and the **biceps femoris** helps both to extend the thigh and flex the leg.

The **sartorius muscle** gets its name from the Latin word **sartor,** which means *tailor.*

Also known as the calf muscle

Other lower leg muscles include the **gastrocnemius,** which flexes the leg and extends the foot and is commonly called the calf muscle (the **Achilles tendon** attaches to this muscle) and the **sartorius,** which flexes and adducts the leg in the "tailor" position.

Foot muscles

Extrinsic foot muscles are located in the leg but pull on tendons that move bones in the ankle and foot. These muscles allow **dorsiflexion** (backward movement at the ankle), **plantar flexion** (movement toward the toes), inversion (turn inward), and eversion (turn outward) of the foot.

Intrinsic foot muscles are located within the foot and produce flexion, extension, abduction, and adduction of the toes. The most important muscles of the foot include:

- **soleus,** which extends and rotates the foot (the Latin word for *sun* is ***sol,*** and as the sun causes the earth to rotate, so does this muscle cause the foot to rotate)
- **tibialis anterior,** which elevates and flexes the foot
- **tibialis posterior,** which extends the foot and turns it inward
- **peroneus longus,** which extends and abducts the foot and turns it outward
- **peroneus brevis,** which extends and abducts the foot
- **peroneus tertius,** which flexes the foot and turns it outward.

Physical examination terms

When a patient seeks medical help for a muscular problem it's usually because of a physical mishap or a chronic ache.

Common complaints

The term **myopathy** refers to any disease of the skeletal muscles. Below are other terms you may need to know when examining a myopathic condition or other muscular complaints:

- **Myalgia** is muscle pain or tenderness. For instance, an athlete with a sore pitching shoulder might have myalgia.
- **Myoclonus** is a spasm of a muscle.
- **Myotasis** is a continual stretching of a muscle, commonly referred to as a "pulled" muscle.
- **Myotonia** is chronic muscle contraction or irritability. Myotonia may be confirmed if there is isometric **contraction** — the muscle length remains the same as the tension on it increases.
- **Tenalgia** is a pain in the tendon, such as tennis elbow.
- **Tetany** is hyperexcitability of nerves and muscles, which results from lessened concentration of extracellular ionized calcium.
- A **tic** is a small muscle spasm.

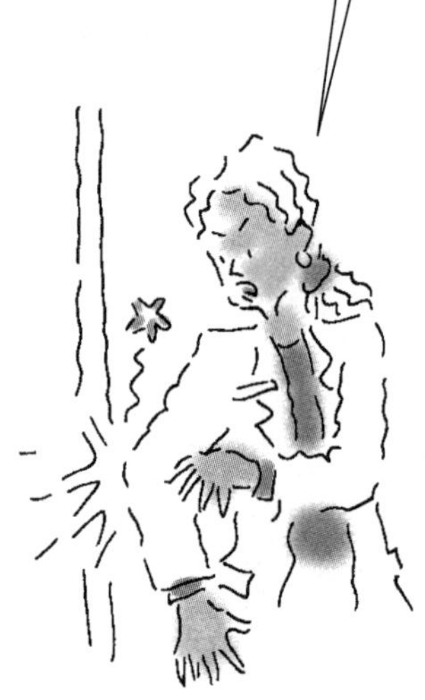

The suffix ***–algia*** comes from the Greek and means *pain.* So **tenalgia** means *pain in the tendon.* I could tell you that!

Common observations

Below are some terms that are useful while giving a physical examination:

- **Myelomalacia** is muscle softening, which may indicate **myoatrophy** (muscle wasting) or **myonecrosis** (death of muscle tissue fibers).
- **Myosclerosis** is muscle hardening.

Action reaction

- **Myobradia** is when a muscle reacts slowly to prodding. This may result if there has been tissue wasting or death.
- **Myospasm** is when a muscle convulses when prodded. This may signal an inflammation of the voluntary muscle tissue, or **myositis.**

Diagnostic tests

Three types of samples—blood, urine, and tissue—may be taken to diagnose muscle disorders. Scanners and other equipment are often necessary as well. Below are some of the terms, tests, and tools that may be used.

Physical tests

There are three common tests used to assess for carpal tunnel syndrome.

Tingle is the signal

Tinel's sign — a tingling over the median nerve on light percussion — is seen in cases of carpal tunnel syndrome.

Flex test

Phalen's maneuver is used to reproduce the symptoms of carpal tunnel syndrome. In this test, the patient extends his forearms vertically while allowing complete flexion at the wrists for 1 minute.

Compression impression

A **compression test** supports a diagnosis of carpal tunnel syndrome. A blood pressure cuff is placed on the forearm and inflated above the patient's systolic blood pressure for 1 to 2 minutes. If carpal tunnel syndrome is present, this intervention produces paresthesia along the distribution of the median nerve.

Blood tests

Enzyme levels or the presence of acids in the blood stream can help diagnose muscular disease. Blood tests are named after the enzyme or acid they're designed to detect:

- Elevated levels of **alanine aminotransferase,** a skeletal enzyme, may indicate muscle tissue damage.
- Elevated levels of **aspartate aminotransferase,** a skeletal muscle enzyme, may indicate muscle damage related to muscle trauma or muscular dystrophy.
- **Creatine kinase,** an isoenzyme found in both skeletal and cardiac muscle, may indicate damage from muscle trauma, I.M. injections, or muscular dystrophy.

Urine tests

Hormone levels or the presence of other substances in the urine can also be key determinants of muscular disorders. A common urine test uses **3-methoxy-4-hydroxymandelic acid** to detect elevated levels of adrenaline and noradrenaline, which may indicate muscle disorders such as muscular dystrophy.

A **myoglobin urine test** detects the presence of myoglobin in the urine, which indicates extensive muscle damage.

Muscle biopsy

In **muscle biopsy,** a needle or incision is used to extract a specimen of muscle tissue for examination. This microscopic evaluation of muscle tissue samples is often required for an accurate diagnosis of muscular disorders.

Tools of the trade

An accurate "image" of the myopathy, which is possible with the use of various equipment, may aid in diagnosis.

The equipment

A **computerized tomography scan** uses multiple X-ray beams that pass through the body at different angles, striking radiation detectors that produce electrical impulses. A computer converts the impulses into digital information that detects tumors in muscle tissue. (See *CAT scan.*)

An **electromyogram** records the electrical activity of skeletal muscles through surface or needle electrodes. It's used to diagnose neuromuscular disorders and pinpoint motor nerve lesions.

Magnetic resonance imaging uses a powerful magnetic field and radiofrequency energy to produce images based on the hydrogen content of body tissues. Also called **nuclear magnetic resonance,** it's used to diagnose muscle disease.

A **myokinesimeter** measures muscular contraction by stimulating the muscles with an electrical current.

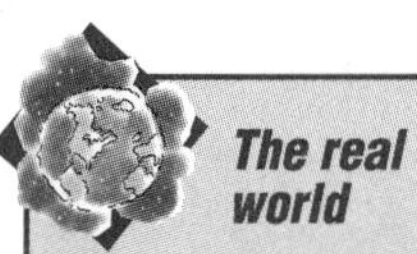

CAT scan

A **computerized tomography scan** was originally known as a **computerized axial tomography scan**. That is why in practice you'll still hear this test referred to as a **CAT scan.**

Disorders

A wide range of problems lead to muscle disorders, including trauma, heredity, autoimmunity, and the normal aging process. This section covers terms associated with muscular disorders.

Muscle conditions

Below are terms for common muscle conditions:
- **Atrophy** is the wasting of muscle.
- **Contractures,** the abnormal flexion and fixation of joints, are typically caused by muscle atrophy and may be permanent.
- **Foot drop** is the failure to maintain the foot in a normally flexed position (dragging of the foot) and is commonly a complication associated with trauma or paralysis.
- **Shin splints** are a strain of the long flexor muscle of the toes caused by strenuous athletic activity.
- **Spastic paralysis** is the involuntary contraction of a muscle with an associated loss of function.
- A **sprain** is a complete or incomplete tear in the supporting ligaments surrounding a joint.

• A **strain** is an injury to a muscle or tendinous attachment.

Tumors and lesions

Below are terms for tumors and lesions of the muscle:

• A **fibroid tumor,** or **leiomyoma,** is a **benign** (noncancerous) tumor found in smooth muscle, usually in the uterus.

• A **leiomyosarcoma** is a malignant tumor of smooth muscle that is usually found in the uterus.

• A **myoblastoma** is a benign lesion of soft tissue.

• A **myofibroma** is a tumor containing muscular and fibrous tissue.

• A **myosarcoma** is a malignant tumor derived from muscle tissue.

• A **rhabdomyoma** is a benign tumor of striated muscle.

• A **rhabdomyosarcoma** is a highly malignant tumor that originates from striated muscle cells.

Infection and inflammation

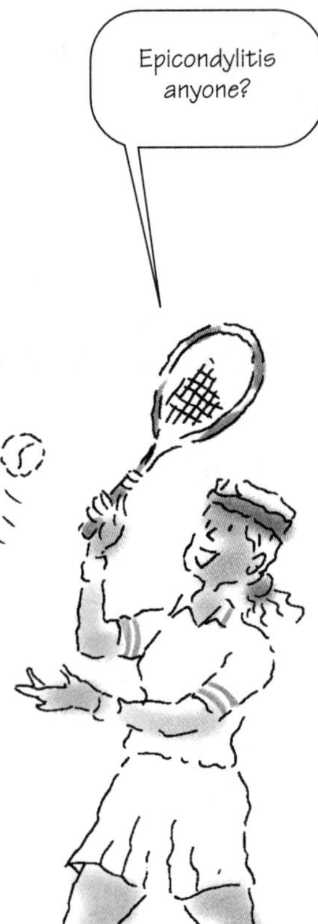

Below are terms for muscular infection and inflammation:

• **Bursitis** is a painful inflammation of one or more of the **bursae,** closed sacs that cushion muscles and tendons over bony prominences such as the knee.

• **Dermatomyositis** is a connective tissue disease marked by itching and skin inflammation in addition to tenderness and weakness of muscles.

• **Epicondylitis,** also known as tennis elbow, is an inflammation of tendons in the forearm at their attachment to the humerus.

• **Fasciitis** is inflammation of the fasciae.

• **Myocellulitis** is inflammation of the cellular tissue within a muscle.

• **Myofibrosis** is an overgrowth of fibrous tissue, which replaces muscle tissue.

• **Myositis purulenta** is any bacterial infection of the muscle tissue that may result in pus formation and ultimately gangrene.

• **Tendinitis,** a painful inflammation of tendons and their muscle attachments to bone, is commonly caused

Beyond the dictionary

Understanding the suffix *-itis*

The suffix ***-itis*** is derived from Greek and means *the inflammation of.* Anyone who has suffered the burning pain of **tendinitis** (inflammation of the tendons and their attachments to the bone) can confirm the accuracy of this suffix.

by trauma, congenital defects, or rheumatic diseases. (See *Understanding the suffix **-itis.***)

Syndromes and diseases

Below are terms for muscular syndromes and diseases:
- An **Achilles tendon contracture** is a shortening of the Achilles tendon. It can cause pain and reduced dorsiflexion.
- **Carpal tunnel syndrome** is a painful disorder of the wrist and hand that results from rapid, repetitive use of the fingers.
- **Dupuytren's contracture** is a progressive, painless contracture of the palmar fascia, causing the last two fingers to contract toward the palm. (See *Dupuytren's contracture*, page 82.)
- **Fibromyalgia syndrome** is a chronic disorder with an unknown cause, producing pain in the muscles, bones, or joints.
- **Muscular dystrophy** is a group of degenerative genetic diseases characterized by weakness and the progressive atrophy of skeletal muscles with no evidence of involvement of the nervous system.
- **Myasthenia gravis** is an abnormal weakness and fatigability, especially in the muscles of the throat and face, resulting from a defect in the conduction of nerve impulses at the myoneural junction.
- **Torticollis** is a neck deformity in which the neck muscles are spastic and shortened, causing the head to bend toward the affected side and the chin to rotate toward the unaffected side.

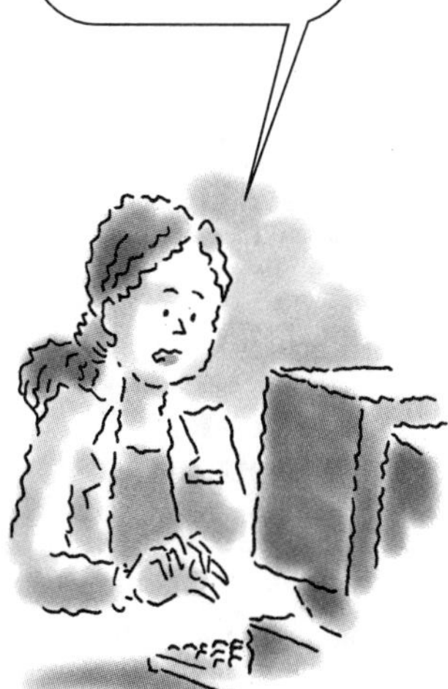

People who do a lot of typing often suffer from carpal tunnel syndrome.

Treatments

Rest is often all that is needed to treat muscle conditions. Other common options include: immobilizing the muscle with a **sling** (bandage that supports an injured body part), **splint** (orthopedic appliance that immobilizes and supports an injured body part), or **cast** (rigid dressing placed around an extremity); undergoing physical therapy; applying cold or hot **compresses** (wet or dry cloths); or medicating with prescription drugs.

Douse the flame

Drug therapy includes nonsteroidal anti-inflammatory drugs to decrease inflammation, muscle relaxants to combat spasticity and relax muscles, and corticosteroids to combat the inflammatory process.

Drain the pain

When inflammation is the problem, as in such conditions as tendinitis and bursitis, fluid is sometimes removed from the joint with a hollow needle. The term for this is **aspiration.**

Free at last

When there is muscular compression on a nerve, as in carpal tunnel syndrome, surgery may be required if more conservative treatments fail. In this case, **neurolysis,** the freeing of the nerve fibers, removes the entire carpal tunnel ligament.

Heat wave

Short-wave diathermy uses a current to generate heat within the muscle. Short-wave diathermy is used to control pain and decrease muscle spasm.

Rub-out

Massage uses manipulation, methodical pressure, friction, and kneading to promote circulation, relieve pain, and reduce tension. Massage is used for patients who have restricted movement.

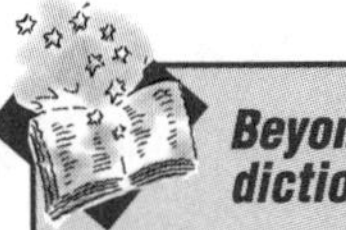

Beyond the dictionary

Dupuytren's contracture

Guillaume Dupuytren (DOO-PWEE-TRAH) (1777-1835) was a French surgeon and clinical teacher. He became intrigued by a peculiar form of **contracture,** *the permanent contraction of a muscle,* that caused the fingers to curl in the hand. After dissection, he discovered the problem was centered in the palmar fascia.

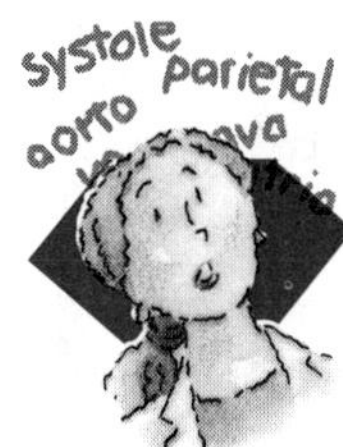

Vocabulary builders

At a crossroads

Here is a little crossword puzzle to help pump up your mental muscle. Good luck!

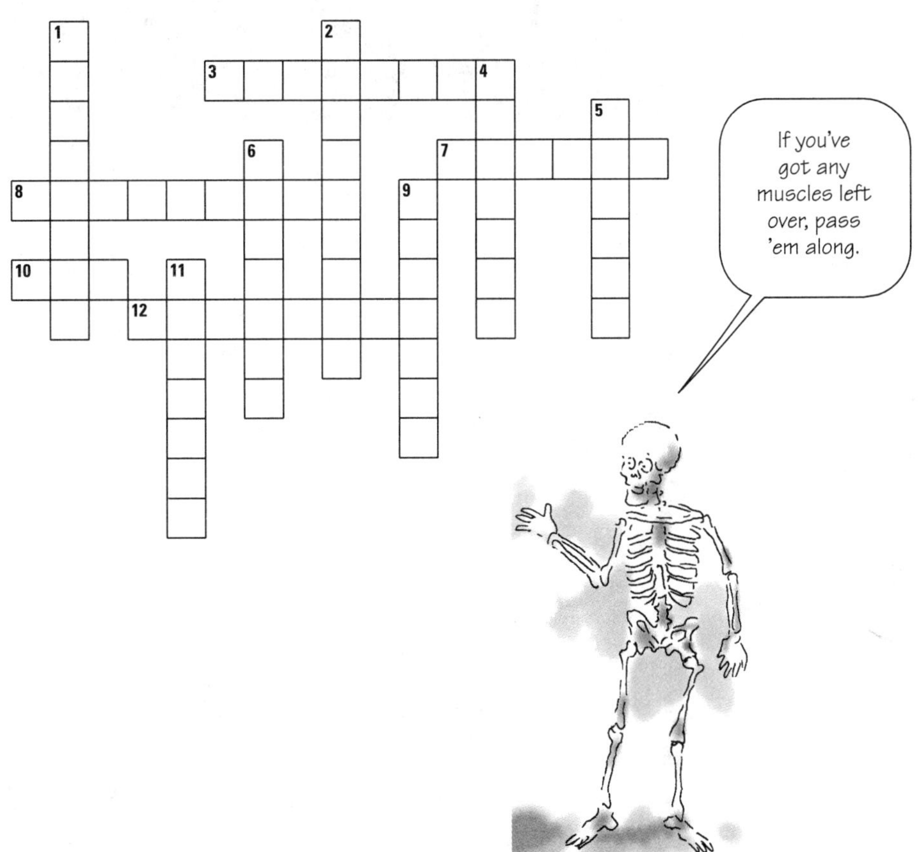
1
2
3
4
5
6
7
8
9
10
11
12
If you've got any muscles left over, pass 'em along.

Across

3. Floor of the pelvis
7. Fibrous membrane sheath
8. Critical for breathing
10. A muscle twitch
12. Muscles composed of thin bands

Down

1. Inflamed bursae
2. Responsible for attaching bones to each other
4. Muscle pain or tenderness
5. Muscle cell groups
6. Adjective for heart muscles
9. Attaches muscles to the periosteum
11. Reduction in the size of muscles

Answers are on page 86.

Finish line

The suffix ***-itis*** comes from the Greek and means *the inflammation of.* Fill in the blanks below to form the correct muscle disorder.

1. Painful inflammation of tendons is called ______________ itis.
2. Painful inflammation of one or more bursae is called ______________ itis.
3. Inflammation of the fascia is called ______________ itis.
4. Inflammation of cellular tissue within a muscle is called ______________ itis.
5. Inflammation of connective tissue and weakness of muscle is called ______________ itis.

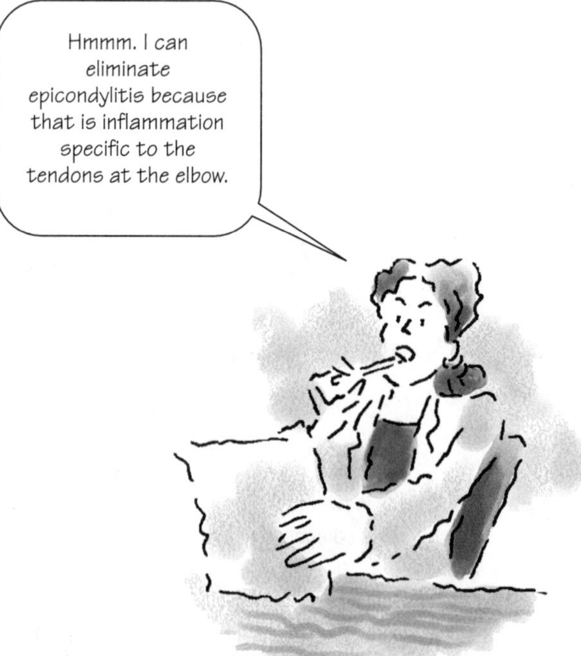
Hmmm. I can eliminate epicondylitis because that is inflammation specific to the tendons at the elbow.

Answers are on page 86.

Scrambled or overeasy

Fill in the answers for the following questions, then unscramble the circled letters to find the answer to the puzzle.

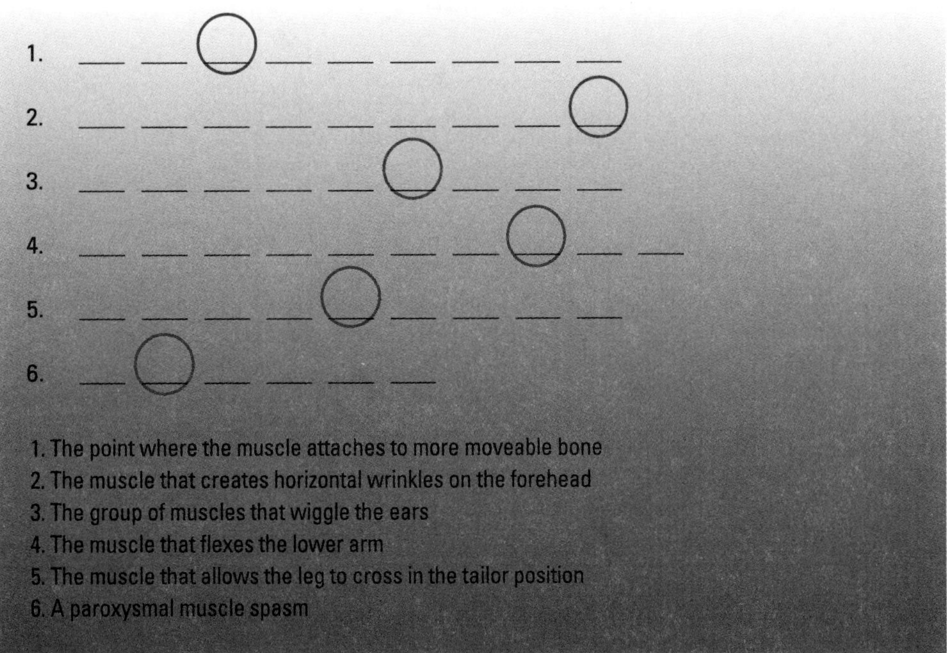

1. The point where the muscle attaches to more moveable bone
2. The muscle that creates horizontal wrinkles on the forehead
3. The group of muscles that wiggle the ears
4. The muscle that flexes the lower arm
5. The muscle that allows the leg to cross in the tailor position
6. A paroxysmal muscle spasm

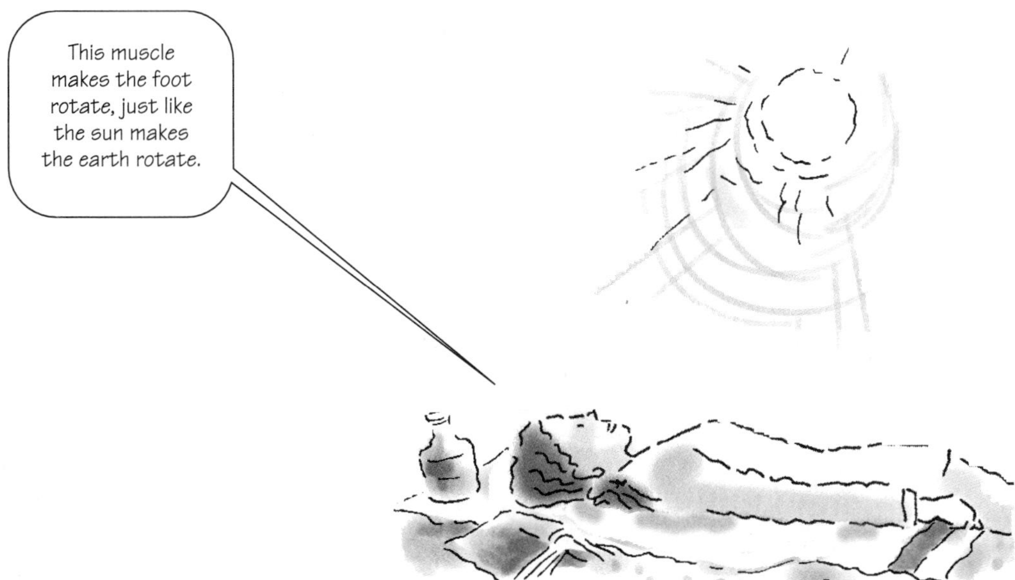

This muscle makes the foot rotate, just like the sun makes the earth rotate.

Answers are on page 86.

Answers

At a crossroads

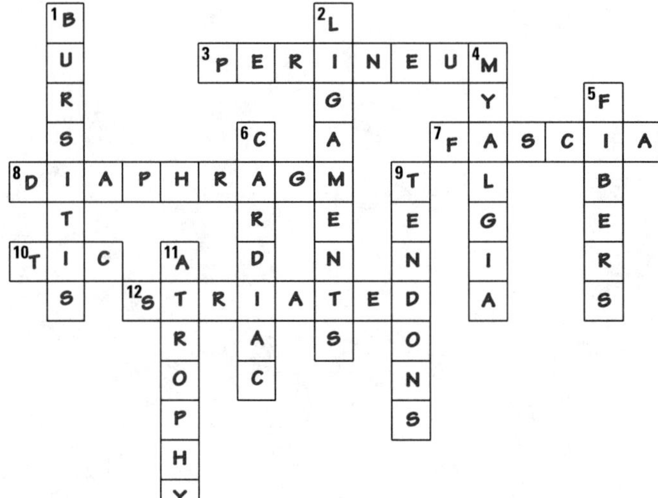

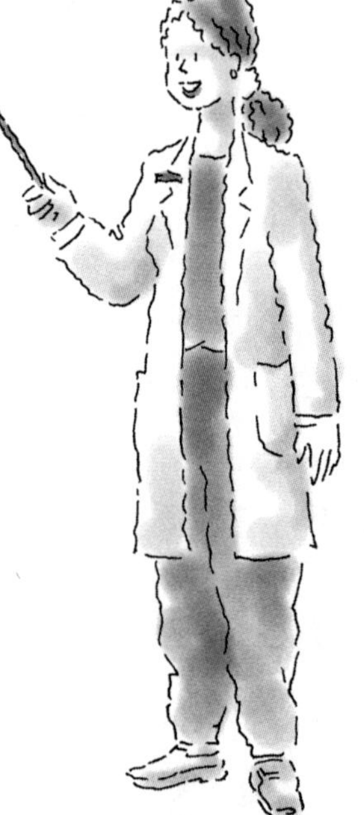
Next, we move out of muscles — and into the integumentary system!

Finish line

1. Tendin; 2. Burs; 3. Fasci; 4. Myocellul; 5. Dermatomyos.

Scrambled or overeasy

1. Insertion; 2. Frontalis; 3. Auricular; 4. Brachialis; 5. Sartorius; 6. Tetany.
Answer to puzzle — Soleus

Integumentary system

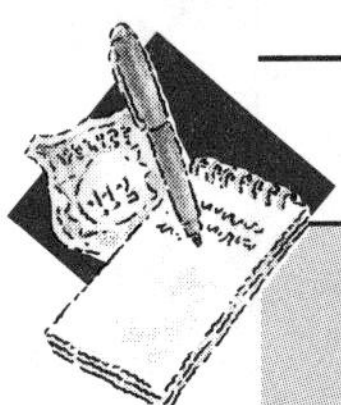

Just the facts

In this chapter, you'll review:

- terminology related to the structure and function of the integumentary system
- terminology needed for physical examination of the integumentary system.
- tests that help diagnose disorders of the integumentary system
- disorders of the integumentary system and their treatments.

Skin structure and function

The largest body system, the integumentary system, includes the skin, or **integument** (from the Latin word ***integumentum,*** which means *covering*), and its appendages — hair, nails, and certain glands. It covers an area that measures 10¾ ft^2 to 21½ ft^2 and accounts for about 15% of body weight. (See *Pronouncing key integumentary system terms*, page 88.)

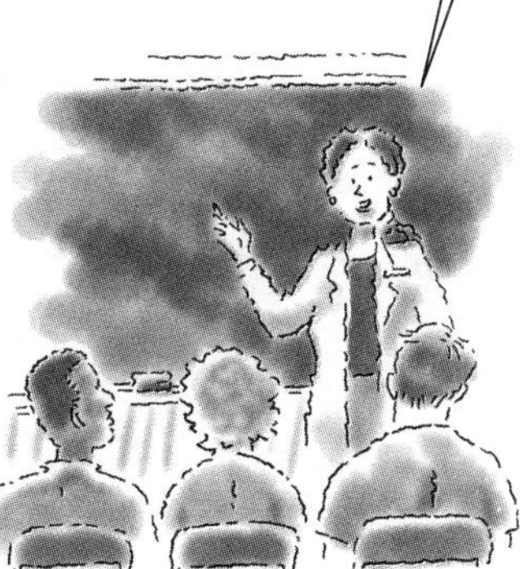

Dermatology, the study of skin, comes from the Greek words derma, which means skin and logos, which means science.

Function

The integumentary system performs many vital functions, including protection of inner body structures, sensory perception, and regulation of body temperature and blood pressure.

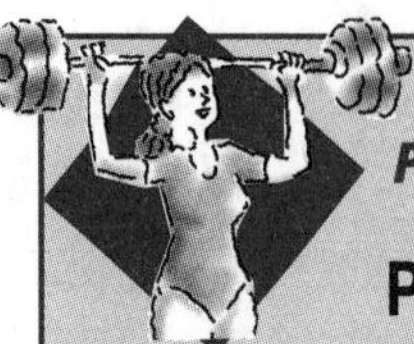

Pump up your pronunciation

Pronouncing key integumentary system terms

Below is a list of key terms, along with the correct way to pronounce them.

Aphthous stomatitis	AFF-THUHS STOH-MAH-TEYE-TISS
Ecchymosis	ECK-IH-MOH-SISS
Erythema	EHR-IH-THEE-MAH
Onychomycosis	AWN-IH-COH-MEYE-COH-SISS
Petechia	PEH-TEE-KEE-AH
Phthirus pubis	THIHR-UHS PYOO-BISS
Rosacea	ROH-ZAY-SHEE-AH
Sebaceous	SEH-BAY-SHUSS
Subcutaneous	SUHB-KYOO-TAY-NEE-UHS
Telangiectasis	TEHL-ANN-JEE-ECK-TAH-SISS
Verrucae	VEH-ROO-SEE

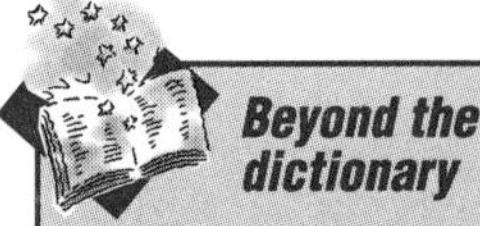

Beyond the dictionary

Calling Doctor Langerhans

Many medical terms are named after the doctors who first brought attention to them.

Langerhans' cells
Paul Langerhans (1847-1888), a German doctor, anatomist, and pathologist, is best known for his research on clusters of pancreatic cells, now known as the **Islets of Langerhans.** He also identified **Langerhans' cells,** which are are specialized cells in the skin layer that help enhance the body's immune system.

More than just a pretty face

The top layer of the skin protects the body against traumatic injury, noxious chemicals, and bacterial and microorganismal invasion.

Langerhans' cells, specialized cells in the top skin layer, enhance the body's immune response by helping process antigens that enter the skin. (See *Calling Doctor Langerhans.*)

Keeping you in touch

Sensory nerve fibers originate in the nerve roots along the spine and terminate in segmental areas of the skin known as **dermatomes.** These nerve fibers carry impulses from the skin to the central nervous system.

An all-weather covering

Abundant nerves, blood vessels, and eccrine glands within the skin's deeper layer aid **thermoregulation,** or control of body temperature. When the skin is too cold, blood vessels constrict, leading to a decrease in blood flow through the skin and conservation of body heat.

When the skin is too hot, small arteries in the second skin layer dilate, increasing blood flow and reducing body heat. If this doesn't adequately lower temperature, the eccrine glands act to increase sweat production, and subsequent evaporation cools the skin.

Pressure cooker

Dermal blood vessels also aid regulation of systemic blood pressure through vasoconstriction.

Other odd jobs

When stimulated by ultraviolet light, the skin synthesizes vitamin D_3 (cholecalciferol).

The skin also excretes sweat, which contains water, electrolytes, urea, and lactic acid, through the sweat glands.

Skin layers

Two distinct layers of skin, the **epidermis** and **dermis,** lie above a third layer of **subcutaneous fat.**

On the face of it

The outermost layer, the **epidermis,** varies in thickness from less than 0.1 mm on the eyelids to more than 1 mm on the palms and soles. It's composed of **avascular** (without a direct blood supply), **squamous** tissue that is **stratified** (arranged in multiple layers). (See *Squamous tissue revealed.*)

The **stratum corneum,** the outermost part of the epidermis, consists of cellular membranes and **keratin,** a protein. Langerhans' cells are interspersed among the keratinized cells below the stratum corneum. Epidermal cells are usually shed from the surface as **epidermal dust.**

Stratum basale, also called the basal or base layer, produces new cells to replace superficial keratinized cells that are continuously shed or worn away. It also

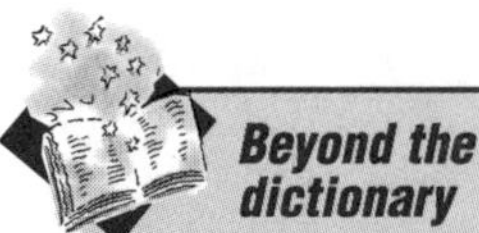

Beyond the dictionary

Squamous tissue revealed

Squamous is derived from the Latin term for the scale of a fish or serpent, ***squama.*** It's used in anatomy to describe thin, flat platelike or scalelike structures — in this case, squamous tissue.

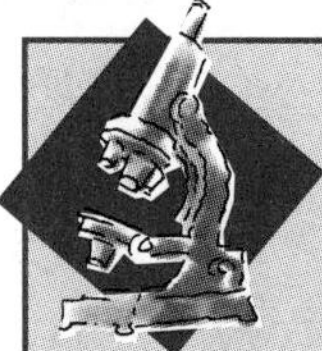

Zoom in

Close-up view of the skin

Major components of the skin include the epidermis, dermis, and epidermal appendages.

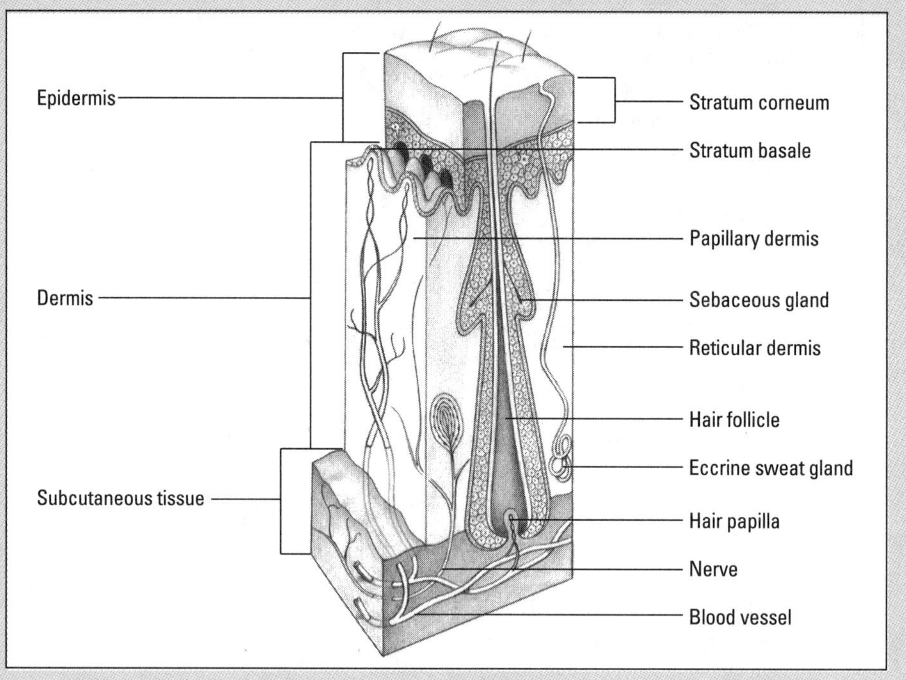

The word **stratum** comes from the Latin ***sternere,*** which means to spread out.

contains specialized skin cells called **melanocytes,** which protect the skin by producing and dispersing **melanin** to surrounding epithelial cells. Melanin is a brown pigment that helps filter ultraviolet light.(See *Close-up view of the skin.*)

Digging beneath the surface

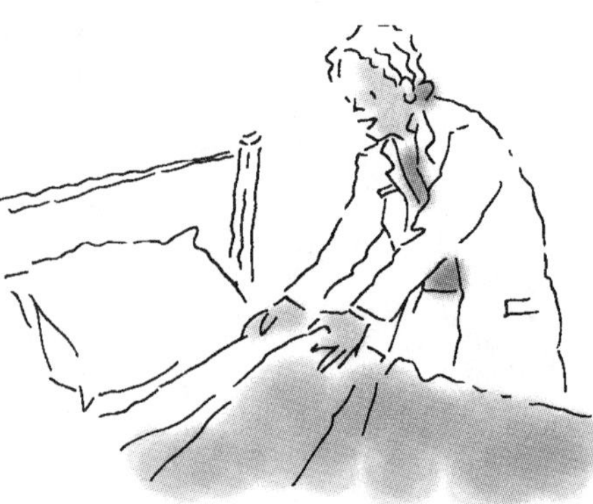

The skin's second layer, the **dermis,** also called the **corium,** is an elastic system that contains and supports blood vessels, lymphatic vessels, nerves, and epidermal appendages.

Most of the dermis is made up of extracellular material called **matrix.** Matrix contains connective tissue fibers, including

Beyond the dictionary

Uncovering panniculus adiposus

Panniculus adiposus is a specialized layer primarily composed of fat cells. In fact, ***panniculus*** is a Latin term that means *a small piece of cloth or covering,* or *a layer.* **Adipose** means *fat.*

collagen, a protein that gives strength to the dermis; **elastin,** which makes the skin pliable; and **reticular fibers,** which bind the collagen and elastin fibers together. These fibers are produced by **dermal fibroblasts,** spindle-shaped connective tissue cells.

The dermis has two layers:

- The **papillary dermis** has fingerlike projections (papillae) that nourish epidermal cells. The epidermis lies over these papillae and bulges downward to fill the spaces. A collagenous membrane known as the **basement membrane** separates the epidermis and dermis and holds them together.
- The **reticular dermis** covers a layer of subcutaneous tissue, the **adipose** or **panniculus adiposus,** that is primarily composed of fat cells. In addition to insulating the body, the reticular dermis provides energy and serves as a mechanical shock absorber. (See *Uncovering panniculus adiposus.*)

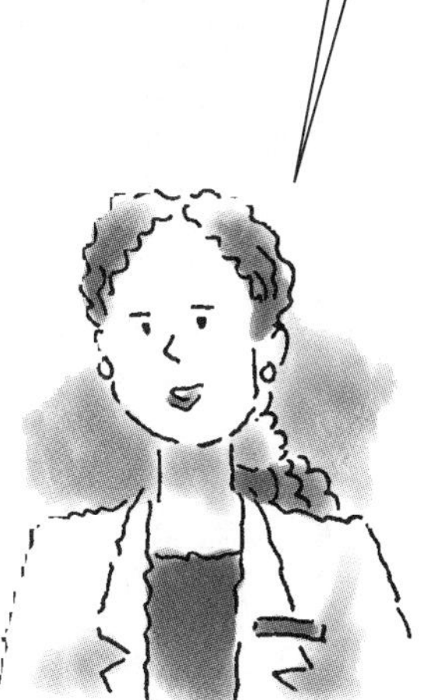
Put the emphasis on the **p.** The **p**apillary dermis has **p**rojections that **p**ush into and nourish the epidermal cells above it.

Epidermal appendages

Numerous epidermal appendages occur throughout the skin. They include the hair, nails, **sebaceous glands,** and two types of sweat glands — the **eccrine** and **apocrine.**

Hair

Hairs are long, slender shafts composed of keratin. At the expanded lower end of each hair is a bulb or root. On its undersurface, the root is indented by a **hair papilla,** a cluster of connective tissue and blood vessels.

A hair-raising experience

Each hair lies within an epithelial-lined sheath called a **hair follicle.** A bundle of smooth-muscle fibers, the **arrector pili,** extends through the dermis to attach to the base of the follicle. When these muscles contract, the hair stands on end.

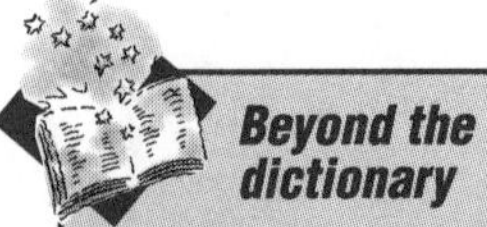

Beyond the dictionary

Lunar expedition

The **lunula** gets its name from its crescent-moon shape. ***Luna*** is the Latin word for *moon* and the suffix ***-ula*** indicates *small.* Another word that shares this root is **lunacy** — literally, *moon-sickness.*

Nails

Situated over the distal surface of the end of each finger and toe, nails are specialized types of keratin. The **nail plate,** surrounded on three sides by the **nail folds** (or **cuticles**), lies on the **nail bed.** The nail plate is formed by the **nail matrix,** which extends proximally about ¼″ (5 mm) beneath the nail fold.

Under the keratin moon

The distal portion of the matrix shows through the nail as a pale crescent-moon-shaped area, called the **lunula.** The translucent nail plate distal to the lunula exposes the nail bed. The **vascular bed** imparts the characteristic pink appearance under the nails. (See *Lunar expedition.*)

The sebaceous glands

Sebaceous glands occur on all parts of the skin except the palms and soles. They are most prominent on the scalp, face, upper torso, and genitalia.

Nature's conditioner

Sebaceous glands produce **sebum,** an oily, lipid substance that helps protect hair and skin. Sebaceous glands secrete sebum into the hair follicle via the sebaceous duct. Sebum then exits through the hair follicle opening to reach the skin surface.

The sweat glands

Widely distributed throughout the body, the **eccrine glands** produce an odorless, watery fluid with a sodium concentration equal to that of plasma. A duct from the coiled secretory portion passes through the dermis and epidermis, opening onto the skin surface.

Located chiefly in the axillary and anogenital areas, the **apocrine glands** have a coiled secretory portion that lies deeper in the dermis than that of the eccrine glands.

A duct connects an apocrine gland to the upper portion of the hair follicle.

A puddle under pressure

Eccrine glands in the palms and soles secrete fluid mainly in response to emotional stress. The other three million eccrine glands respond primarily to thermal stress, effectively regulating temperature.

Apocrine glands begin to function at puberty. However, they have no known biological function. As bacteria decompose the fluids produced by these glands, body odor occurs.

Physical examination terms

The skin can provide useful information about the body's overall condition. Below are terms associated with a complete skin examination.

Skin color

Decreased hemoglobin level and oxygen in the blood cause changes in skin color. Skin color also responds to changes in the quality and amount of blood circulating through superficial blood vessels.

Blue in the face

Cyanosis is a bluish color caused by an excess of oxygen-starved hemoglobin molecules in the blood. Pale skin is called **pallor,** and pale, cyanotic skin around the lips is known as **circumoral pallor.**

Seeing red

Ecchymosis is a reddish purple discoloration caused by hemorrhages in the dermal or intradermal spaces. **Erythema** refers to redness or inflammation of the skin resulting from congestion of the superficial capillaries.

Purpura is purple-red or brown-red discoloration on the skin due to hemorrhage in the tissues. Small discolored areas are called **petechiae,** while large ones are **ecchymoses.**

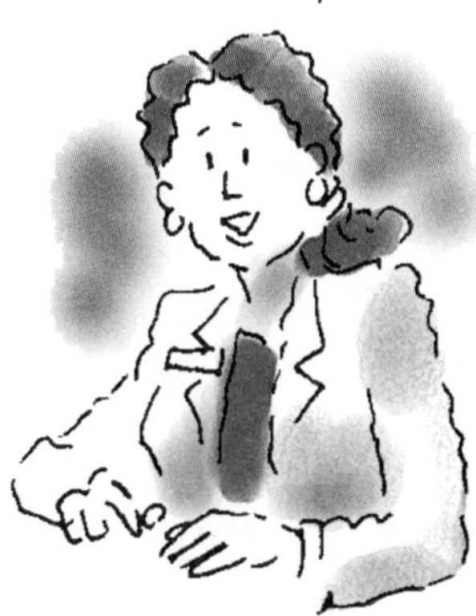
Cyanosis is Greek to me no longer. **Cyan-** comes from the Greek word ***kuanos***, meaning *dark blue.*

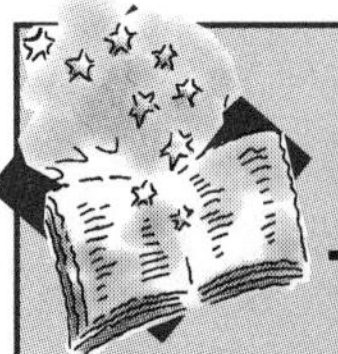

Beyond the dictionary

Turgor and its Latin root

Turgid and **turgor** come from the Latin word ***turgidus,*** which means *swollen.* However, **turgor** refers to the normal tension of the skin or the lack of excessive swelling.

Feeling yellow — not mellow

Yellowing of the skin, known as **jaundice,** is caused by elevated bilirubin levels.

Carotenemia is a yellow-orange skin discoloration that is caused by excess levels of **carotene** in the blood stream.

Skin turgor

Turgor is a condition of normal tension in the skin and reflects the skin's elasticity.

Keeping its shape

Turgor is assessed by gently grasping and pulling up a fold of skin. Normal skin returns to its flat shape within 3 seconds. Abnormal turgor may be a sign of dehydration or connective tissue disorders. (See *Turgor and its Latin root.*)

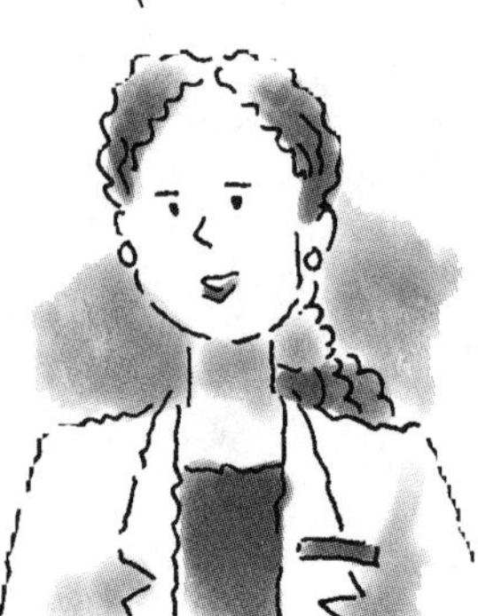
Carotene is an enzyme also found in carrots. When you have **carotenemia,** an excess of carotene in your bloodstream, you turn orange like a carrot.

Lesions

Allergens, weather, injury, and various diseases can produce **lesions,** or abnormal changes in the skin. Types of lesions include wounds, sores, tumors, and rashes.

First signs of trouble

Primary lesions are the first lesions of an onsetting disease. Below are examples:

- A **bulla** is a fluid-filled lesion, also called a **blister** or **bleb.**
- A **cyst** is a semisolid encapsulated mass that extends deep into the dermis.

- A **macule** is a flat, pigmented area less than 3/8″ in diameter such as a **freckle.**
- A **papule** is a firm, raised lesion up to 1/4″ in diameter that may be the same color as the skin or pigmented.
- A **plaque** is a flat, raised patch on the skin.
- A **pustule** is a lesion that contains pus, which gives it a yellow-white color.
- A **tumor** is an elevated solid lesion larger than 3/4″ that extends into the dermal and subcutaneous layers.
- A **vesicle** is a raised, fluid-filled lesion less than 1/4″ in diameter. Chickenpox produces vesicles.
- A **wheal** is a raised, firm lesion with intense, usually temporary, swelling around the area. **Urticaria,** or hives, are a type of wheal.

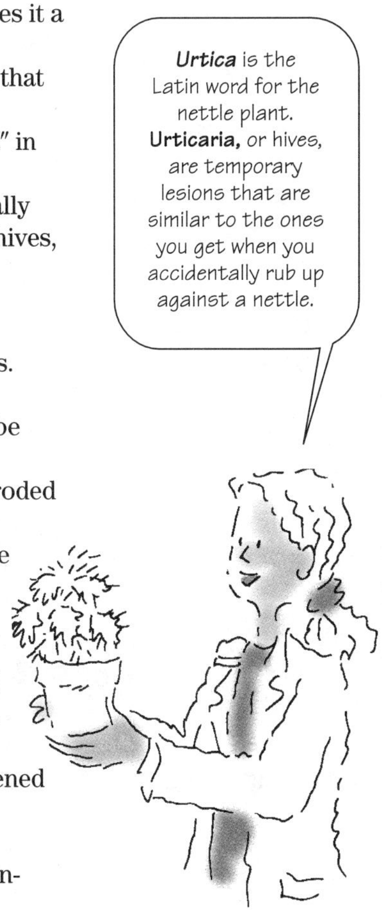

> ***Urtica*** is the Latin word for the nettle plant. **Urticaria,** or hives, are temporary lesions that are similar to the ones you get when you accidentally rub up against a nettle.

As if that wasn't bad enough

Secondary lesions are the result of primary lesions. Below are examples:

- **Atrophy** is thinning of the skin surface that may be caused by a disorder or aging.
- **Crust** is dried **exudate** (drainage) covering an eroded or weeping area of skin.
- An **erosion** is a lesion that is caused by loss of the epidermis.
- **Excoriation** is a linearly scratched or abraded area.
- **Fissures** are linear cracks in the skin that extend into the dermal layer. Chapped skin causes fissures.
- A **keloid** is a hypertrophied scar.
- **Lichenification** is characterized by thick, roughened skin with exaggerated skin lines.
- **Scales** are thin, dry flakes of shedding skin.
- **Scars** are fibrous tissue caused by trauma, deep inflammation, or a surgical incision.
- An **ulcer** is an epidermal and dermal destruction that may extend into the subcutaneous tissue.

Diagnostic tests

Many skin conditions are diagnosed on sight, but several studies are used to diagnose skin disorders and systemic problems.

Allergy testing

The **patch test** identifies allergies to such substances as dust, mold, and foods. During this test, paper or gauze that has been saturated with a possible **allergen** (substance capable of producing an allergic reaction) is applied to the skin. The test is positive if redness or swelling develops.

Scratching the surface

Another method for detecting allergies is the **scratch test.** This test involves inserting small amounts of possible allergens into scratches on the skin surface and watching for a sensitivity reaction.

Cultures

Gram stains rapidly provide diagnostic information about which organism is causing an infection. A gram stain separates bacteria into two categories based on cell wall composition. **Gram-positive** organisms retain crystal violet stain after decoloration. **Gram-negative** organisms lose the violet stain but stain red with safranine.

The **Tzanck test** requires smearing vesicular fluid or drainage from an ulcer on a glass slide, then staining the slide with several chemicals. Herpes virus infection is confirmed by examining the fluid under a microscope. (See *How do I say Tzanck?*)

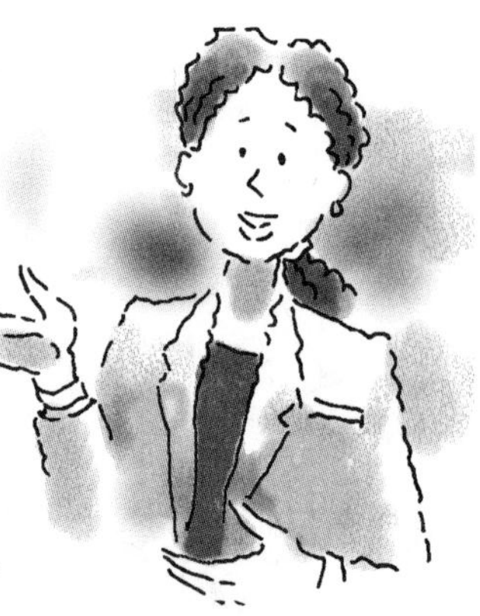

Whenever these terms begin to get you down, just think of a couple of my favorite terms: **a good movie** and **a bucket of popcorn.** That should cheer you up!
Take a break!

Prescriptions are a sensitive matter

A **culture** is used to isolate and identify an infectious agent. In a culture, a sample of tissue or fluid is placed in a jellylike medium that provides nutrients for microorganisms. If an organism is present, it may multiply rapidly or may take several weeks to grow.

A **sensitivity** test determines the drug that will best treat an infection. Drugs are added to a cultured sample to see which ones kill the offending organism.

Biopsies and smear tests

A **biopsy** is the removal of tissue for microscopic examination. Below are types of biopsies used for skin disorders:

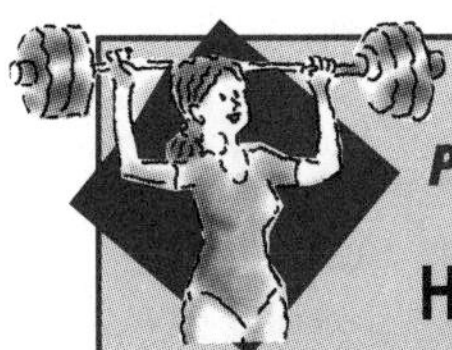

Pump up your pronunciation

How do I say Tzanck?

The **Tzanck test** requires smearing vesicular fluid or drainage from an ulcer on a glass slide, then staining the slide with several chemicals. Arnault Tzanck (1886-1954) was a Russian dermatologist who worked in Paris. The ***t*** sound in **Tzanck** is silent as is the ***t*** sound in **tsar.** Therefore, **Tzanck** is pronounced ZANK.

- A **skin biopsy** tests a small piece of tissue from a lesion suspected of malignancy or other disorder.
- A **shave biopsy** cuts the lesion above the skin line, leaving the lower layers of dermis intact.
- A **punch biopsy** removes an oval core from the center of a lesion.
- An **excision biopsy** may remove an entire lesion that is small.

A smear campaign

A somewhat less invasive method than biopsy is the **smear test,** in which cells are spread on a slide and studied under a microscope. In the **buccal smear** test, cells are scraped from the inner surface of the cheek to detect hereditary abnormalities.

Tools of the trade

During **phototesting,** small areas of skin are exposed to ultraviolet light to detect photosensitivity (acute sensitivity to light). A **Wood's light** is an ultraviolet light used to diagnose **tinea capitis.** Hairs infected by this fungus appear fluorescent under Wood's light.

Disorders

Skin forms a barrier against the environment and also reflects problems within the body, so it's an easy target for infection, injury, and infestation.

Bacterial infections

Below are some common bacterial infections:

- **Impetigo** is a contagious, superficial skin infection that is usually caused by the *Staphylococcus aureus* organism. Impetigo lesions start as macules, then develop into vesicles that become pustular with a honey-colored crust. When the vesicle breaks, a thick yellow crust forms from the exudate.
- **Cellulitis** is an inflammation of subcutaneous tissue that often appears around a break in the skin, such as an insect bite or a puncture wound. Fever, chills, headache, and tiredness often accompany cellulitis.
- **Folliculitis** is a bacterial infection of the hair follicles that is usually caused by the *S. aureus* bacteria. A **furuncle,** or **boil,** begins deep in the hair follicles. When a boil spreads to surrounding tissue and produces a cluster of furuncles, it's called a **carbuncle.**
- A **stye** is an abscess in the eyelash follicle caused by a staphylococcal infection.

Carbuncle means a small *live coal* in Latin. The burning and glowing of hot coals is an apt image for a carbuncle, which is a cluster of angry, painful boils.

Viral infections

Two common manifestations of viral infections are the sores associated with different types of **herpes** and **warts.**

A not-so-simple(x) infection

The word **herpes,** often used as a singular word, actually refers to a variety of viruses. Below are some common types of herpes:

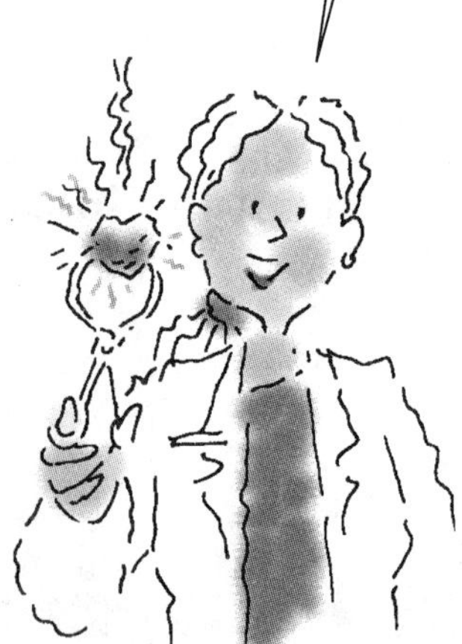

- **Herpes simplex virus type 1** causes painful cold sores and fever blisters on the skin and mucous membranes. After initial infection, patients are susceptible to recurrent bouts with the virus. Outbreaks are accompanied by burning pain, swelling, redness, and fatigue.
- **Herpes simplex virus type 2,** also known as genital herpes, produces lesions in the genital area. Patients complain of flulike symptoms, including headache, fatigue, muscle pain, fever, and loss of appetite. Both herpes simplex types 1 and 2 are caused by contact with an infected lesion.
- **Herpes zoster,** also known as **shingles,** is caused by **varicella-zoster,** the chickenpox virus. Lesions appear

along spinal nerve fibers outside the central nervous system called **spinal ganglia.** The virus is dormant until the patient's resistance is low, then a row of vesicular skin lesions erupts along a spinal nerve pathway, accompanied by severe pain, fever, and weakness. (See *A creeping virus.*)

As common as a toad

Verrucae (warts) are common, harmless infections of the skin and mucous membranes. They're caused by the human **papillomavirus** and can be transmitted by direct contact. Diagnosed by their appearance, warts are divided into the following categories:

- **common** (also called **verruca vulgaris**) — rough, elevated wart appearing most often on extremities, especially hands and fingers
- **filiform** — stalklike, horny projection commonly occurring around the face and neck
- **flat** — multiple groupings of up to several hundred slightly raised lesions with smooth, flat, or slightly rounded tops
- **genital** (also called **condyloma acuminatum**) — sexually transmitted infection appearing on the penis, scrotum, vulva, and anus
- **periungual** — rough wart appearing around the edges of fingernails and toenails
- **plantar** — appearing singularly or in large clusters, primarily at pressure points of the feet, with lesions that are slightly elevated or flat.

Beyond the dictionary

A creeping virus

Hippocrates used the term ***herpes,*** which was the Greek word for *creeping,* to describe a spreading cutaneous infection. Galen later revived the term during the 2nd century and diagnosed three types of the infection. Until the 18th century, the term was used for a number of conditions, including varieties of eczema and psoriasis. Around this time, English doctor Robert Willan restricted its use to the definition used today.

Parasitic infections

Pediculosis results from the infestation of bloodsucking lice. These lice feed on human blood and lay their eggs, or **nits,** in body hair or clothing fibers. When a louse bites, it injects a toxin into the skin that produces mild irritation and a reddened spot. Repeated bites can lead to serious inflammation. Three types of lice attack humans:

- ***Pediculus humanus capitis,*** or head louse
- ***Pediculus humanus corporis,*** or body louse
- ***Phthirus pubis,*** or pubic louse. (See *Crabs*, page 100.)

The nesting instinct

Scabies, another common parasitic infection, is caused by a female mite that penetrates and burrows into the skin. Under the skin, the mite lays eggs that mature and rise to the surface. A scabies infestation produces intense itching and secondary infections from the excoriation caused by scratching. Wavy, brown, threadlike lines appear on the hands, arms, body folds, and genitals.

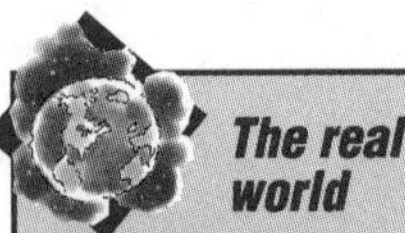

The real world

Crabs

In nonmedical settings, you'll often hear pubic lice called **crabs.** This makes sense figuratively because pubic lice move in a crablike manner. Thus, the term **crabs** has become common slang for cases of sexually transmitted pubic lice.

Fungal infections

Dermatophytosis is the general name for a fungal infection. Mushrooms, molds, and yeasts are common **fungi** (plural of fungus). Fungi are present in the air, soil, and water, but only a few species of fungi cause disease.

One of the most common fungal disorders is **tinea,** or **ringworm.** Each type of tinea is named according to the body part it affects:

- **Tinea barbae** affects the bearded facial hair of men. This infection produces raised areas that have marked crusting.
- **Tinea capitis** is characterized by small, spreading papules on the scalp that cause patchy hair loss with scaling.
- **Tinea corporis** affects the body and produces lesions with a ring-shaped appearance.
- **Tinea cruris,** commonly called **jock itch,** produces red, raised itchy lesions on the groin and surrounding areas.
- **Tinea pedis** is also called athlete's foot. This infection causes scaling and blisters between the toes, severe itching, and pain.
- **Tinea unguium,** also called **onychomycosis,** usually starts at the tip of one or more toenails and produces gradual thickening, discoloration, and crumbling of the nail.

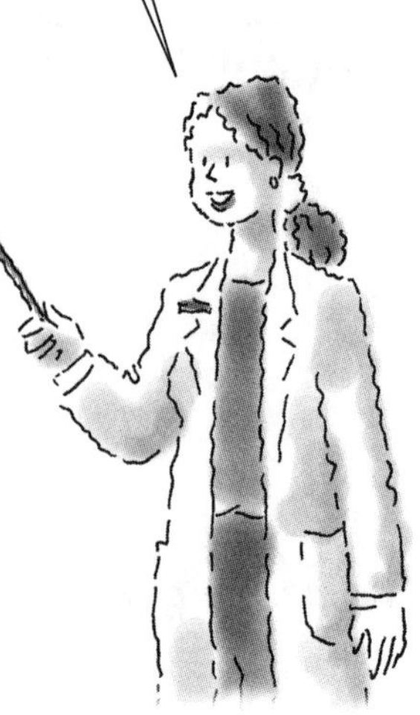

Remember to break down seemingly difficult words such as **dermatophytosis.** In Greek, ***derma*** means skin, ***phyto*** means plant, and ***osis*** means disease.

The red on a baby's bottom

Candidiasis, also called **moniliasis,** is a mild superficial fungal infection of the skin, nails, or mucous membranes. The patient develops a scaly, reddened papular rash with severe itching and burning. This fungus is often the culprit in diaper rash and vaginal infections. It's diagnosed through skin scrapings.

The white on another set of cheeks

Thrush is a fungal infection of the oral mucous membranes caused by ***Candida albicans.*** This infection develops most often in patients whose defenses are weakened by illness, malnutrition, infection, or prolonged treatment with antibiotics. White patches develop on a red, moist, inflamed surface inside the mouth, usually the inner cheeks. Thrush is accompanied by pain and fever.

Inflammatory disorders

Different types of dermatitis make up the most common inflammatory disorders.

Dermatitis

Superficial skin infections are known as **dermatitis** and can be caused by numerous things, such as drugs, plants, chemicals, and food.

Don't touch that!

Contact dermatitis occurs when direct contact with an irritant causes the epidermis to become inflamed and damaged. Touching such substances as poison ivy, poison oak, detergents, and industrial chemicals can lead to pain, burning, itching, and swelling — signs of dermatitis.

Other types of dermatitis include:

- **atopic dermatitis** — a chronic inflammatory response to other atopic diseases such as asthma. The skin is reddened, oozing, crusting, and intensely **pruritic** (itchy)
- **exfoliative dermatitis** — a severe chronic inflammation characterized by peeling of the skin
- **localized dermatitis** — a superficial inflammation characterized by redness and widespread erythema and scaling
- **nummular dermatitis** — a chronic form of dermatitis characterized by vesicular, crusted scales
- **seborrheic dermatitis** — an acute or subacute skin disease that primarily affects the skin and face, characterized by dry or moist greasy scales and yellowish crusts
- **stasis dermatitis** — typically caused by impaired circulation. Appears as tan pigmentation, patchy redness, and petechiae, with hardening of the skin.

Other inflammatory disorders

Here are some other inflammatory disorders, including allergies.

Don't eat that!

Angioedema is characterized by urticaria and edema that occurs as an allergic reaction, usually to a certain food. It occurs in the subcutaneous tissues of isolated areas, such as the eyelids, hands, feet, tongue, larynx, GI tract, or lips.

Don't do what?

Psoriasis is a chronic skin disorder, commonly with unknown causes, that is characterized by periods of remission and worsening. Psoriasis usually starts between ages 25 and 30. Lesions appear as reddened papules and plaques covered with silvery scales and vary widely in severity and location.

Skin tumors

Most skin tumors are **benign** (noncancerous), but they can be a starting point for skin cancer.

An **angioma** is formed by a group of blood vessels that dilate and form a tumorlike mass. The port-wine birthmark is a typical angioma. **Spider angiomas,** also called **telangiectases,** are made up of tiny, dilated veins that spread outward with a spiderlike appearance. (See *Caught in a web.*)

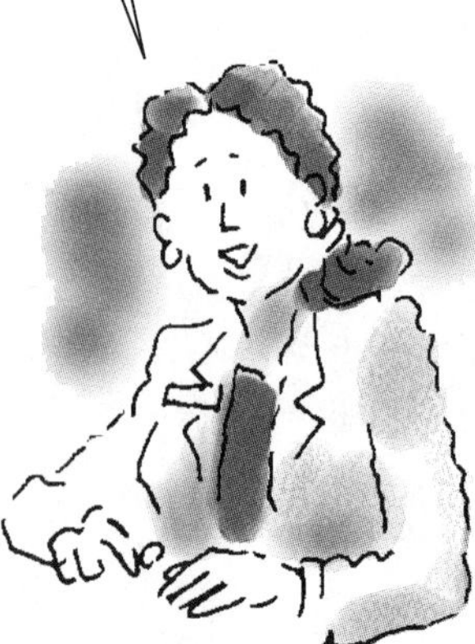

To pronounce **psoriasis**, think of the word "sore." The ***p*** is silent.

Not so benign...

Basal cell carcinoma is a type of skin cancer arising in the basal cell layer of the epidermis. Commonly found on the face and upper trunk, these tumors are painless and may go unnoticed by the patient.

Squamous cell carcinoma begins in the epidermis and produces a firm, **nodular** (knotlike) lesion covered with a crust or a central ulceration.

...and malignant

In **malignant melanoma,** cancer arises from the **melanocytes** (pigment cells) of the skin and its underlying structures. There are three types of malignant melanomas, which are categorized by location and description.

- **Superficial spreading melanoma** arises from an area of chronic irritation and is characterized by irregular colors and margins.
- **Nodular melanoma** grows vertically, invading the dermis and metastasizing early.
- **Lentigo maligna melanoma** arises from a lentigo maligna on an exposed skin surface and features a large lesion with scattered black nodules.

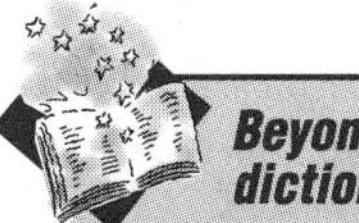

Beyond the dictionary

Caught in a web

The word **telangiectases** derives from Greek. ***Tela*** is the Greek term for *weblike*, ***angi-*** is a Greek affix for *vessels*, and ***ectasia*** is the Greek word for *distended*. Put them all together and you have a good description of **telangiectases** — distended weblike veins.

Cutaneous ulcers

An **ulcer** is an open sore. Ulcers on the skin are usually caused by a lack of circulation to a vulnerable area. Ulcers may be superficial, caused by local skin irritation, or deep, originating in the underlying tissue.

Pressure cooked

Pressure ulcers are localized areas of cellular death that occur most often in the skin and subcutaneous tissue over bony prominences.

Not in a good flow

Stasis ulcers are caused by chronic **venous stasis** (poor blood flow) due to varicose veins or blood clots. Prolonged standing in one position and obesity are predisposing factors for stasis ulcers.

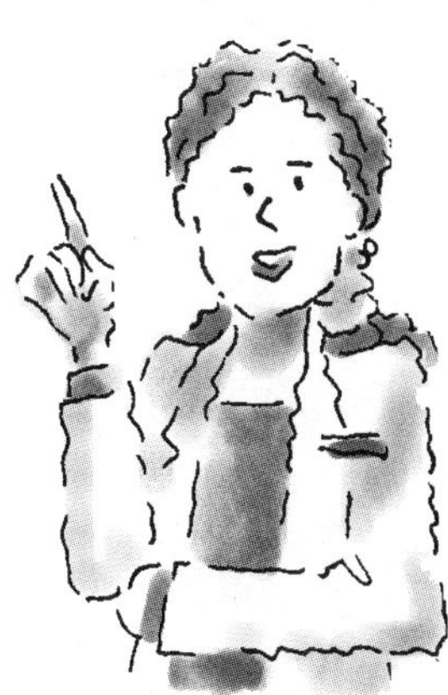
Remember, **ulcer** comes from the Latin word ***ulcus,*** which means *sore*.

Burns and cold injury

The skin is an effective protective covering. It can, however, be severely damaged when it comes in contact with excessive heat or cold.

Too hot

A burn is injury to tissue caused by contact with dry heat (fire), moist heat (steam), electricity, chemicals, lightning, or radiation. Categorized according to depth, burns are referred to as **superficial, partial-thickness,** or **full-thickness.** When named according to severity, burns are called **first, second, third,** or **fourth degree.** (See *Assessing burns*, page 104.)

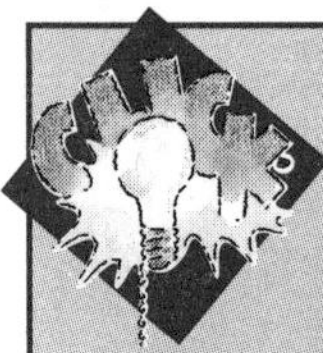

Now I get it!

Assessing burns

Assessing a burn means determining the depth of skin and tissue damage. It's traditional to describe burn depth by degrees, although most burns are a combination of different degrees and thickness.

First-degree, or superficial burn
In a first-degree burn, damage is limited to the epidermis, causing redness and pain. The skin is dry, with no blisters or drainage. A sunburn is typical of a first degree burn.

Second-degree, or partial thickness burn
In second-degree burns, the epidermis and part of the dermis are damaged, producing blisters and mild-to-moderate edema and pain. Large, moist blisters may occur, and the skin is mottled with dull white, tan, pink, or cherry red areas. Spilling a hot cup of coffee on the skin could produce a second-degree burn.

Third-degree, or full-thickness burn
In third-degree burns, the dermis and epidermis are damaged. No blisters appear, but white, brown, or black leathery tissue and thrombosed vessels are visible. There is little or no pain with this burn because the nerves are damaged, and the skin doesn't blanche with pressure. Contact with hot liquids, flames, chemical, or electricity may cause a third-degree burn.

Fourth-degree burn
In fourth-degree burns, damage extends through deeply charred subcutaneous tissue to muscle and bone.

Too cold

Cold injury, or **frostbite,** results from overexposure to cold air or water. Upon returning to a warm place, a person with superficial frostbite will experience burning, tingling, numbness, swelling, and a mottled, blue-gray skin color. Deep frostbite causes pain, blisters, tissue death, and gangrene. The skin appears white until it thaws and then appears purplish-blue.

Other skin disorders

Below are some other common skin disorders:
- **acne** — an inflammatory skin eruption caused by plugged sebaceous glands, resulting in papules and pustules
- **albinism** — an inherited condition with defective melanin production, causing lack of pigmentation to the skin
- **alopecia** — hair loss
- **aphthous stomatitis (canker sores)** — recurring ulcers on the mucous membrane of the mouth, with small, white lesions

• **chiggers** — the larvae of a mite, which attach to the host's skin, causing severe itching and dermatitis
• **chilblains** — redness and swelling of the skin caused by exposure to cold, damp conditions
• **eczema** — superficial dermatitis caused by reaction to a causative agent
• **nevus** — a benign birthmark
• **rosacea** — dilated and inflamed surface blood vessels causing reddening of the nose and adjoining areas and often accompanied by acne (**acne rosacea**)
• **vitiligo** — irregularly shaped patches of lighter or white skin caused by the loss of pigment-producing cells.

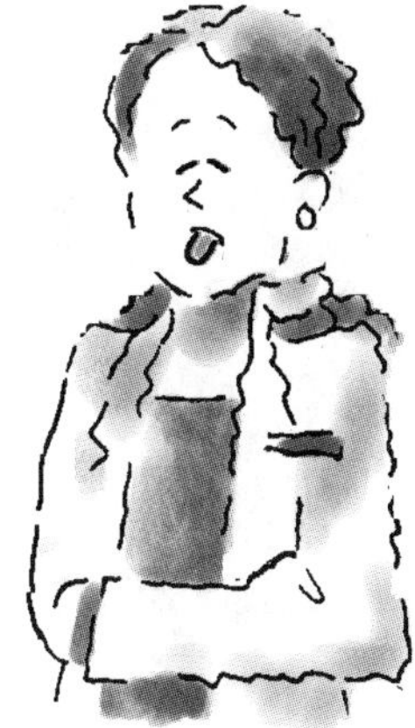
Chilblain is a combination of the English word ***chill*** and the Old English word for *sore*, ***blain.***

Treatments

Treating skin disorders is an example of hands-on health care. Most medicines are applied **topically** (to the affected area only). Surgery is typically performed with only a local anesthetic, and monitoring depends mostly on simple observation.

Drug therapy

Drugs used to treat skin disorders include **local anti-infectives, topical corticosteroids** to reduce inflammation, **protectants** to prevent skin breakdown, **keratolytics** to loosen thickened layers of skin, **astringents** to shrink tissues, and **emollients** and **demulcents** to soothe the skin.

Laser surgery

The highly focused and intense light of **lasers** is used to treat many types of skin lesions. Performed on an outpatient basis, laser surgery typically spares normal tissue (with the exception of CO_2 lasers), promotes healing, and helps prevent postsurgical infection.

Set your lasers on...

Three types of lasers are used in dermatology:
• The blue-green light of **argon lasers** is absorbed by the red pigment in hemoglobin. It coagulates small blood vessels and treats superficial vascular lesions.

• The CO_2 **laser** emits an invisible beam in the far-infrared wavelength; water absorbs this wavelength and converts it to heat energy. This laser helps treat warts and malignancies.
• The **tunable dye laser** is also absorbed by hemoglobin and has successfully treated port-wine stains.

Other surgery

Cryosurgery causes epidermal-dermal separation above the basement membranes, which prevents scarring. In this common dermatologic procedure, the application of extreme cold leads to tissue destruction. It can be performed simply by applying liquid nitrogen to the skin with a cotton-tipped applicator or may involve a complex cryosurgical unit.

Mohs' micrograph surgery involves excising cancerous tissue in a step-by-step manner, which minimizes scarring and helps prevent recurrence by removing all malignant tissue.

No more childhood scars

Dermabrasion removes superficial scars on the skin using revolving wire brushes or sand paper. Dermabrasion is typically used to reduce facial scars caused by acne.

Skin grafts

Skin grafts cover defects caused by burns, trauma, or surgery. They are used when primary closure of the skin isn't possible or cosmetically acceptable, when the defect is on a weight-bearing surface, when primary closure would interfere with functioning, and when a skin tumor is **excised** (cut out) and the site needs to be monitored for recurrence.

Types of skin grafts include:
• **split-thickness grafts,** which consist of the epidermis and a small portion of dermis
• **full-thickness grafts,** which include all of the dermis as well as the epidermis
• **composite grafts,** which also include underlying tissues, such as muscle, cartilage, and bone.

Cryosurgery sounds complicated but it's often just liquid nitrogen applied to the skin with a cotton-tipped applicator.

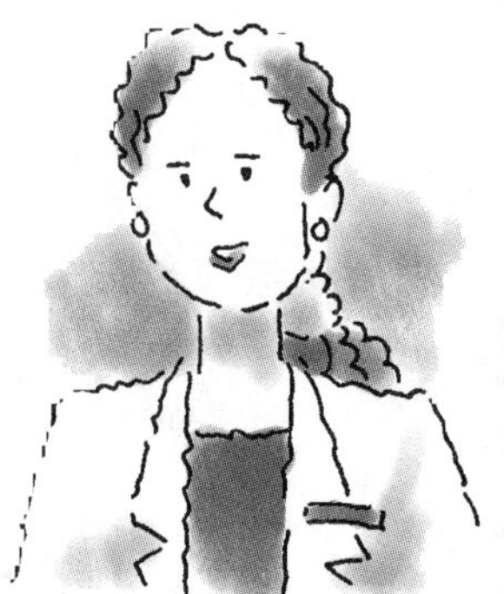

The gift of the graft

An **autologous graft,** or **autograft** (***auto-*** means *self*), is taken from the patient's own body and is the most successful type of skin graft. A graft from a genetically similar person, such as a twin, is an **isologous** graft, or **isograft** (***iso-*** means *alike*).

Patching it up

Biological dressings function like skin grafts to ease pain and prevent infection and fluid loss. However, they're only temporary; eventually the body rejects them. If the underlying wound hasn't healed, these dressings must be replaced with a graft of the patient's own skin. There are four types of biological dressings:

- **Homograft (allograft),** which is harvested from cadavers, is rejected in 7 to 10 days. Homografts are used to debride wounds, protect new tissue growth, serve as a test graft before skin grafting, and temporarily cover burns. (***Allo*** is Greek for *deviating from normal* and ***homo*** refers to *human beings.*)
- **Heterograft (xenograft),** a graft harvested from animals (usually pigs), is also rejected after 7 to 10 days. It's used for the same purposes as the homograft and is also used to cover exposed tendons and burns that are only slightly contaminated.
- **Amnion,** made from amnion and chorionic membranes (fetal membranes), is used to protect burns and temporarily cover new tissue while awaiting an autograft.
- **Biosynthetic grafts,** which are woven from man-made fibers, are used to cover donor graft sites, protect wounds awaiting autografts, and cover meshed autografts.

Debridement is borrowed from the French and means *to unbridle.* Originally a medical term, it was used to describe the cutting of constricting bands — similar to a horse's bridle.

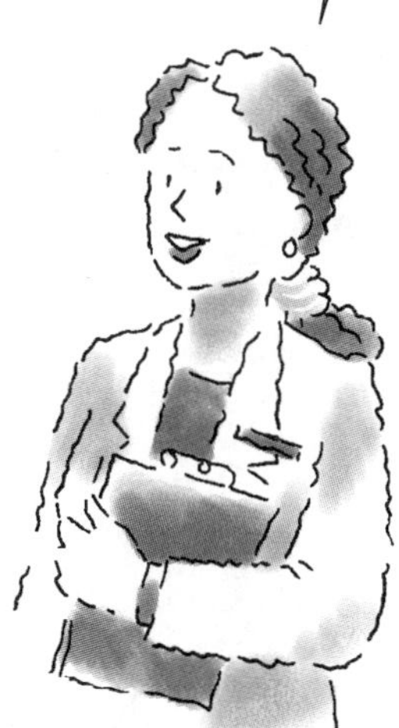

Debridement

Debridement uses mechanical, chemical, or surgical techniques to remove **necrotic** (dead) tissue from a wound. Although it can be extremely painful, debridement is necessary to prevent infection and promote healing of burns and skin ulcers. There are three types of debridement:

- **Chemical debridement** calls for special wound-cleaning beads or topical medications, which absorb drainage and debris from a wound. These agents also absorb bacteria, reducing the risk of infection.

- **Mechanical debridement** uses dressings, irrigation, **hydrotherapy** (whirlpool baths), and bedside debridement to remove necrotic tissue. During bedside debridement, dead tissue is scraped off or cut away with a scalpel or scissors.
- **Surgical debridement** requires anesthesia and is usually reserved for burn patients or those with extremely deep or large ulcers.

Therapeutic baths

Also known as **balneotherapy,** baths are used to treat many skin conditions, including psoriasis, eczema, exfoliative dermatitis, and bullous diseases that cause blisters.

The four types of baths commonly used are **antibacterial, colloidal, emollient,** and **tar.** In addition to promoting relaxation, these baths permit treatment of large areas. Therapeutic baths are limited to 30 minutes because they can cause dry skin, itching, scaling, and fissures. (See *The baths.*)

The baths

There are four types of therapeutic baths:

- **Antibacterial baths** treat infected eczema, dirty ulcerations, and furunculosis. Acetic acid, hexachlorophene, potassium permanganate, and povidone iodine are commonly used.
- **Colloidal baths** are great to relieve itching and soothe irritated skin. They're indicated for any irritating or oozing skin condition such as atopic eczema. Oatmeal, starch, and baking soda are used for colloidal baths.
- **Emollient baths** use bath oils and mineral oil to clean and hydrate the skin. They're helpful for any dry skin condition.
- **Tar baths** utilize special bath oils with tar or coal tar concentrate to treat scaly skin disorders. This bath loosens scales and relieves itching.

Phototherapy

Used to treat skin conditions by exposure to ultraviolet radiation, **phototherapy** slows the growth of epidermal cells, most likely by inhibiting the synthesis of deoxyribonucleic acid. Two different ultraviolet light wavelengths are used; ultraviolet A (UVA) is the component of sunlight that tans skin and ultraviolet B is the component that causes sunburn.

Light plus drugs equals . . .

Photochemotherapy combines light with a drug called **psoralen,** making the skin more sensitive to UVA. The combination of psoralen with UVA is also known as **PUVA therapy.**

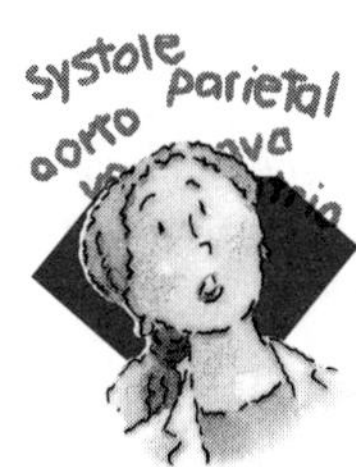

Vocabulary builders

Get ready to toughen up! These puzzles are pretty tough.

At a crossroads

Hopefully, this is a crossword puzzle that won't get under your skin. Good luck!

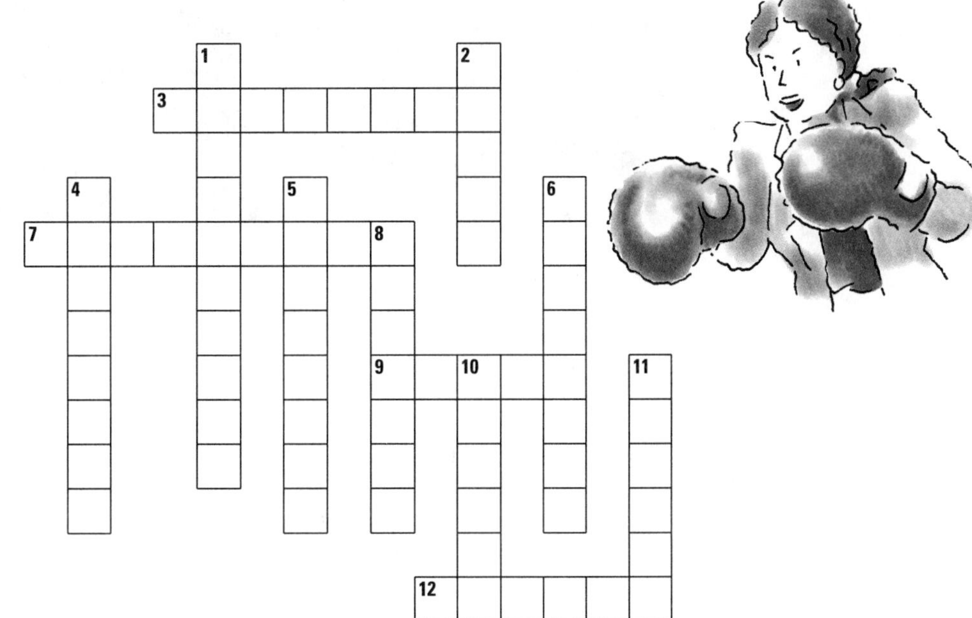

Across

3. An excess of this enzyme turns the skin yellow-orange
7. The outermost layer of skin
9. A fluid filled lesion
12. Word that describes pale skin

Down

1. The specialized cells in the skin layer that enhance the immune system are named after this doctor
2. The Greek word for skin
4. Glands that begin to function at puberty
5. A contagious, superficial skin infection
6. A protein that gives strength to the dermis
8. Caused by female mites
10. Crescent-moon-shaped area on the nail
11. Condition of normal tension in the skin

Answers are on page 112.

Finish line

One of the most common fungal disorders is tinea. Each specific type of tinea is named according to the body part it affects. Fill in the blanks to complete each type of this fungal disorder.

1. Tinea _______________ affects the bearded facial hair of men.
2. Tinea _______________ produces raised itchy lesions in the groin area.
3. Tinea _______________ is also called athlete's foot.
4. Tinea _______________ usually starts at the tip of one or more of the toenails.
5. Tinea _______________ affects the body.
6. Tinea _______________ is characterized by small papules on the scalp.

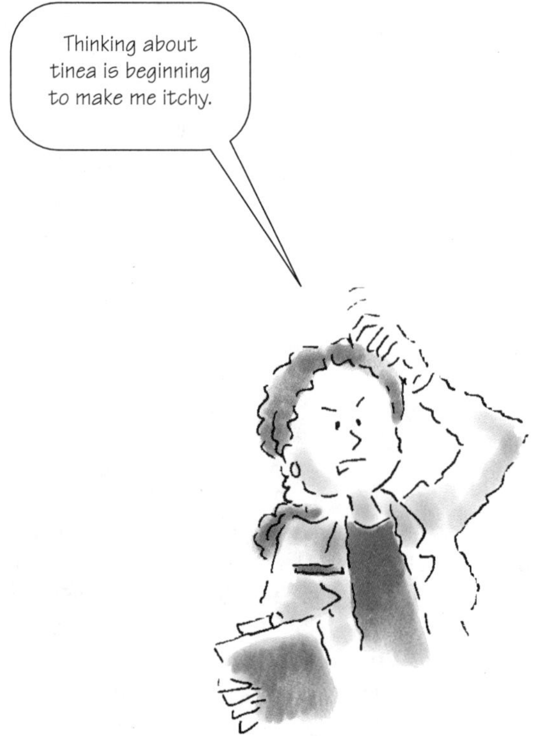

Thinking about tinea is beginning to make me itchy.

Answers are on page 112.

Scrambled or overeasy

Fill in the answers for the following questions, then unscramble the circled letters to find the answer to the puzzle.

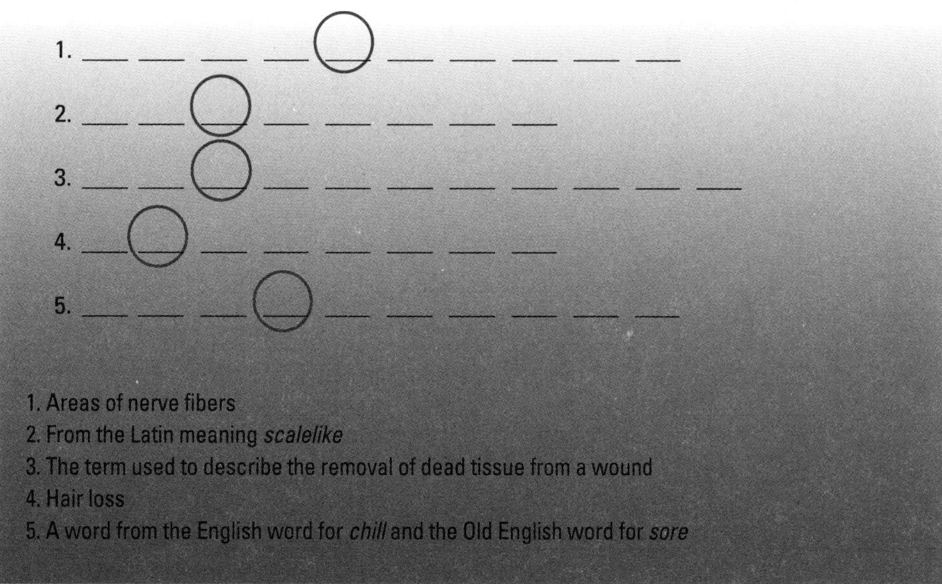

1. ___ ___ ___ ___ (◯) ___ ___ ___ ___ ___
2. ___ ___ (◯) ___ ___ ___ ___ ___
3. ___ ___ (◯) ___ ___ ___ ___ ___ ___ ___ ___
4. ___ (◯) ___ ___ ___ ___ ___ ___
5. ___ ___ ___ (◯) ___ ___ ___ ___ ___ ___

1. Areas of nerve fibers
2. From the Latin meaning *scalelike*
3. The term used to describe the removal of dead tissue from a wound
4. Hair loss
5. A word from the English word for *chill* and the Old English word for *sore*

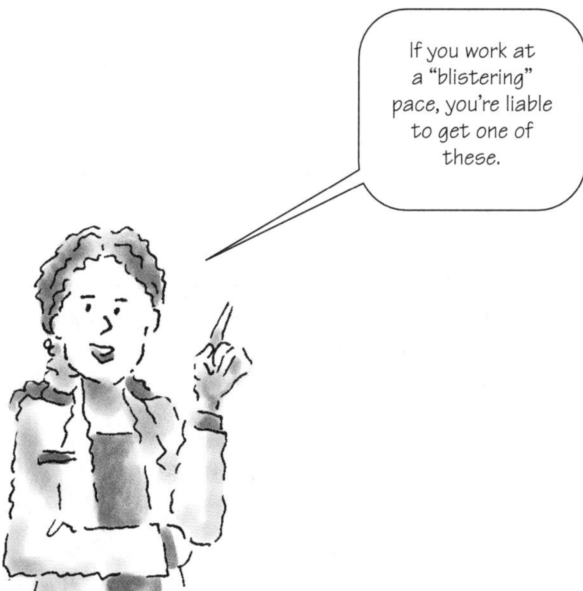

If you work at a "blistering" pace, you're liable to get one of these.

Answers are on page 112.

Answers

At a crossroads

				1 L						2 D				
			3 C	A	R	O	T	E	N	E				
				N						R				
	4 A			G		5 I				M		6 C		
7 E	P	I	D	E	R	M	I	8 S		A		O		
	O			R		P		C				L		
	C			H		E		A				L		
	R			A		T		9 B	U	10 L	L	A		11 T
	I			N		I		I		U		G		U
	N			S		G		E		N		E		R
	E					O		S		U		N		G
										L				O
									12 P	A	L	L	O	R

Finish line

1. Barbae; 2. Cruris; 3. Pedis; 4. Unguium; 5. Corporis; 6. Capitis.

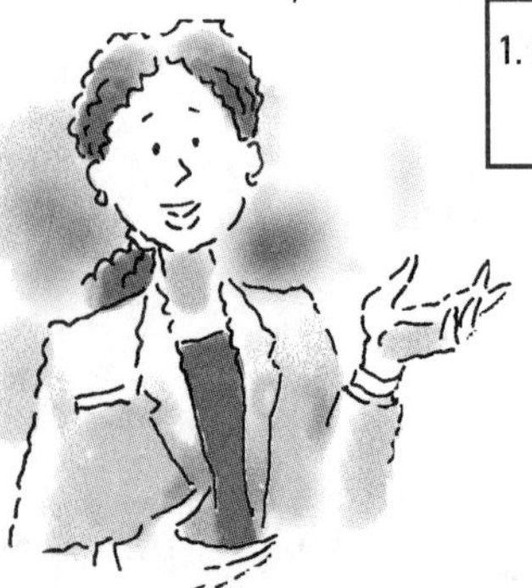

Scrambled or overeasy

1. Dermatomes; 2. Squamous; 3. Debridement; 4. Alopecia; 5. Chilblains.
Answer to puzzle — Bulla

Cardiovascular system

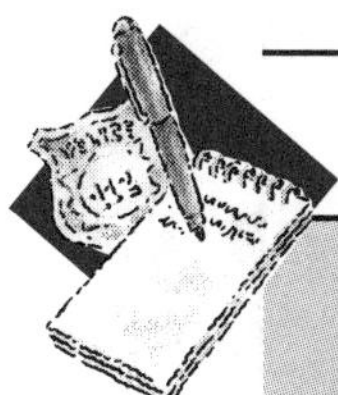

Just the facts

In this chapter, you'll review:

- terminology related to the structure and function of the cardiovascular system
- terminology needed for physical examination of the cardiovascular system
- tests that help diagnose cardiovascular disorders
- disorders of the cardiovascular system and their treatments.

Heart structure and function

A key to learning terminology related to the cardiovascular system is knowing the medical word for *heart:* it's the Latin word ***cardium,*** which is borrowed from the Greek word ***kardia.*** Cardium is often combined with other words in the forms ***cardi*** or ***cardio.*** Some examples include *cardiology, electrocardiogram,* and *tachycardia.* (See *Cardiac versus heart* and *Pronouncing key cardiovascular system terms,* page 114.)

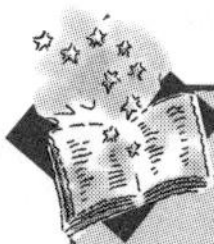

Beyond the dictionary

Cardiac versus heart

The word **cardiac** is nearly as familiar to most English-speaking people as the word **heart.** Because Greek and Latin were the primary languages of universities up until the 1900s, terms from those languages were adopted for scientific use. Some of those terms, like **cardiac,** have migrated into ordinary English speech as well.

The heart's protector

The heart is protected by a thin sac called the **pericardium.** ***Peri-*** is a Greek suffix that means *around.* ***Cardi*** comes from the Latin word that means *heart.* The pericardium has an inner, or **visceral,** layer that forms the **epicardium** and an outer, or **parietal,** layer.

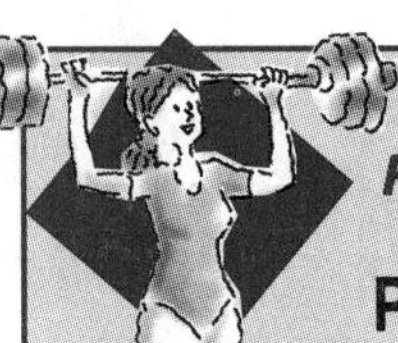

Pump up your pronunciation

Pronouncing key cardiovascular system terms

Below is a list of key terms, along with the correct ways to pronounce them.

Aneurysm	ANN-YOO-RIHZ-UHM
Angina	ANN-JEYE-NAH
Arrhythmia	AH-RIHTH-MEE-AH
Arteriosclerosis	AHR-TEER-EE-OH-SKLEH-ROH-SISS
Coarctation	COH-ARK-TAY-SHUNN
Defibrillation	DEE-FIHB-BRIH-LAY-SHUNN
Diuretic	DEYE-YOO-REHT-IHK
Ischemia	IHS-KEE-MEE-AH
Paroxysmal atrial tachycardia	PAHR-AWK-SIHZ-MAHL AY-TREE-AHL TACK-IH-KAHR-DEE-AH
Pericardiocentesis	PEHR-IH-KAHR-DEE-OH-SEHN-TEE-SISS
Sphygmomanometer	SFIGG-MOH-MAH-NAWM-EH-TEHR
Thrombophlebitis	THRAWM-BOH-FLEH-BEYE-TISS

A three-layered heart

The heart wall is composed of three layers. The outer layer is the **epicardium.** The **myocardium** is the heart muscle itself, and the **endocardium** is the innermost layer, which lines the heart's chambers and covers its valves.

Welcome to my chambers

The heart consists of four chambers. Each of the two upper chambers is called an **atrium** (plural: **atria**). The atria are thin-walled chambers that serve as reservoirs for blood. Each atrium is connected by its own valve to a chamber below it. The two lower chambers are called **ventricles** (also called **ventriculi**). The ventricles have thick walls and are responsible for pumping blood throughout the body. (See *Why the atria are called atria.*)

Beyond the dictionary

Why the atria are called atria

It's fitting that the upper chambers of the heart are called **atria** because, in a Roman house, the atrium was an entrance where a person was greeted before moving into other rooms. The atria are the first chambers in the heart to receive blood before it empties into the ventricles and is pumped throughout the body.

And those ventricles? The word **ventricle** derives from the Latin word ***ventriculus,*** which means *little stomach,* and refers to any small cavity of the body. There are two ventricles in the heart and four in the brain.

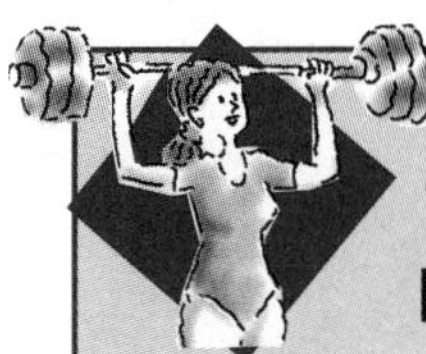

Pump up your pronunciation

How do I say *vena cava*?

In the term **vena cava,** the first word looks like the word **vein,** and that is exactly what it means. It's pronounced VEE-NAH. The second word is pronounced with a long first ***a*** and a short final ***a*** sound, CAY-VAH. The plural **venae cavae,** pronounced VEE-NAY KAH-VAY, refers to both veins.

The blood's path

Blood is carried into the heart through several major vessels, all of which empty into either the **superior vena cava** or **inferior vena cava** (plural: **venae cavae**). The superior vena cava carries blood from the upper body to the right atrium; it's called **superior** because that means *near the top*. **Inferior** means *situated below*, and the inferior vena cava carries blood from the lower body to the right atrium. (See *How do I say vena cava?*)

Through the pulmonary artery and into the lungs

Blood in the right atrium empties into the right ventricle mostly by gravity. When the ventricle contracts, the blood is ejected into the **pulmonary artery** (called such because ***pulmon*** is Latin for *lung*). The blood is pushed through the pulmonary arteries to the lungs.

Beyond the dictionary

Why call it the aorta?

Aorta means *that which is hung.* Because of the arching curve in the aorta as it exits the heart and its subsequent descent into the body, it looks something like a modern clothes hanger. Apparently, Aristotle had a similar notion; he was the first to apply the name to this artery.

The final trip

From the lungs, blood travels to the left atrium through the **pulmonary veins.** The left atrium empties blood into the left ventricle. The left ventricle pumps the blood into the **aorta** and from there, it travels throughout the body. (See *Why call it the aorta?*)

The heart's valves

The heart contains two **atrioventricular (AV)** valves (the tricuspid and mitral) and two **semilunar** valves (the pulmonic and aortic). The **tricuspid** valve separates the right atrium from the right ventricle. It has three flaps or cusps, which is why it is called the tricuspid valve.

The **pulmonic** valve separates the right ventricle from the pulmonary artery.

Zoom in

Inside the heart

This illustration shows a cross-sectional view of the structures and blood flow of the heart and major blood vessels.

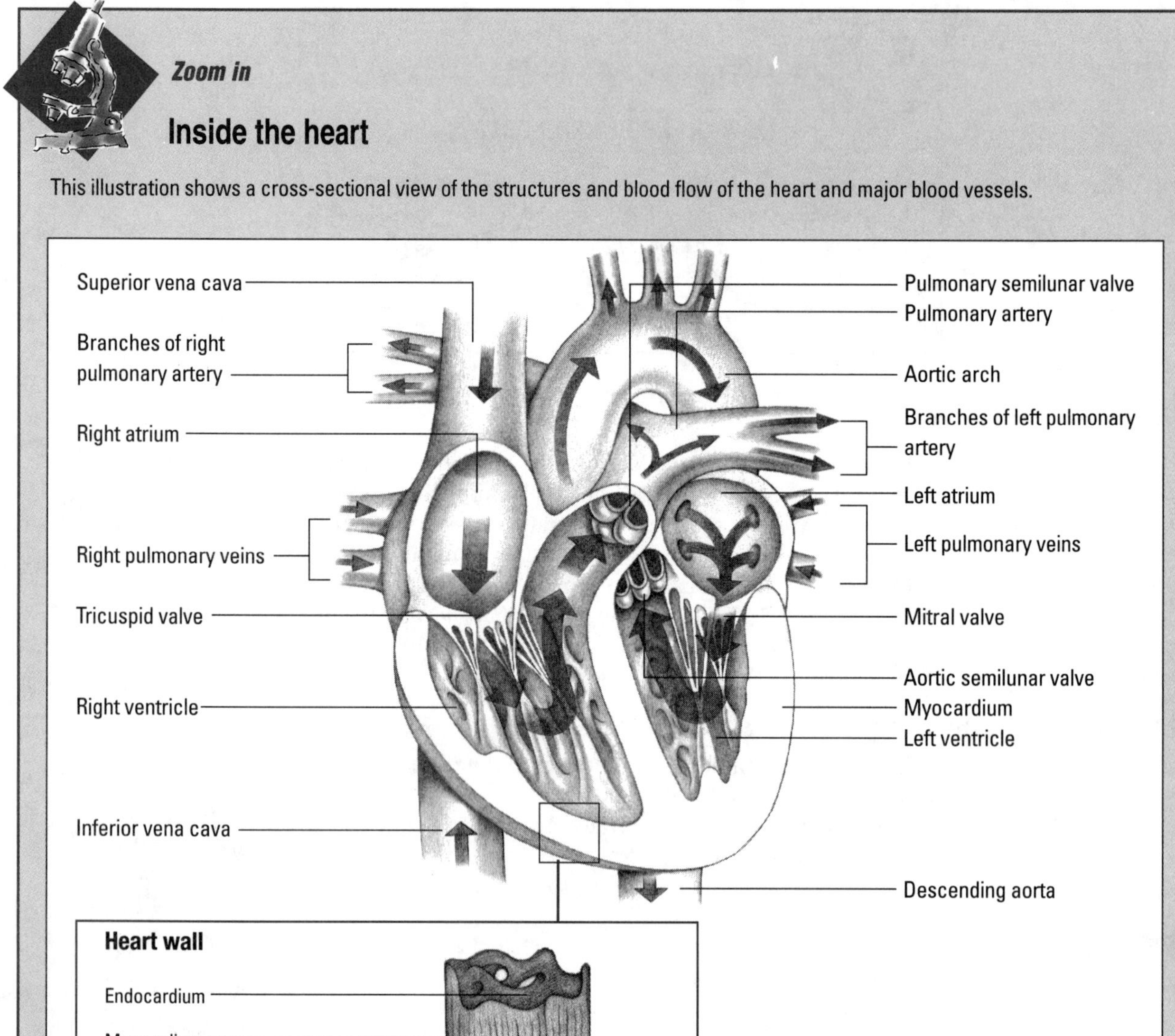

The **mitral** valve separates the left atrium from the left ventricle. It has two flaps or cusps and is also known as the **bicuspid** valve. (See *Inside the heart.*)

The heart's rhythm

Contractions of the heart occur in a rhythm — the cardiac cycle — and are regulated by impulses that normally begin at the **sinoatrial (SA) node,** the heart's pacemaker. The impulses are conducted from there through the **AV node,** down through the **AV bundle,** or the **bundle of His** (pronounced HIHS), and through the **Purkinje fibers,** where the impulse stimulates ventricular contraction. (See *What is a Purkinje?*)

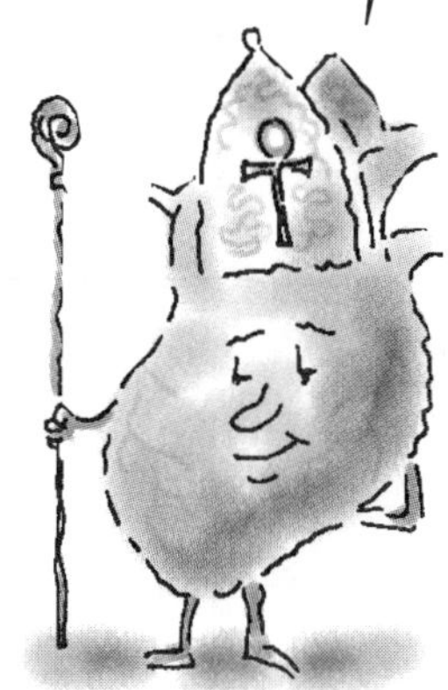

The **mitral valve** looks like a bishop's miter — thus the name mitral valve.

For every opposite action

The autonomic nervous system has two divisions that have opposite actions on the heart. The **parasympathetic** division acts on the SA and AV nodes. This division slows heart rate, reduces impulse conduction, and dilates coronary arteries.

The **sympathetic** division also acts on the SA and AV nodes but with an opposite effect. This division increases heart rate and impulse conduction and constricts and dilates the coronary arteries.

The cardiac cycle

No discussion of heart functions would be complete without an explanation of the **cardiac cycle,** the period from the beginning of one heart beat to the beginning of the next. During this cycle, electrical and mechanical events must occur in proper sequence and to the proper degree to provide adequate blood flow to all body parts. (See *Cardiac conduction route*, page 118.)

The two phases

The cardiac cycle has two phases, systole and diastole. Systole is the period when the ventricles contract and send blood on an outward journey to the aorta or the pulmonary artery. Diastole, the second period, is when the heart relaxes and fills with blood. During diastole, the mitral valve and tricuspid valves are open, and the aortic and pulmonic valves are closed. (See *Systole and diastole*, page 118.)

Diastole — passive then active

Diastole consists of two parts, **ventricular filling** and **atrial contraction.** During the first part of diastole, 70%

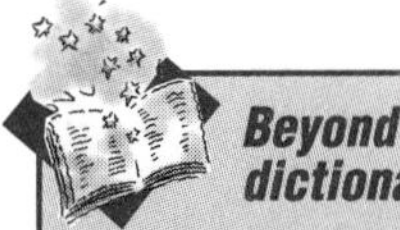
Beyond the dictionary

What is a Purkinje?

The Purkinje (PUHR-KIHN-JEE) fibers are microscopic muscles first distinguished from ordinary heart muscle tissue by the Czech physiologist Jan Purkinje (1787-1869). He also originated the analysis and classification of fingerprints.

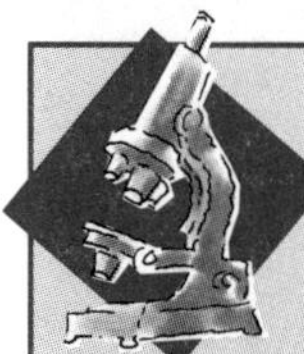

Zoom in

Cardiac conduction route

Specialized fibers propagate electrical impulses throughout the heart's cells, causing the heart to contract. This illustration shows the elements of the cardiac conduction system.

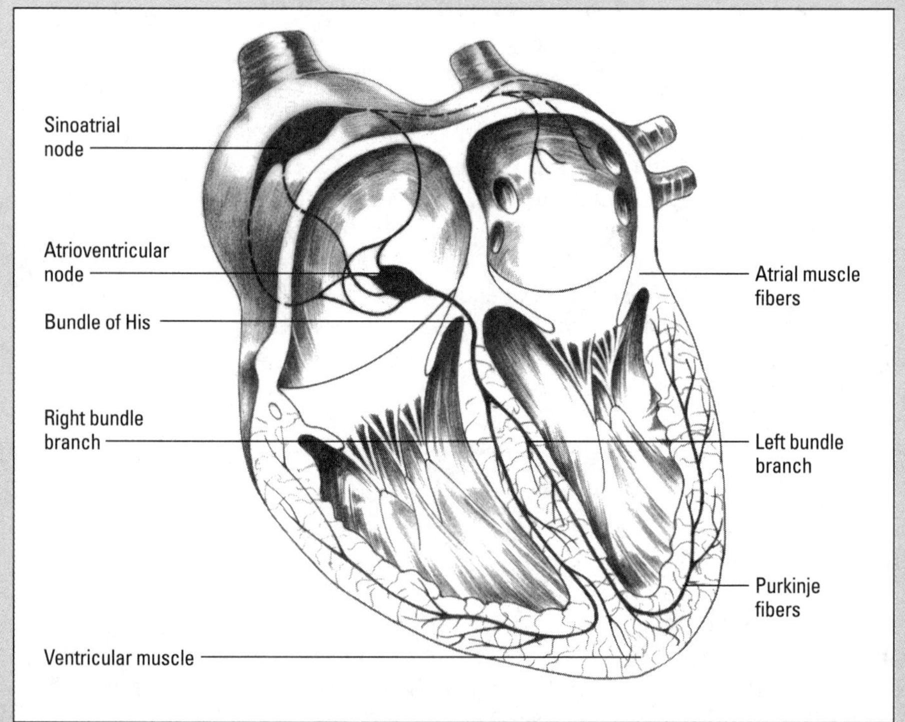

of the blood in the atria drains into the ventricles as a result of gravity, a passive action.

The active period of diastole, atrial contraction (also called atrial kick), accounts for the remaining 30% of blood that passes into the ventricles. Diastole is also the period in which the heart muscle receives its own supply of blood, which is transported there by the **coronary arteries.**

Lub...

Systole is the period of ventricular contraction. As pressure within the ventricles rises, the mitral and tricuspid

Beyond the dictionary

Systole and diastole

Systole (pronounced SIHS-TOH-LEE) and ***diastole*** (pronounced DEYE-AH-STOH-LEE) have the same Greek root, ***stole,*** which means *to send.*

Apart or together?
The prefixes are the keys to these words. The prefix ***dia-*** means *apart;* and ***sy-***, a contraction of ***syn-***, means *together.* If you think about the interior wall of the ventricles contracting, coming closer together, you'll remember **systole.** If you think about the relaxation of the muscle and the walls moving apart, you'll remember **diastole.**

valves snap closed. This closure leads to the first heart sound, S_1 (the **lub** of ***lub-dub***).

When the pressure in the ventricles rises above the pressure in the aorta and pulmonary artery, the aortic and pulmonic valves open. Blood then surges from the ventricles into the pulmonary artery to the lungs and into the aorta to the rest of the body.

Coronary arteries got their name because they encircle the heart like a crown. The word **coronary** comes from the Greek ***koron,*** which means *crown.*

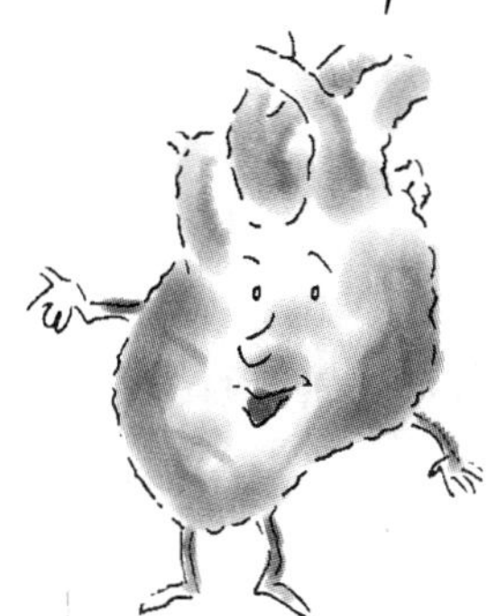

...then dub

At the end of ventricular contraction, pressure in the ventricles drops below the pressure in the aorta and the pulmonary artery. That pressure difference forces blood to back up toward the ventricles and causes the aortic and pulmonic valves to snap shut, which produces the second heart sound, S_2 (the **dub** of **lub-dub**). As the valves shut, the atria fill with blood in preparation for the next period of diastolic filling, and the cycle begins again.

Pumping it out

Cardiac output refers to the amount of blood pumped out by the heart in 1 minute and is determined by the **stroke volume,** the amount of blood ejected with each heartbeat multiplied by the number of beats per minute. Stroke volume, in turn, depends on three factors: contractility, preload, and afterload.

- **Contractility** refers to the ability of the myocardium to contract normally.
- **Preload** is the stretching of muscle fibers in the ventricles. This stretching results from the volume of blood in the ventricles at the end of diastole. The more muscles stretch, the more forcefully they contract during systole.
- **Afterload** refers to the pressure the ventricular muscles must generate to overcome the higher pressure in the aorta.

Vascular network

The peripheral vascular system consists of a network of arteries, arterioles, capillaries, venules, and veins.

Keep air in there

Artery comes from the Greek words ***aer,*** which means *air,* and ***terein,*** which means *to keep,* because the ancients believed that arteries contained air. Arteries carry blood away from the heart. Nearly all arteries carry oxygen-rich blood from the heart to the rest of the body. The only exception is the pulmonary artery, which carries oxygen-depleted blood to the lungs.

Smaller and smaller

The exchange of fluid, nutrients, and metabolic wastes between blood and cells occurs in the **capillaries.** Capillaries are connected to arteries and veins through intermediary vessels called **arterioles** and **venules,** respectively. (See *Call it a capillary.*)

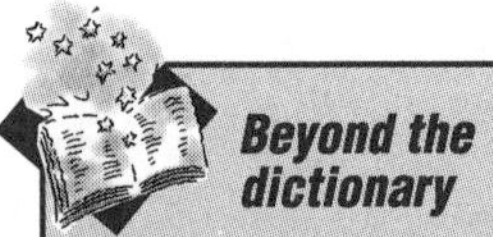

Call it a capillary

Capillary is a Latin word that means *hairlike* and refers to the minute size of these vessels.

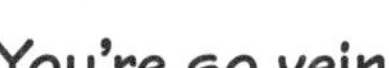

You're so vein

Veins carry blood toward the heart. Nearly all veins carry oxygen-depleted blood. The sole exception to this is the pulmonary vein which carries oxygen-rich blood from the lungs to the heart.

Physical examination terms

Below are the terms associated with examination of the heart and abnormalities an examination might reveal.

The vital signs

The physiologic condition of a patient is reflected in his vital signs. The vital signs that are directly related to the cardiovascular system are pulse and blood pressure.

Stay on the beat

A patient's **pulse** is the expansion and contraction of an artery in a regular, rhythmic pattern; this happens when the left ventricle of the heart ejects blood as it contracts, causing waves of pressure.

We thrive on pressure

A person's **blood pressure** is maintained by the complex interaction of the homeostatic mechanisms of the body and is influenced by the volume of blood, the lumen of the arteries and arterioles, and the force of the cardiac contraction.

When you take a blood pressure, you're measuring the pressure exerted by the circulating volume of blood on the walls of the arteries, the veins, and the chambers of the heart.

Systole and diastole again

A typical blood pressure reading consists of the systolic blood pressure and the diastolic blood pressure; the pulse pressure is a third measurement that depends on the other two pressures. Here is a description of each:

- **Systolic blood pressure** is the blood pressure caused by the contraction phase or systole of the left ventricle of the heart. It's the top number given in a blood pressure measurement. For example, the systolic blood pressure in a measurement of 120/80 mm Hg is 120.
- **Diastolic blood pressure** is the pressure during the heart's relaxation phase, or diastole. It's the bottom number given in a blood pressure measurement. For example, the diastolic blood pressure in a measurement of 120/80 mm Hg is 80.
- **Pulse pressure** is the numerical difference between the systolic and diastolic blood pressures. For example, if the patient's blood pressure reading is 120/80 mm Hg, his pulse pressure is 40 mm Hg.

Tools of the trade

To take a blood pressure, you use a **sphygmomanometer,** an instrument that consists of an inflatable cuff, an inflatable bulb, and a gauge, which is designed to measure arterial blood pressure.

You also listen to the sound of flowing blood with a **stethoscope.** The word **stethoscope** comes from the Greek words ***stethos,*** which means chest, and **skopein,** which means *to examine.* A stethoscope is an instrument used for auscultation of respiratory, cardiac, intestinal, uterine, fetal, arterial, and venous sounds; it consists of two earpieces that are connected by flexible tubing to a diaphragm, which is placed against the patient's chest or back.

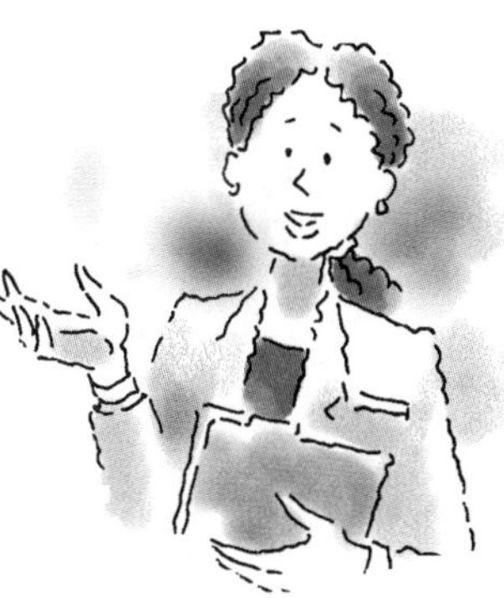
Sphygmoma- ...what? Oh, it's just a jazzed-up name for a blood pressure cuff.

What you hear

In determining blood pressure, you should listen for **Korotkoff's sounds,** which are typically the first faint sounds heard as the pressure in the cuff is released and blood begins to flow and the last sound heard before silence as blood flows. These two points correspond to the systolic and diastolic pressures, respectively.

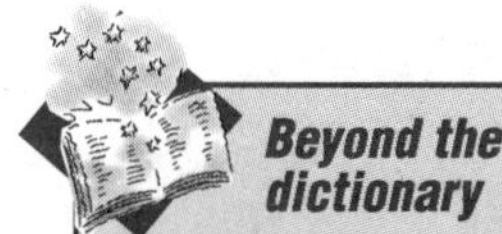

Beyond the dictionary

What is all the bruit about?

It's easy to mispronounce **bruit** because it's a French word. It means *noise, din,* or *racket.* It's pronounced BROOEE; the ***t*** sound is dropped.

Abnormalities in the physical examination

Auscultation may reveal a **murmur,** a soft blowing or fluttering sound of cardiac or vascular origin, or a **bruit,** an abnormal sound heard over peripheral vessels that indicates turbulent blood flow. (See *What is all the bruit about?*)

Color matters, too

Other signs of cardiovascular problems include **cyanosis,** a bluish discoloration of the skin and mucous membranes that results from an excessive amount of deoxygenated hemoglobin in the blood or a structural defect in the hemoglobin molecule. The word **cyanosis** comes from the Greek word ***cyanos,*** which means *dark blue.* You may also encounter patients with **pallor.** Pallor is a fancy term for paleness, or a decrease or absence of color in the skin.

Too much liquid

The examination can also reveal **edema,** the accumulation of abnormal amounts of fluid in the intercellular tissues, pericardial sac, pleural cavity, peritoneal cavity, or joint capsules. Any of these conditions may be accompanied by **diaphoresis,** a perfuse perspiration associated with an elevated body temperature, physical exertion, heat exposure, and mental or emotional stress. (See *Edema! That's just swell!*)

Too much pain

Angina, also called **angina pectoris,** is severe chest pain that lasts several minutes and results from an inadequate supply of oxygen to the heart muscle.

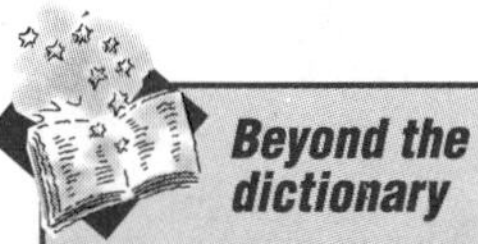

Beyond the dictionary

Edema! That's just swell!

The word **edema** is a recent borrowing from Greek. It means *swelling.*

Diagnostic tests

No single test can diagnose cardiovascular disease. Therefore, your patient will undergo more than one — sometimes several — tests if a cardiovascular disease or disorder is suspected. These tests are described below.

Incredibly Easy miniguide: The heart

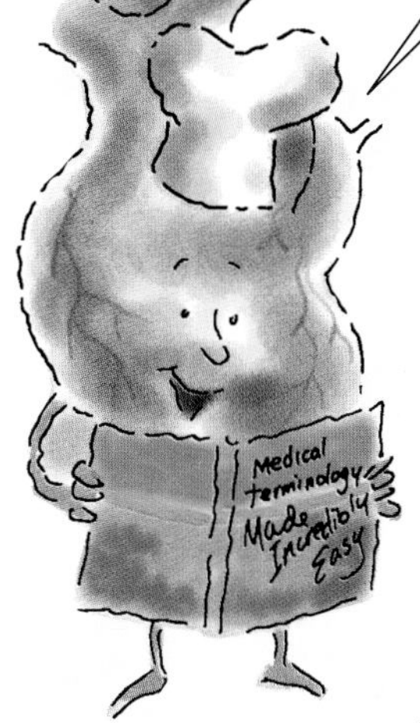

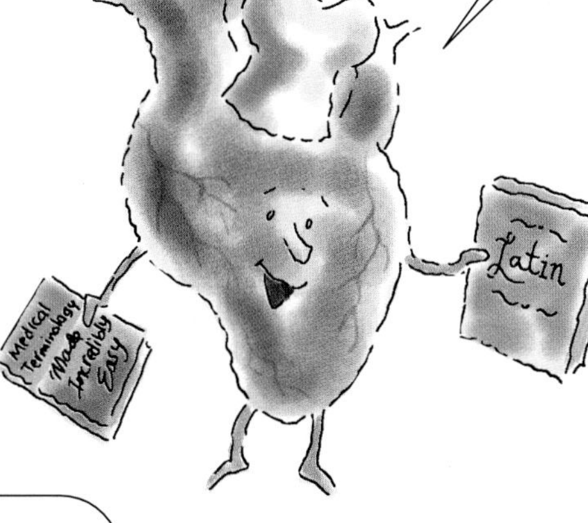
The Latin word **cardium,** which is borrowed from the Greek word **kardia,** is the medical word for *heart.*
Medical Terminology Made Incredibly Easy
Latin

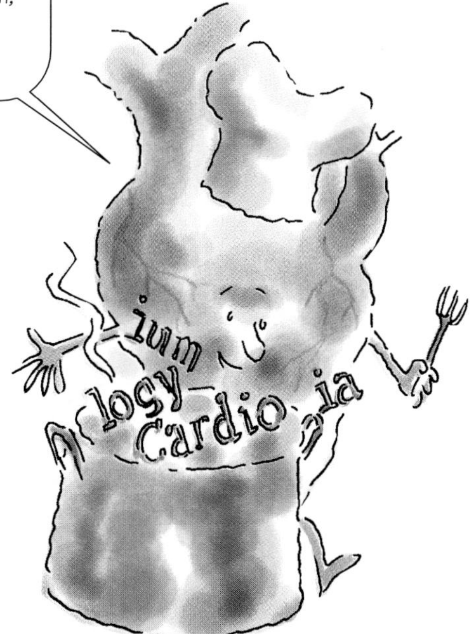

Incredibly Easy miniguide: The heart

Within the heart lie four chambers (two atria and two ventricles). A system of blood vessels carries blood to and from the heart.

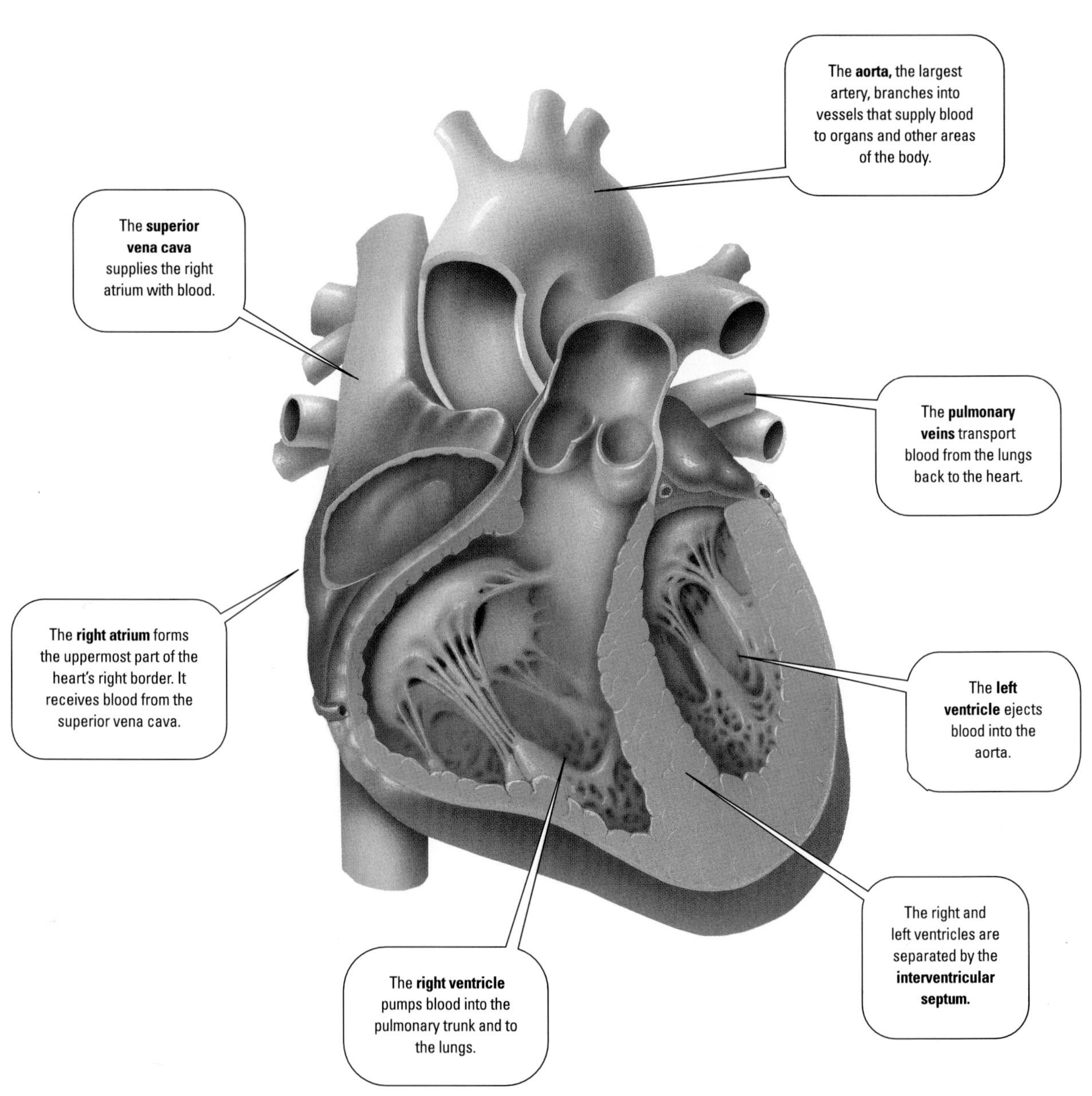

The **aorta,** the largest artery, branches into vessels that supply blood to organs and other areas of the body.
The **superior vena cava** supplies the right atrium with blood.
The **pulmonary veins** transport blood from the lungs back to the heart.
The **right atrium** forms the uppermost part of the heart's right border. It receives blood from the superior vena cava.
The **left ventricle** ejects blood into the aorta.
The right and left ventricles are separated by the **interventricular septum.**
The **right ventricle** pumps blood into the pulmonary trunk and to the lungs.

Incredibly Easy miniguide: The heart

The semilunar valves of the heart have three cusps that are shaped like half-moons. The two atrioventricular valves separate the atria from the ventricles.

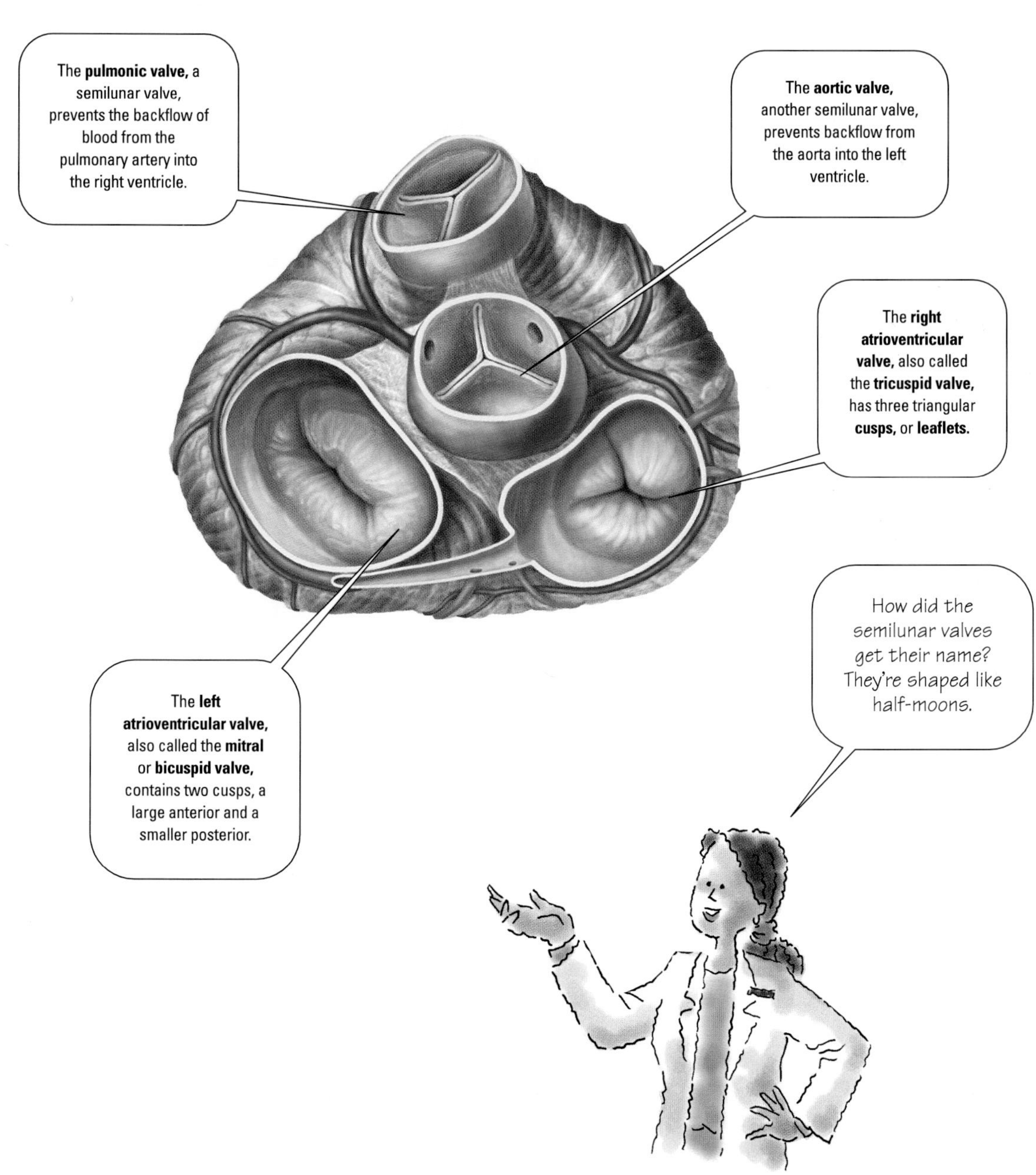

The **pulmonic valve,** a semilunar valve, prevents the backflow of blood from the pulmonary artery into the right ventricle.
The **aortic valve,** another semilunar valve, prevents backflow from the aorta into the left ventricle.
The **right atrioventricular valve,** also called the **tricuspid valve,** has three triangular **cusps,** or **leaflets.**
The **left atrioventricular valve,** also called the **mitral** or **bicuspid valve,** contains two cusps, a large anterior and a smaller posterior.
How did the semilunar valves get their name? They're shaped like half-moons.

Incredibly Easy miniguide: The heart

The heart relies on the coronary arteries and their branches for its supply of oxygenated blood.

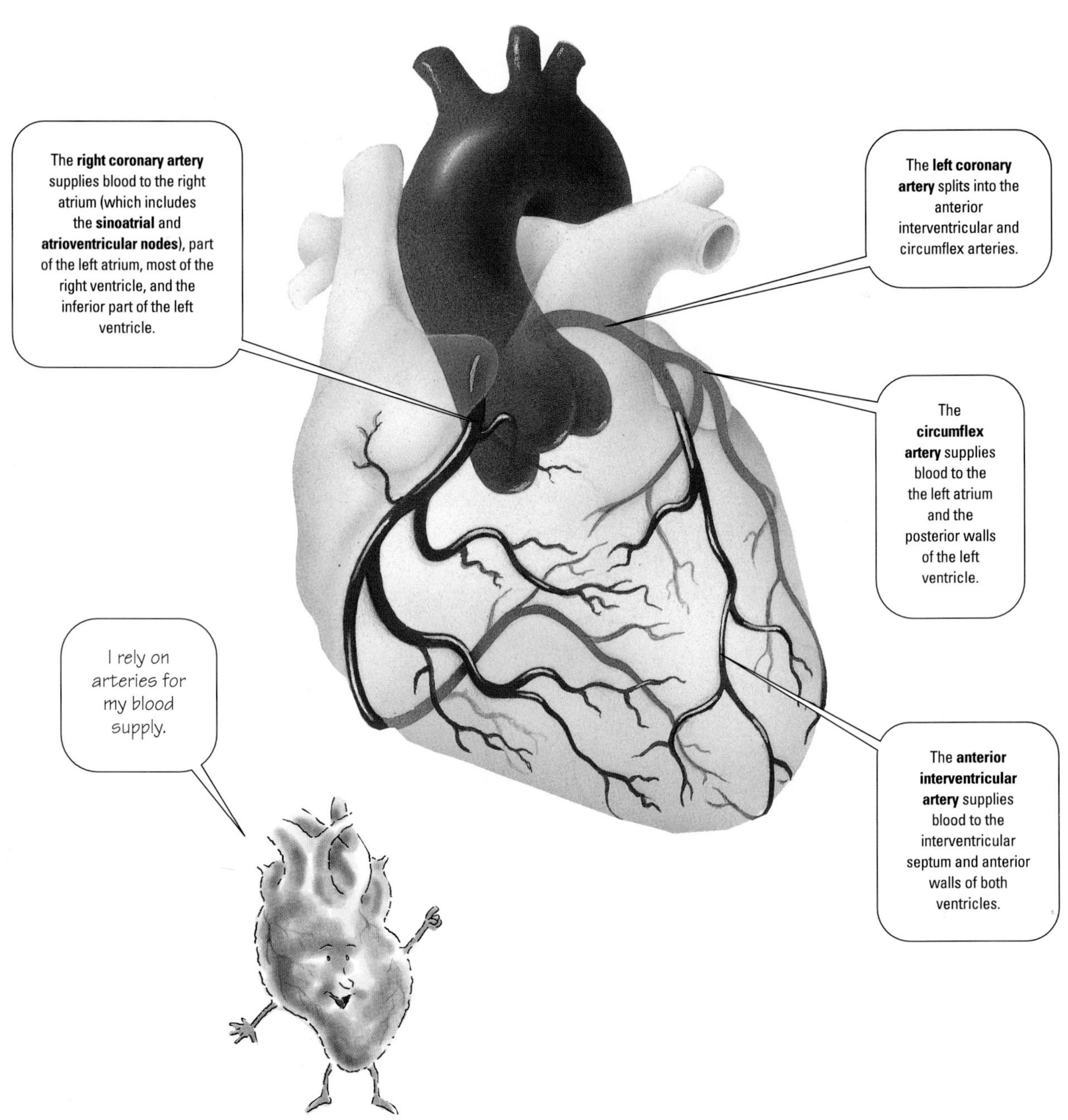

The **right coronary artery** supplies blood to the right atrium (which includes the **sinoatrial** and **atrioventricular nodes**), part of the left atrium, most of the right ventricle, and the inferior part of the left ventricle.
The **left coronary artery** splits into the anterior interventricular and circumflex arteries.
The **circumflex artery** supplies blood to the the left atrium and the posterior walls of the left ventricle.
The **anterior interventricular artery** supplies blood to the interventricular septum and anterior walls of both ventricles.
I rely on arteries for my blood supply.

Blood tests

There are three important blood tests that may be used to diagnose cardiovascular problems.

Clotting by the clock

Activated partial thromboplastin time, the test to measure the time required for formation of a fibrin clot, requires a blood sample to evaluate all the clotting factors (except platelets) of the intrinsic pathway.

Any damage here?

The **cardiac enzyme** test determines if cardiac tissue has been damaged. Normally present in high concentrations in the heart, cardiac enzymes are released into the bloodstream from their normal intracellular area during cardiac trauma and create an elevation of the serum cardiac enzyme levels. Elevated levels of the enzyme creatine kinase (CK) and the CK-MB isoenzyme over a 72-hour period usually confirm a myocardial infarction (MI).

Did I have an MI?

The **cardiac troponin** test uses a blood sample to measure the cardiac protein called troponin. This is the most precise way to diagnose an MI.

Radiologic tests

Here are terms for common radiologic tests:

- **Cardiac catheterization** is a diagnostic procedure in which a catheter is inserted into a large vein (usually in an arm or leg) and then threaded through the vein to the patient's heart. After injection of a radiopaque contrast medium, X-rays are taken to detect heart anomalies.
- **Angiocardiography** creates an X-ray of the heart and great vessels after injection of contrast medium into a blood vessel or one of the heart chambers. (See *Angiocardiography*, page 128.)
- **Angiography** produces an X-ray of the blood vessels after injection of a radiopaque contrast medium.

Let's see what's going on in there

A **radionuclide scan** is a test that helps to measure heart function and damage. During this

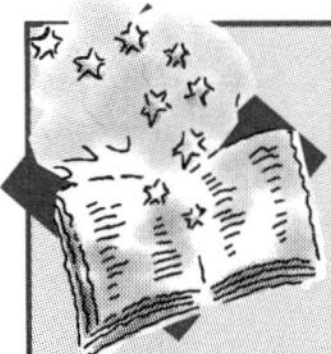

Beyond the dictionary

Two troublesome terms

Pericardiocentesis and **transesophageal** look like hard words, but they're easy to understand if broken apart.

Around the heart + puncture

The prefix ***peri-*** means *around,* the root ***cardio-*** means *heart,* and ***pericardiocentesis*** comes from the Greek word ***kentesis,*** which means *to puncture.* Put it all together and you have the meaning — *a procedure that requires puncturing the sac around the heart.*

Through the esophagus

The first part of **transesophageal,** ***trans-,*** means *through;* therefore, **transesophageal** means *through the esophagus.* Transesophageal echocardiography is an echocardiogram performed through the esophagus.

test, a mildly radioactive material is injected into the patient's bloodstream. Computer-generated pictures are used to locate the radioactive element in the heart.

Running hot and cold

The **thallium stress test** diagnoses coronary artery disease. For this test, the patient is given a thallium isotope I.V. after a treadmill stress test. The isotope doesn't collect in areas of poor blood flow and damaged cells, so these areas show up as "cold spots" on a scanner.

Other invasive tests

Electrophysiologic studies are invasive tests that help diagnose conduction system disease and serious heart rhythm disturbances. The **cardiologist** (heart specialist) induces a rhythm disturbance by using different medications or procedures. After identifying the source of the rhythm disturbance, the cardiologist either administers medications to terminate the disturbance or eliminates the abnormal pathway in the heart by treatment with high-frequency waves.

Pericardiocentesis is a surgical procedure in which the pericardium cavity is punctured for the aspiration of fluid from the pericardial sac. This procedure can be performed for both diagnosis and treatment of some cardiac disorders.

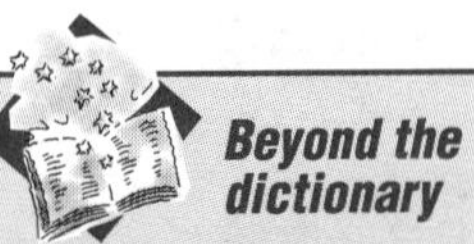

Beyond the dictionary

Angiocardiography

The word **angiocardiography** looks overwhelming but it becomes easier if you break it down. ***Angio-*** comes from the Greek word for *vessel,* ***cardi-*** means *heart,* and ***-graphy*** comes from the Greek word ***graphein,*** which means *to write.*

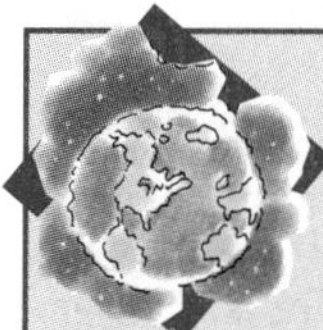

The real world

Did you hear an echo?

In practice, you'll commonly hear **echocardiography** referred to as an **echo.** You'll also hear **cardiac catheterization** referred to as **cath.** For example, you might hear someone say, "Mrs. Heartman is scheduled for her **cath** today."

Transesophageal echocardiography is a technique in which a probe is passed through the mouth and down the esophagus to study the structure and motion of the heart using an echo obtained from beams of ultrasonic waves directed through the esophagus. (See *Two troublesome terms.*)

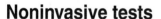

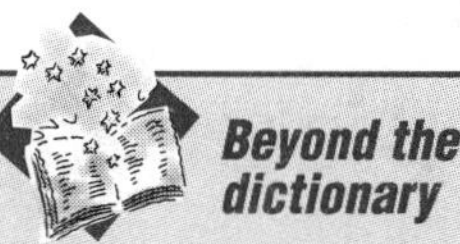

Beyond the dictionary

Electrocardiogram

The prefix ***electro-*** comes from the Greek word ***elektron,*** which refers to the semiprecious stone amber. (Rubbing amber produces an electric charge.) **Cardiogram** comes from the Latin word ***cardium,*** which means *heart,* and the Greek term ***gramma,*** which means *mark.*

Noninvasive tests

An **electrocardiogram** is a graphic record that is produced by an electrocardiograph and shows variations in electrical potential, as detected at the body surface, resulting from excitation of the heart muscle. Electrocardiogram displays a wave that represents phases of the cardiac cycle. (See *Electrocardiogram.*)

In a normal rhythm, the P wave is the first wave seen in the cardiac cycle. Atrial depolarization is represented on the ECG by the P wave. After atrial depolarization an absence of electrical activity is noted for a brief period. This is labeled the PR interval.

Next, ventricular depolarization is represented on the ECG by the waveform labeled QRS. After ventricular activation, ventricular repolarization begins. The ST segment is a flat T wave and it represents the actual recovery or repolarization of the ventricular muscle. The T wave represents the actual recovery.

Let me sound you out

Echocardiography is a diagnostic technique that studies the structure and motion of the heart by the echo obtained from beams of ultrasonic waves directed through the chest wall. The waves are then recorded on a strip chart. (See *Did you hear an echo*?)

Disorders

Some cardiovascular problems occur suddenly and without warning, while others are long-term problems. Either way, when the heart is sick, the entire body is affected. Types of cardiac disorders include:
• cardiac complications
• congenital heart defects
• degenerative disorders
• inflammatory heart disease
• vascular disorders
• valvular heart disease.

Cardiac complications

Many types of injury or illness cause problems for the heart, resulting in serious cardiac complications:
• **Cardiac arrest** is when the heart stops abruptly with an absence of blood pressure or pulse.
• In **cardiac tamponade,** blood or fluid fills the pericardial space and presses against the heart, compressing the heart chambers and obstructing venous return to the heart
• **Cardiogenic shock,** also called **pump failure,** results when over 40% of the heart muscle is damaged by MI. As a result, body tissues don't receive the necessary amounts of oxygen and nutrients.
• **Hypotension** refers to blood pressure below normal limits.
• **Hypovolemic shock** occurs when reduced intravascular blood volume causes circulatory dysfunction and inadequate blood flow to tissues.
• **Pulmonary edema** is an accumulation of excess fluid in the lungs.
• **Ventricular aneurysm** is an outpouching of the ventricular wall that is most often seen in the left ventricle.

Who's got rhythm?

Arrhythmia, as the prefix ***a-*** indicates, refers to a lack of normal heart rhythm. It's an irregular heartbeat that is caused by a disruption in the heart's electrical conduction system. There are a number of types of arrhythmia:

- **Atrial flutter** is an arrhythmia in which the atrial rhythm is regular, but the rate is 250 to 400 beats/minute. The P waves have a sawtooth appearance. The ventricular rate is variable, typically 60 to 100 beats/minute.
- **Bradycardia** is an abnormally slow heartbeat.
- **Fibrillation** refers to an uncoordinated, irregular contraction of the heart muscle, which may originate in the atria (atrial fibrillation) or in the ventricles (ventricle fibrillation).
- **Heart block** describes an impaired conduction of the heart's electrical impulses, which often leads to a slow heartbeat.
- **Paroxysmal atrial tachycardia** is an arrhythmia in which the atrial and ventricular rates are regular and exceed 160 beats/minute. There is typically a sudden onset and termination of this arrhythmia.
- **Premature atrial contraction** is an arrhythmia in which there are premature, abnormal looking P waves that differ in configuration from normal P waves.
- **Premature ventricular contraction** is characterized by a regular atrial rate and an irregular ventricular rate. The QRS complex is premature, usually followed by a complete compensatory pause. Premature QRS complexes may occur singly, in pairs, or in threes, alternating with normal beats or originating from one or more sites.
- **Tachycardia** refers to an abnormally rapid heartbeat.
- **Ventricular tachycardia** is an arrhythmia in which P waves are discernible and the ventricular rate is 140 to 220 beats/minute. QRS complexes are wide and bizarre.

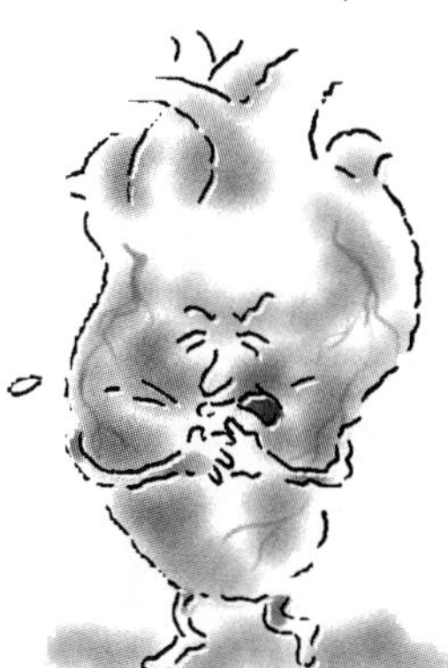

It seems like so many things can go wrong. It just breaks my heart to think about it!

Congenital heart defects

Congenital means *present at birth*, and infants with congenital heart problems have structural defects of the heart or its blood vessels. The term **blue baby** describes cyanosis that is caused by several of these congenital defects:

- **Atrial septal defect** is an opening between the two atria. Because left atrial pressure is slightly higher than right atrial pressure, blood shunts from left to right. This shunting causes right heart overload, and the right side of the heart enlarges to accommodate the increased volume.

• **Coarctation of the aorta** is narrowing of the **lumen** *(opening of the aorta)*, which results in high pressure above and low pressure below the stricture.

• **Patent ductus arteriosus** occurs when the **ductus arteriosus,** a passage between the aorta and pulmonary artery that normally closes at birth, remains open, sending oxygenated blood back through the lungs.

• The **Tetralogy of Fallot** got its name because it involves four (hence ***tertra-***) major defects of the heart and great vessels and it was first described by the French doctor Etienne Fallot (1850-1911).

• In **ventricular septal defect,** an opening between the two ventricles allows blood to shunt between them. Depending on the anomaly's size, spontaneous closure may occur (if small); if closure doesn't occur, right- and left-sided heart failure and cyanosis occur.

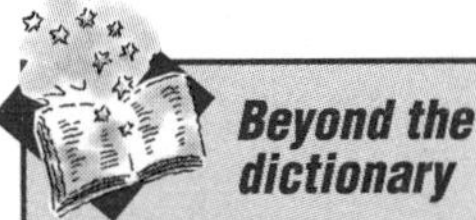

Atherosclerosis: The hard facts

Breaking apart the word **atherosclerosis** is easy. The Greek word ***athere*** means *soft, fatty,* and *gruel-like* and ***scler-*** means *hard.* Put them together and these terms accurately describe the material deposited on the inner lining of an artery that causes atherosclerosis.

Degenerative heart conditions

Degenerative heart disease is a progressive deterioration of heart structures, tissue, and function. Some forms of degenerative heart disease are listed below:

• **Coronary artery disease** (**CAD**) occurs when the arteries that serve the heart are obstructed or narrowed. The most common cause of CAD is **atherosclerosis** (deposits of plaque inside the arteries). In addition to slowing blood flow, atherosclerosis damages and deforms the muscular arterial walls, increasing the risk of aneurysm. (See *Atherosclerosis: The hard facts.*)

• In **dilated cardiomyopathy,** the heart dilates and takes on a round shape as a result of extensively damaged heart muscle fibers.

• **Heart failure** develops when the heart can't effectively pump blood and becomes congested with extra fluid.

• **Hypertension** refers to blood pressure above normal limits.

• **Hypertrophic cardiomyopathy** is a primary disease of cardiac muscle that is characterized by disproportionate thickening of the interventricular septum.

• In **MI,** commonly called a **heart attack,** reduced blood flow through one of the coronary arteries results in myocardial **ischemia** (lack of blood supply) and **necrosis** (tissue death).

• **Restrictive cardiomyopathy** is characterized by restricted ventricular filling (the result of left ventricular hypertrophy) and endocardial fibrosis.

Inflammatory heart disease

Types of heart inflammation, caused by injury or tissue destruction, are described below:

• **Endocarditis** is a bacterial or fungal infection of the heart valves or endocardium.

• **Myocarditis** is an inflammation of the heart muscle that can be acute or long term.

• **Pericarditis** is an inflammation of the pericardium, the protective sac that encloses the heart. In **constrictive** pericarditis, the pericardium thickens and constricts the heart, causing heart failure.

• **Rheumatic fever** is a childhood disease caused by streptococcal bacteria.

Vascular disorders

The following terms are associated with disorders of the vascular system.

• **Arterial occlusive disease** is caused by the obstruction of the lumen of the aorta and its major branches, causing **ischemia**, usually to the legs and feet.

• **Raynaud's disease** is an arteriospastic disease characterized by episodic vasospasm in the arteries or arterioles precipitated by cold or stress.

• **Thrombophlebitis** is an acute condition characterized by inflammation and thrombus formation. Thrombophlebitis may occur in deep (intermuscular or intramuscular) or superficial (subcutaneous) veins. Deep vein thrombophlebitis affects small veins, such as the soleal venus sinuses or large veins such as the vena cava.

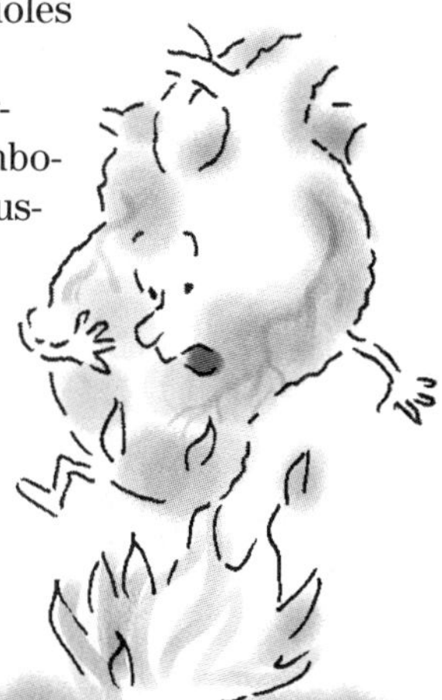
Inflammation can be pretty serious business.

Weak walls

An **aneurysm** (a weakening of the walls of a vessel) occurs most often in the aorta but can happen in any vessel and can take a number of different forms:

• **Abdominal aortic aneurysm**, an abnormal dilation in the arterial wall, generally occurs in the aorta between the renal arteries and iliac branches.
• **Thoracic aortic aneurysm** is an abnormal widening of the ascending, transcending, or descending part of the aorta.

Aneurysms may be **saccular** (unilateral pouch-like bulge with a narrow neck), **fusiform** (spindle-shaped bulge encompassing the entire diameter of the vessel), **dissecting** (hemorrhagic separation of the medial layer of the vessel wall, which creates a false lumen), or **false** (a pulsating hematoma resulting from trauma and often mistaken for an abdominal aneurysm.)

Valvular disorders

When a valve fails, several different disorders can result.

Stenosis, a thickening of valvular tissue that results in narrow valve openings, can occur as one of three types:
• **Aortic stenosis,** or narrowing of the aortic valve, creates elevated pressure in the left ventricle.
• **Mitral stenosis,** or narrowing of the mitral valve, obstructs blood flow from the left atrium to the left ventricle, causing enlargement of the left atrium as a form of compensation.
• **Tricuspid stenosis** obstructs blood flow from the right atrium to the right ventricle, causing the right atrium to enlarge.

Four types of **coronary insufficiency,** the incomplete closure of a valve, that may also result are described here:
• **Aortic insufficiency** occurs when blood leaks back into the left ventricle during the diastolic phase of the heartbeat, when the ventricles rest. The left ventricle enlarges and fluid builds up in the left atrium and the pulmonary system, leading to left-sided heart failure and pulmonary edema.
• **Mitral valve insufficiency** occurs when blood from the left ventricle flows back into the left atrium, causing the left atrium and ventricle to enlarge as compensation for the heart's decreased efficiency.
• **Pulmonary valve insufficiency** allows blood from the pulmonary artery to flow back into the right ventricle during diastole.

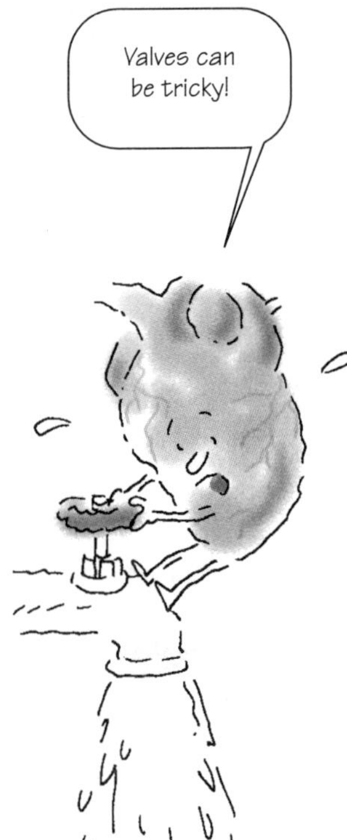

• In **tricuspid insufficiency,** blood flows back into the right atrium as the ventricles contract during systole. This reduces blood flow to the lungs and the left side of the heart and also decreases cardiac output.

Treatments

Cardiovascular disorders can be treated with drug therapy and surgery. Here is a list of treatments and surgical interventions.

Drug therapy

These drugs may be used alone or in combination to treat cardiovascular disorders:

• **Adrenergics** help treat serious hypotension.
• **Angiotensin-converting enzyme inhibitors** are used to treat hypertension.
• **Antianginal** drugs treat or prevent pain.
• **Antiarrhythmics** can prevent or treat arrhythmias.
• **Antihypertensives** reduce cardiac output or decrease peripheral vascular resistance to lower blood pressure.
• **Digitalis glycosides** are used to manage heart failure and certain types of arrhythmia
• **Diuretics** treat edema and hypertension by reducing circulating fluid volume.
• **Thrombolytic therapy** is used to dissolve clots.

Surgery

Below are common surgical procedures used to correct functional or structural heart problems:

• **Cardiac conduction surgery** is done to treat atrial and ventricular tachycardias that can't be controlled by drug therapy or pacing.
• **Coronary artery bypass graft (CABG)** surgery restores circulation when occluded coronary arteries prevent normal blood flow to the heart muscle. Occluded arteries are replaced with segments (grafts) from other vessels, most often the saphenous veins in the leg. (See *Cabbage is slang for CABG,* page 136.)

• **Heart transplantation** is a complex and controversial procedure that involves replacing a diseased heart with the healthy heart of a brain-dead donor.

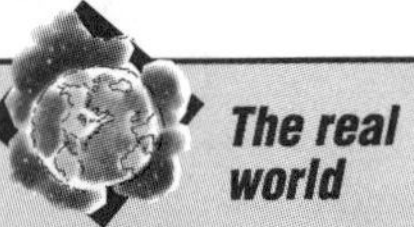

The real world

Cabbage is slang for CABG

You may hear **coronary artery bypass surgery** referred to as **cabbage. Cabbage** is slang for CABG, the abbreviation for coronary artery bypass graft. A **triple cabbage** is a three vessel bypass procedure.

Other treatments

• **Cardiopulmonary resuscitation** is a basic life support procedure performed on victims with cardiac arrest.
• **Defibrillation** uses an electric shock to terminate tachyarrhythmias.
• **Implantable cardioverter-defibrillator** is an implanted device that senses arrhythmias and delivers an electric shock to the myocardium, automatically terminating the arrhythmia.
• In **intra-aortic balloon counterpulsation,** used to temporarily reduce the left ventricle's workload, an inflatable balloon is inserted into the patient's aorta. A pump inflates the balloon while the ventricle rests and deflates it at the start of each ventricular contraction. The inflated balloon forces blood into the major arteries and reduces the heart's workload during contraction.
• During **laser-enhanced angioplasty,** the physician threads a laser-containing catheter into the diseased artery. Rapid laser pulses destroy the occlusion, and balloon angioplasty is later performed.

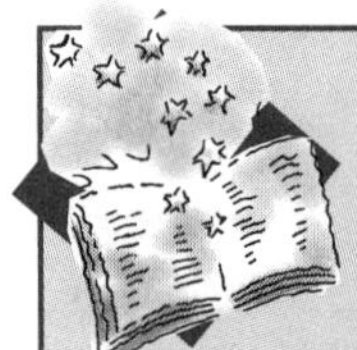

Beyond the dictionary

PTCA

The term **percutaneous transluminal coronary angioplasty** is abbreviated **PTCA.**

First half

The first component of the term, ***per-*** means *through;* ***cutaneous*** means *the skin* — so *through the skin.* The prefix ***trans-*** means *through;* ***luminal*** refers to *a blood vessel.*

Second half

Coronary refers to the two arteries and their branches that stem from the aorta, which supply the heart tissue with blood. ***Angio-*** also means *blood vessel* and ***plasty*** is a suffix that means *the repair of.* So PTCA really means: *repair of a coronary blood vessel by way of the skin and another blood vessel.*

• **Pacemakers** use electrical impulses to regulate cardiac rhythm. Pacemakers can be permanent, transvenous or transcutaneous, or external.
• **Percutaneous transluminal coronary angioplasty** is a nonsurgical alternative to CABG surgery. During this procedure, a guide catheter is threaded into the coronary artery and positioned at the site of an occlusion. A doctor then inserts a small balloon catheter through the guide catheter and positions the balloon inside the occlusion. When the balloon is inflated, the coronary artery dilates and blood flow improves (See *PTCA.*)
• In some cases, a **stent,** or tube is placed inside the artery to support it and prevent further occlusion.
• **Synchronized cardioversion** delivers an electric charge to the myocardium at the peak of the R wave on the ECG. This causes immediate termination of the tachyarrhythmia.
• **Valve replacement surgery** replaces faulty valves in patients with severe symptoms who don't respond to more conservative approaches. Both mechanical and biological prosthetic valves are commonly used.
• The **ventricular assist device** is a temporary, life-sustaining treatment that diverts systemic blood flow from a diseased ventricle into a centrifugal pump.

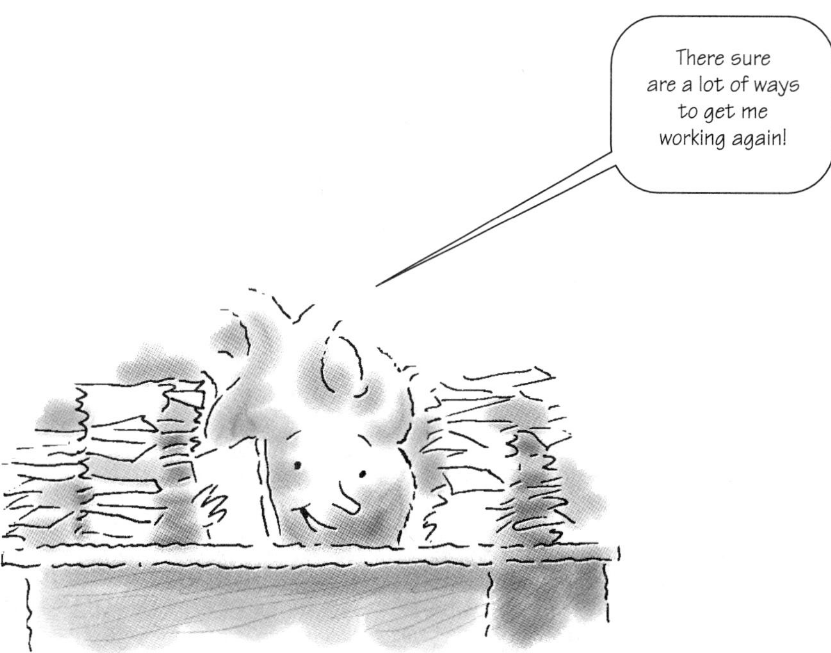
There sure are a lot of ways to get me working again!

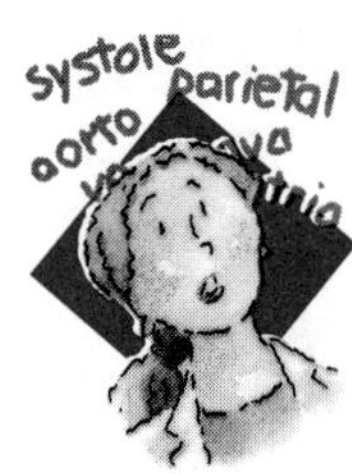

systole
parietal
aorta

Vocabulary builders

At a crossroads

Here is a puzzle that is sure to tug at your heartstrings. Good luck!

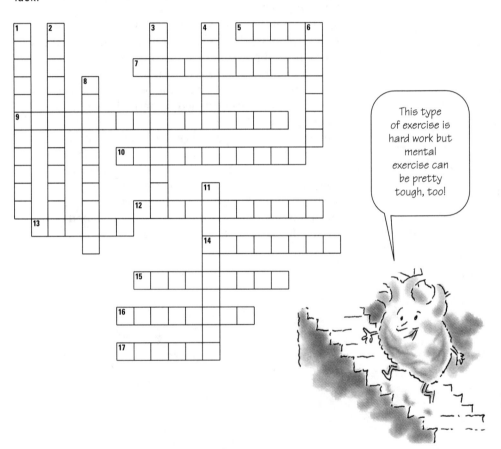

This type of exercise is hard work but mental exercise can be pretty tough, too!

Across

5. Return blood to the heart
7. Smallest blood vessels
9. Hardening of the arteries
10. Thin sac that protects the heart
12. Rapid heartbeat
13. Chest pain
14. Blue-colored skin
15. Lower chamber of the heart
16. Carry blood away from the heart
17. Upper chamber of the heart

Down

1. Lining of the heart's chambers
2. High blood pressure
3. Slow heartbeat
4. Word for abnormal paleness
6. When the heart contracts
8. Deviation from normal rhythm
11. Heart muscle

Answers are on page 142.

Finish line

The Latin word ***cardium,*** which means *heart,* appears in almost all medical terminology relating to that structure. Fill in each of the blanks below with the affix, suffix, or root that finishes the heart-related term.

1. A heart doctor is a cardi ____________.
2. A patient with ____________ cardia has a slow heart beat.
3. Another name for the condition of an enlarged heart is cardio ____________.
4. Inflammation of the heart muscles due to infection is called card ____________.
5. The ____________ cardio ____________ is a device for recording the electrical activity of the myocardium.

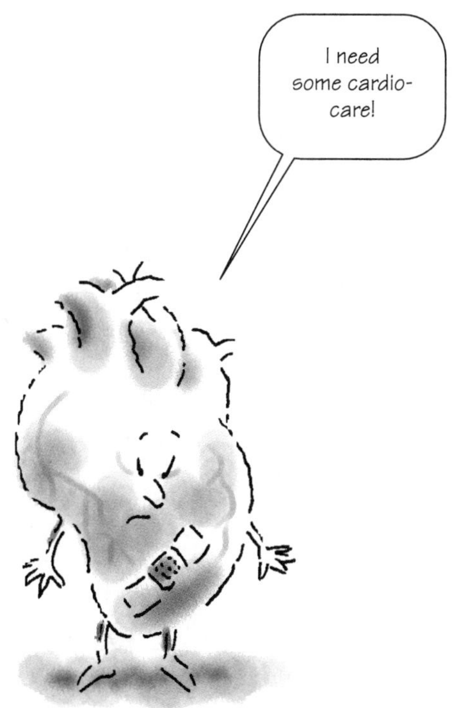

Answers are on page 142.

Match game

Match the choices below to the appropriate answers.

Clues

1. Add the prefix that means ***rapid*** to the correct form of the root **cardium.** ________

2. Add the prefix that means ***around*** and the affix that means ***puncture*** to the correct form of the root **cardium.** __________

3. Add the prefix that means ***muscle*** to the correct form of the root ***cardium.*** _________

4. Add the affix that refers to the ***lungs*** to the correct form of the root **cardium.** _________

Choices

A. Cardiocentesis

B. Tachycardia

C. Cardiopulmonary

D. Myocardial

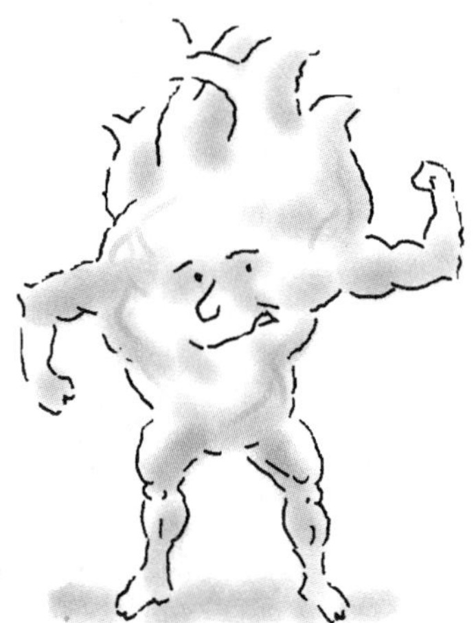

Add muscle to cardium? You've got it!

Answers are on page 142.

Scrambled or overeasy

Fill in the answers for the following questions, then unscramble the circled letters to find the answer to the puzzle.

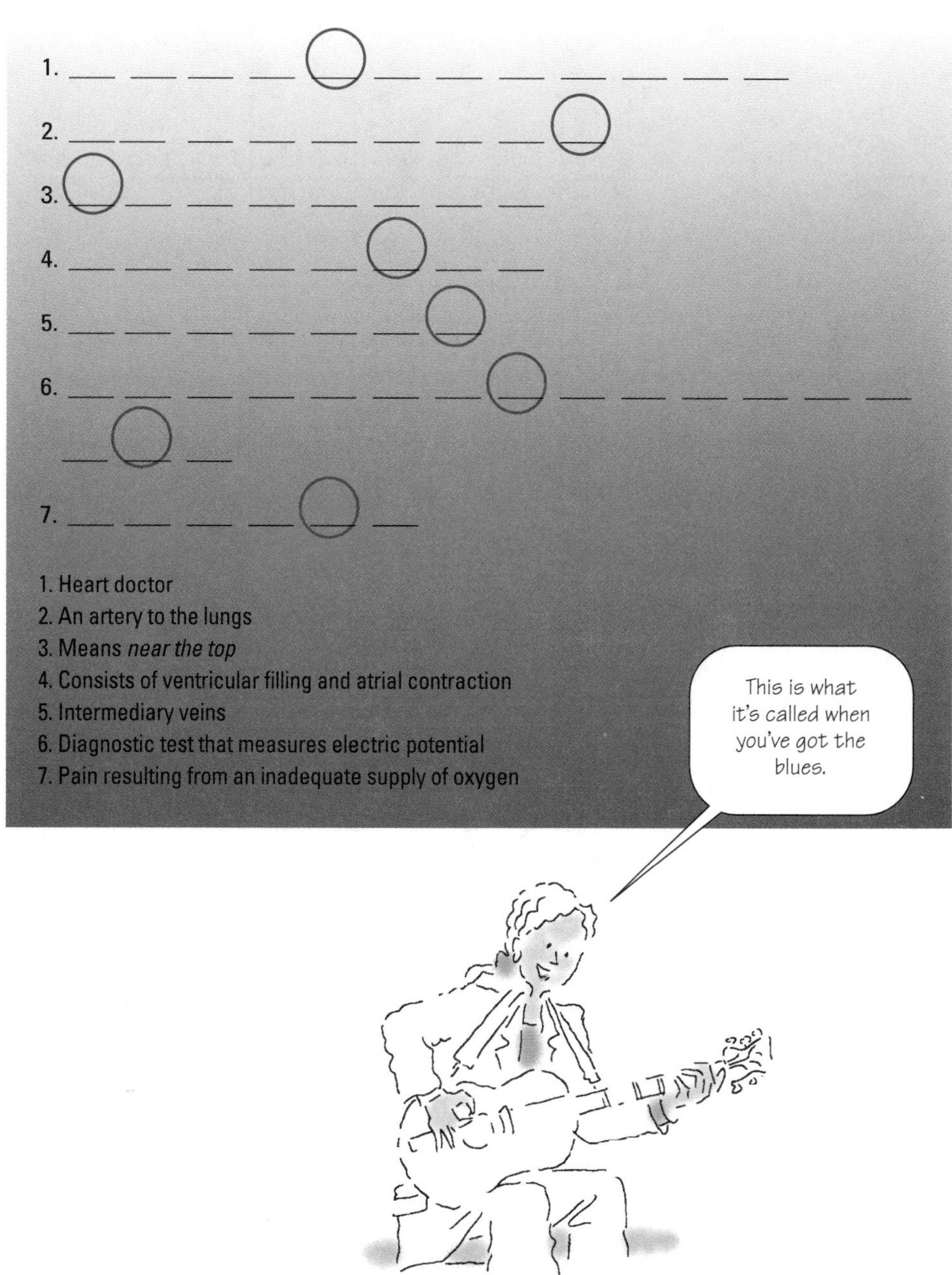

1. ___ ___ ___ ___ (___) ___ ___ ___ ___ ___ ___ ___
2. ___ ___ ___ ___ ___ ___ ___ (___)
3. (___) ___ ___ ___ ___ ___ ___ ___
4. ___ ___ ___ ___ ___ (___) ___ ___
5. ___ ___ ___ ___ ___ ___ (___)
6. ___ ___ ___ ___ ___ ___ ___ (___) ___ ___ ___ ___ ___ ___ ___ (___) ___
7. ___ ___ ___ ___ (___) ___
1. Heart doctor
2. An artery to the lungs
3. Means *near the top*
4. Consists of ventricular filling and atrial contraction
5. Intermediary veins
6. Diagnostic test that measures electric potential
7. Pain resulting from an inadequate supply of oxygen
This is what it's called when you've got the blues.

Answers are on page 142.

Answers

At a crossroads

1 E		2 H						3 B			4 P		5 V	E	I	N	6 S	
N		Y						R			A						Y	
D		P					7 C	A	P	I	L	L	A	R	I	E	S	
O		E		8 A				D			L						T	
C		R		R				Y			O						O	
9 A	R	T	E	R	I	O	S	C	L	E	R	O	S	I	S		L	
R		E		H				A									E	
D		N		Y		10 P	E	R	I	C	A	R	D	I	U	M		
I		S		T				D										
U		I		H				I			11 M							
M		O		M			12 T	A	C	H	Y	C	A	R	D	I	A	
	13 A	N	G	I	N	A					O							
				A							14 C	Y	A	N	O	S	I	S
											A							
							15 V	E	N	T	R	I	C	L	E			
											D							
						16 A	R	T	E	R	I	E	S					
											U							
						17 A	T	R	I	U	M							

Finish line

1. Ologist; 2. Brady; 3. Megaly; 4. Itis; 5. Electro, graph.

Match game

1. B; 2. A; 3. D; 4. C.

Scrambled or overeasy

1. Cardiologist; 2. Pulmonary; 3. Superior; 4.Diastole; 5. Venules; 6. Electrocardiogram; 7. Angina.
Answer to puzzle — Cyanosis

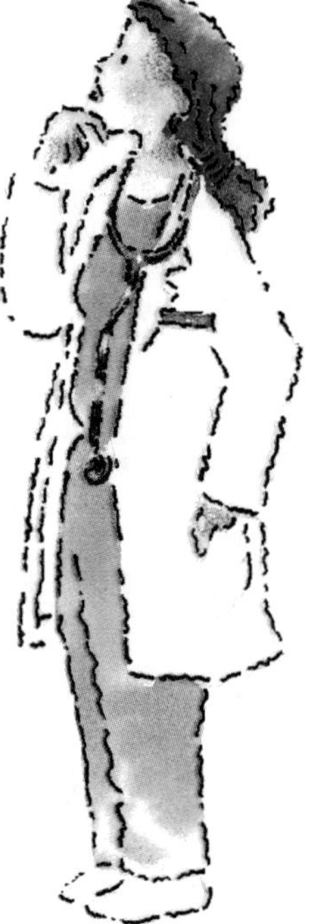

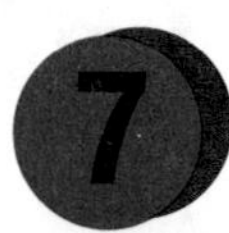

Respiratory system

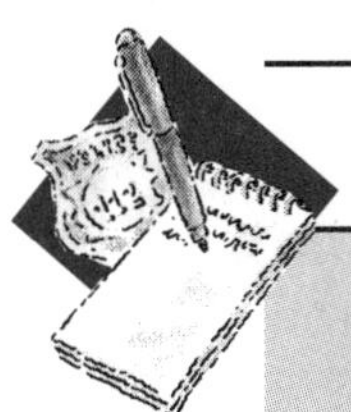

Just the facts

In this chapter, you'll review:

- terminology related to the structure and function of the respiratory system
- terminology needed for physical examination
- tests that help diagnose respiratory disorders
- respiratory system disorders and their treatments.

Respiratory structure and function

The **respiratory system** consists of the upper and lower respiratory tracts, lungs, and thoracic cage. In addition to maintaining the exchange of oxygen (O_2) and carbon dioxide (CO_2) in the lungs and tissues, the respiratory system helps regulate the body's acid-base balance. (See *Pronouncing key respiratory system terms*, page 144.)

Upper respiratory tract

The **upper respiratory tract** consists primarily of the nose, mouth, nasopharynx, oropharynx, laryngopharynx, and larynx. Besides warming and humidifying inhaled air, these structures enable taste, smell, and the chewing and swallowing of food. (See *Structures of the respiratory system*, page 145.)

Nose

Air enters the respiratory tract through the mouth and **nares** (nostrils). In the nares, small hairs filter out dust

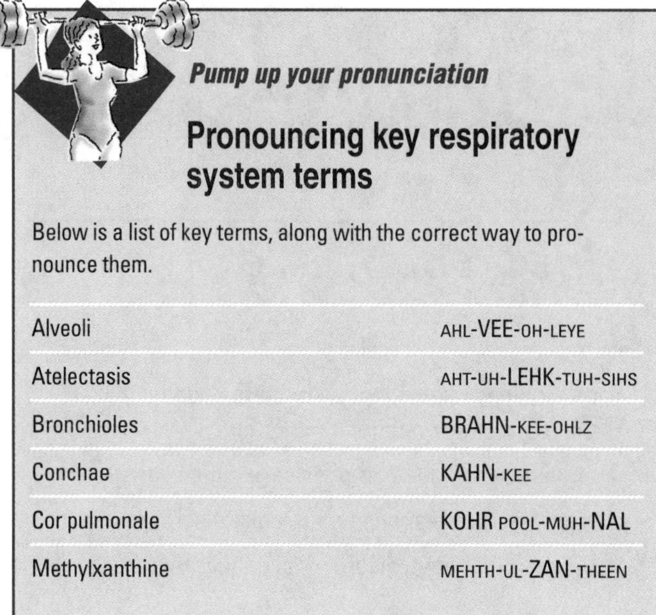

Pump up your pronunciation

Pronouncing key respiratory system terms

Below is a list of key terms, along with the correct way to pronounce them.

Alveoli	AHL-VEE-OH-LEYE
Atelectasis	AHT-UH-LEHK-TUH-SIHS
Bronchioles	BRAHN-KEE-OHLZ
Conchae	KAHN-KEE
Cor pulmonale	KOHR POOL-MUH-NAL
Methylxanthine	MEHTH-UL-ZAN-THEEN

and large foreign particles. Air then passes into the two **nasal passages,** which are separated by the **septum.** Cartilage forms the anterior walls of the nasal passages.

Humidifiers

Bony structures, **conchae** (singular: **concha**), form the posterior walls of the nasal passages. The conchae warm and humidify air before it passes into the **pharynx** (plural: **pharynges**) or **throat,** which serves as a passageway for the digestive and respiratory tracts.

Pharynx

The pharynx consists of three sections:

- The **nasopharynx** extends from the posterior nares to the soft palate.
- The **oropharynx** extends from the soft palate to the upper portion of the epiglottis.
- The **laryngopharynx** extends to the esophagus and larynx. (See *The three pharynges.*)

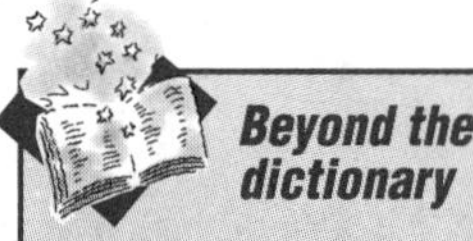

Beyond the dictionary

The three pharynges

Notice that the words for the three parts of the pharynx are all connected by the common root ***pharynx,*** which is Greek for *throat.* **Nasopharynx** uses the word for *nose,* ***naso,*** and the root ***pharynx*** to describe the upper portion of the pharynx. **Oropharynx** uses the Latin word for *mouth,* ***or,*** from which we also get *orifice.* **Laryngopharynx** adds **laryngo,** which is a form of ***larynx*** that is used when combining it with another word.

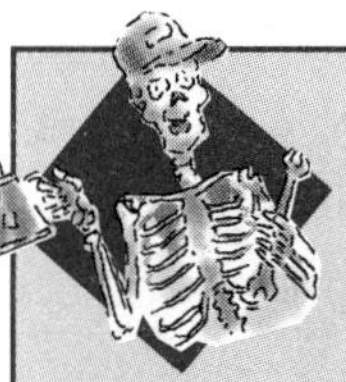

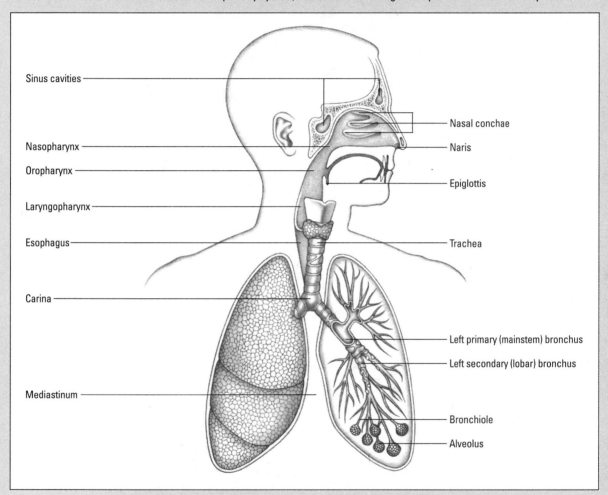

Body shop

Structures of the respiratory system

This illustration shows the structures of the respiratory system, which include the organs responsible for external respiration.

Sinus cavities
Nasal conchae
Nasopharynx
Naris
Oropharynx
Epiglottis
Laryngopharynx
Esophagus
Trachea
Carina
Left primary (mainstem) bronchus
Left secondary (lobar) bronchus
Mediastinum
Bronchiole
Alveolus

Larynx

The **larynx,** which contains the **vocal cords,** connects the pharynx with the trachea. (See *Learn to say larynx,* page 146.)

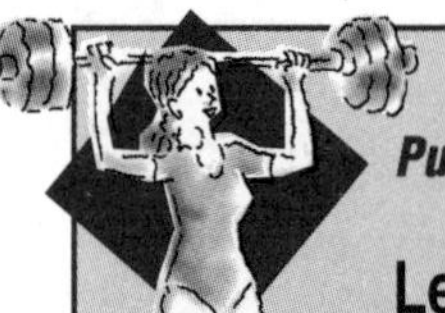

Pump up your pronunciation

Learn to say larynx

It's likely you'll hear larynx (LAHR-INKS) pronounced LAHR-NIKS with the sounds of the *L* and the *N* reversed. Although this reversal of sounds, called ***metathesis,*** is a common mix-up in all languages, you may save yourself some embarrassment if you say LAHR-INKS.

Epiglottis... let's see. The prefix ***epi-*** comes from Greek, meaning *upon.* ***Glottis*** comes from the Greek word ***glossa,*** which means *tongue.*

Speaking of the voice box

The larynx is also called the **voice box.** It's the main organ of speech. Air passing through the **glottis** — a slitlike opening between the vocal cords — causes vibration of the cords during expiration, creating the sound of the voice. The larynx is protected during swallowing by the **epiglottis,** a flexible cartilage that bends reflexively to close the larynx to swallowed substances.

Lower respiratory tract

The **lower respiratory tract** is contained within the **thoracic cavity** and consists of the **trachea, bronchi,** and **lungs.** This space within the chest wall is bounded below by the diaphragm, above by the scalene muscles and fascia of the neck, and around the circumference by the ribs, intercostal muscles, vertebrae, sternum, and ligaments.

Trachea

The tubular **trachea,** also called the **windpipe,** lies half in the neck and half in the thorax. C-shaped cartilage rings reinforce and protect the trachea, preventing its collapse. The trachea is lined with a mucous membrane covered with small hairlike projections called **cilia.** The cilia continuously sweep foreign material out of the breathing passages toward the mouth.

Bronchi

The trachea branches at the **carina** (also known as the tracheal bifurcation) into two smaller airways, the left and right **mainstem bronchi** (primary bronchi). (See *Careening with the carina.*)

The right mainstem bronchus — shorter, wider, and more vertical than the left — supplies air to the right lung; the left mainstem bronchus delivers air to the left lung.

A way in

The mainstem bronchi — along with blood vessels, nerves, and lymphatics — enter the **pleural cavity** (the space between the visceral and parietal pleurae) at the hilum. Located behind the heart, the **hilum** is a slit on the lungs' medial surface. In the lung, the mainstem bronchi divide into five **lobar bronchi** (secondary bronchi), so called because they enter into the **lobes** of the lung, one for each of the three lobes of the right lung and two for the left.

First branches, now twigs

The lobar bronchi divide into smaller and smaller branches, until they become **bronchioles.** Each bronchiole branches into a **lobule.** The lobule includes **terminal bronchioles** and the **acinus** — the chief respiratory unit for gas exchange. (See *Looking at a lobule*, page 148.)

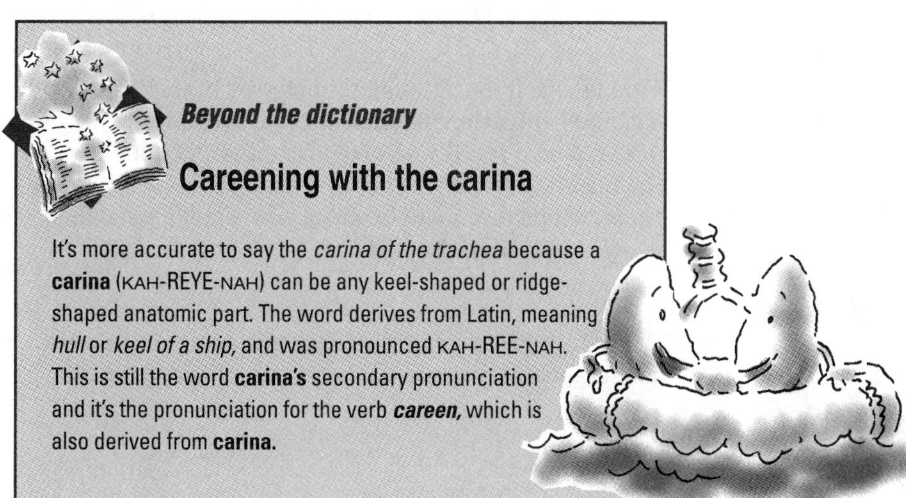

Beyond the dictionary

Careening with the carina

It's more accurate to say the *carina of the trachea* because a **carina** (KAH-REYE-NAH) can be any keel-shaped or ridge-shaped anatomic part. The word derives from Latin, meaning *hull* or *keel of a ship,* and was pronounced KAH-REE-NAH. This is still the word **carina's** secondary pronunciation and it's the pronunciation for the verb ***careen,*** which is also derived from **carina.**

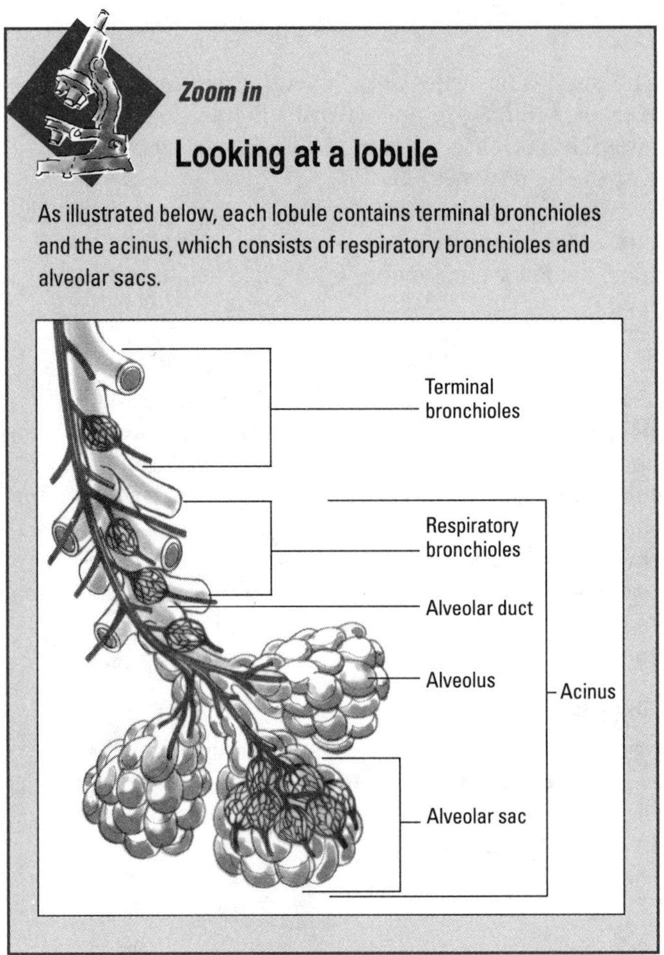

Zoom in
Looking at a lobule
As illustrated below, each lobule contains terminal bronchioles and the acinus, which consists of respiratory bronchioles and alveolar sacs.
Terminal bronchioles
Respiratory bronchioles
Alveolar duct
Alveolus
Acinus
Alveolar sac

Ducts and sacs

Within the acinus, terminal bronchioles branch into yet smaller **respiratory bronchioles.** The respiratory bronchioles feed directly into alveoli at sites along their walls. The respiratory bronchioles eventually become **alveolar ducts,** which terminate in clusters of capillary-swathed alveoli called **alveolar sacs.**

Fruit of the vine

The walls of the ducts contain **alveoli** (singular: **alveolus**), grapelike clusters where O_2 is exchanged for CO_2.

Capillary network

Surrounded by networks of tiny blood vessels called **capillaries,** alveoli have thin walls through which gas exchange occurs. The average pair of lungs has about 300 million alveoli.

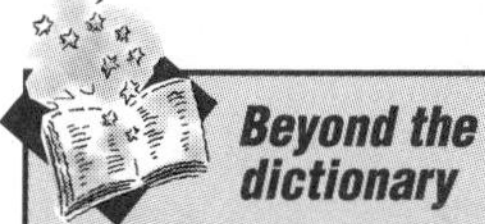

Beyond the dictionary

Studying the lungs

Pulmonology, which comes from the Latin word ***pulmo,*** meaning *lung,* and the suffix ***-ology,*** meaning *the study of,* is the science that studies the lungs.

Lungs

The cone-shaped lungs differ slightly from one another. The right lung is shorter, broader, and larger than the left. The right lung has three lobes and handles 55% of gas exchange. The left lung has only two lobes; it shares the left side of the thoracic cavity with the heart. Each lung's concave base rests on the **diaphragm.** The **apex** (extreme top) of each lung extends about ⅓″ (1 cm) above the first rib. (See *Studying the lungs.*)

Remember the membrane

The **pleura** is the membrane that totally encloses the lungs. It's composed of a visceral layer and parietal layer.

Hugging the lung surface

The **visceral pleura** hugs the entire lung surface, including the areas between the lobes.

The **parietal pleura** extends from the roots of the lungs and covers the sides of the pericardium to the chest wall and backward to the spine.

Fluid space

The **pleural cavity**—the tiny area between the visceral and parietal pleural layers—contains a thin film of **serous fluid.** This fluid has two functions:

- It lubricates the pleural surfaces so that they slide smoothly against each other during respiration.
- It creates a bond between the layers that causes the lungs to move within the chest wall during breathing.

A cage around it all

Several structures support and protect the lungs and aid in respiration. Composed of bone and cartilage, the **thoracic cage** supports and protects the lungs and permits them to expand and contract. The anterior portion of the thoracic cage consists of the **manubrium, sternum, xiphoid process,** and 10 pairs of **ribs.** The posterior portion of the thoracic cage consists of the **vertebral**

column, the same 10 pairs of ribs, and 2 pairs of floating **ribs.**

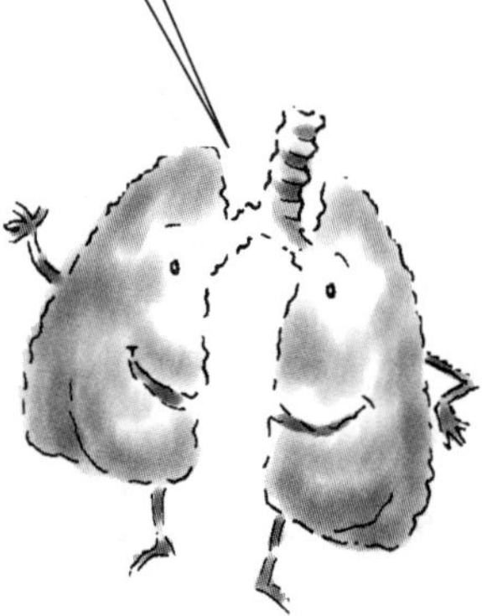

See the space between my lobes? It's called the **mediastinum.**

In the middle

The **mediastinum** (the space between the lungs) contains the following organs and structures:
- heart and pericardium
- thoracic aorta
- pulmonary artery and veins
- venae cavae and azygos veins
- thymus, lymph nodes, and lymphatic vessels
- trachea, esophagus, and thoracic duct
- vagus, cardiac, and phrenic nerves.

At the base

The most important muscle for respiration is the **diaphragm,** a dome-shaped organ composed of muscle and membrane that separates the thoracic and abdominal cavities. During inspiration, the diaphragm moves down and expands the volume of the thoracic cavity; during expiration, it moves up, reducing the volume.

Respiration

Effective respiration consists of a gas exchange in the lungs, called **external respiration,** and a gas exchange in the tissues, called **internal respiration.** External respiration occurs through three processes:
- **diffusion** — gas movement through a semipermeable membrane from an area of greater concentration to one of lesser concentration (Internal respiration occurs only through diffusion.)
- **pulmonary perfusion** — blood flow from the right side of the heart, through the pulmonary circulation, and into the left side of the heart
- **ventilation** — gas distribution into and out of the pulmonary airways.

Air supply

Adequate ventilation depends on the proper working of the nervous, musculoskeletal, and respiratory systems to accomplish the necessary changes in lung pressure. (See *Ventilation and perfusion.*)

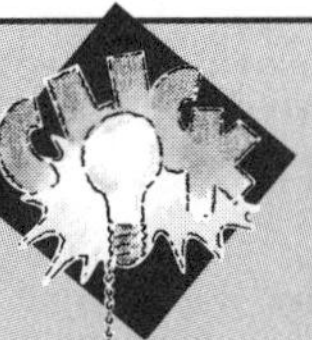

Now I get it!

Ventilation and perfusion

Effective gas exchange depends on a stable relationship between ventilation and perfusion. You'll see this called the **$\dot{V}/\dot{Q}$ ratio.** A **$\dot{V}/\dot{Q}$ mismatch** accounts for many respiratory disorders and can affect all body systems. The following types of mismatch can occur.

Need more oxygen

Inadequate ventilation, also called a **shunt,** occurs when the pulmonary circulation is adequate but not enough oxygen (O_2) is available in the lungs. As a result, a portion of the blood flowing through the pulmonary capillaries doesn't receive O_2. Perfusion without ventilation usually results from airway obstruction, particularly that caused by acute diseases, such as atelectasis and pneumonia, which produce a low $\dot{V}/\dot{Q}$ ratio.

Need more blood

Inadequate perfusion, also called **dead-space ventilation,** produces a high $\dot{V}/\dot{Q}$ ratio. Ventilation is normal, but blood flow in the pulmonary capillaries isn't adequate. Narrowed capillaries, decreased cardiac output, and pulmonary emboli (blood clots) often cause this condition.

Need both!

Inadequate ventilation and perfusion, also referred to as a **silent unit,** describes a lack of O_2 in the lungs (ventilation) and in the pulmonary circulation (perfusion). When entire sections of the lung become "silent," the body compensates by delivering blood flow to better ventilated lung areas. Chronic alveolar collapse and pulmonary emboli can create silent units.

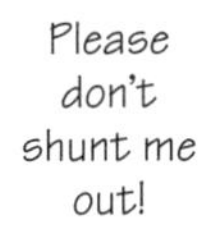
Please don't shunt me out!

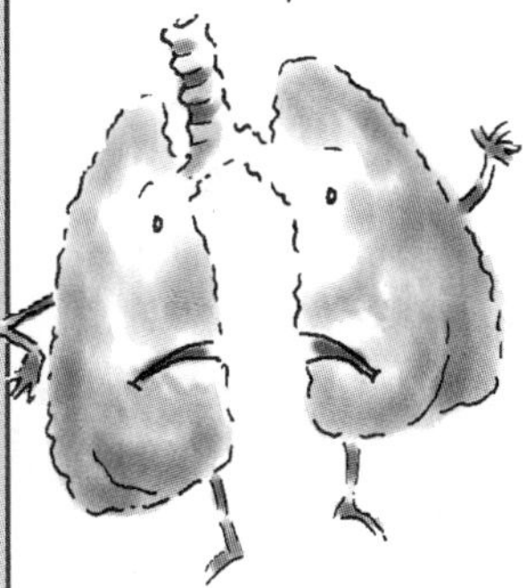

Respiration chemistry

The body depends on a delicate balance between acids and bases to sustain life. The lungs help maintain this balance by altering the rate and depth of respiration in response to changes in blood pH.

Acids and bases

To understand acid-base balance, you need to know three important terms:

- **acids,** which are substances that dissociate (become fragmented, or separate) in solution, releasing hydrogen ions (carbonic acid is an example of an acid found in the body)
- **bases,** such as bicarbonate, which are substances that dissociate to yield hydroxide ions in aqueous solutions
- **pH,** which represents the relative concentration of hydrogen ions in a solution compared to the hydrogen ion concentration of a standard solution (normally, blood pH level measures 7.35 to 7.45).

A solution with more base than acid contains fewer hydrogen ions, resulting in a higher pH. A solution that contains more acid than base has more hydrogen ions, resulting in a lower pH.

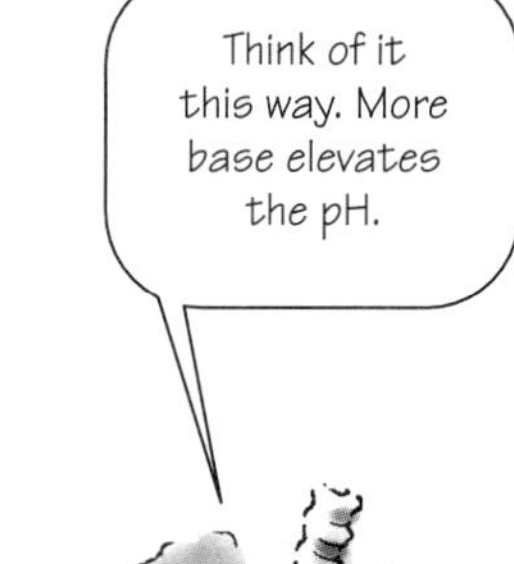

Think of it this way. More base elevates the pH.

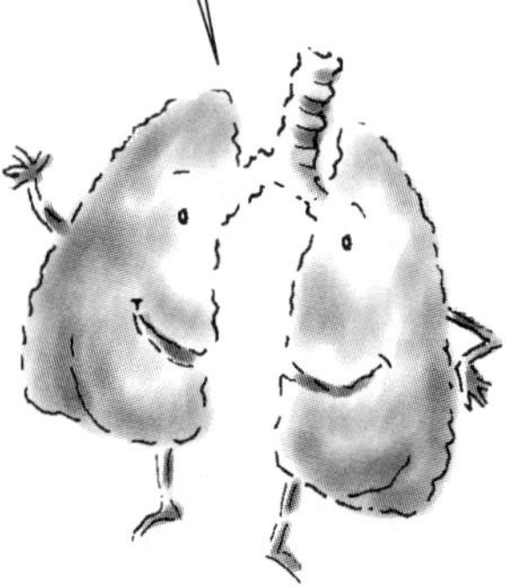

Staying in balance

A deviation in pH level can compromise essential body functions, including electrolyte balance, the activity of critical enzymes, muscle contraction, and basic cellular function. The body normally maintains a pH level within a narrow range by carefully balancing acidic and alkaline elements. When one aspect of that balancing act breaks down, the body can't maintain a healthy pH level as easily, and problems arise.

Regulating method

The lungs use **hyperventilation** (increased ventilation) or **hypoventilation** (decreased ventilation) to regulate blood levels of CO_2, a gas that combines with water to form **carbonic acid.** Increased carbonic acid levels lead to a decrease in pH level.

Eliminate CO_2, increase pH

Chemoreceptors in the brain sense pH changes and vary the rate and depth of breathing to compensate. Breathing faster or more deeply eliminates more CO_2 from the lungs. The more CO_2 is expelled, the less carbonic acid is made and, as a result, the pH level rises. (See *CO_2 and hyperventilation.*)

Increase CO_2, reduce pH

The body normalizes such a change in pH by slowing the rate or decreasing the depth of breathing, thus reducing

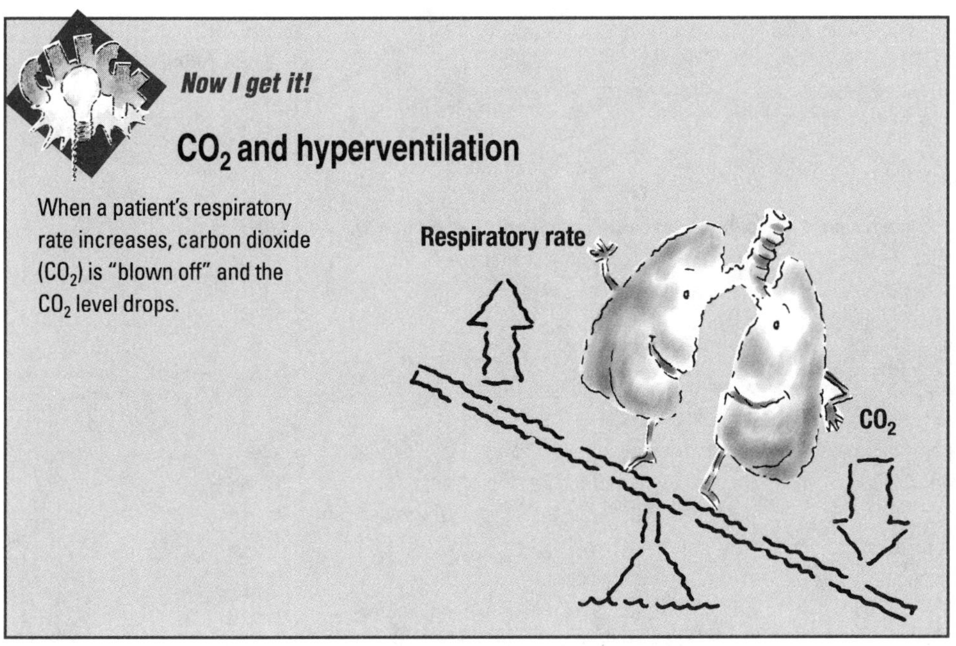
Now I get it!
CO_2 and hyperventilation
When a patient's respiratory rate increases, carbon dioxide (CO_2) is "blown off" and the CO_2 level drops.
Respiratory rate
CO_2

CO_2 excretion. CO_2 and pH move in opposite directions. If pH rises, CO_2 falls, and vice versa.

Physical examination terms

Examining a patient's respiratory status requires observation, palpation, and the ability to identify breath sounds. (See *Name that breath sound*, page 154.) Before you can perform a complete physical examination you need to understand these essential respiratory terms:

- **anoxia** — absence or near absence of O_2 in inhaled air, body tissues, or arterial blood
- **auscultation** — assessment step; listening, either directly or with a stethoscope, for sounds within the body
- **bronchospasm** — sudden, forceful, involuntary contraction of the smooth muscle of the bronchi, causing narrowing and obstruction of the airway
- **chest retraction** — visible depression of soft tissues of the chest between and around the cartilaginous and bony ribs, occurring with increased inspiratory effort
- **clubbing** — enlargement of the soft tissues of the distal phalanges that occurs in children with congenital

Name that breath sound

Listed below are normal and abnormal breath sounds, including their characteristics and where they are heard.

Normal sounds

Normal breath sounds reflect air movement through the tracheobronchial tree. Normal breath sounds are described below:

- **Tracheal** breath sounds are harsh, discontinuous sounds heard over the trachea. They occur when a patient inhales or exhales.
- **Bronchial** breath sounds are loud, high-pitched sounds normally heard next to the trachea. They're discontinuous and loudest when the patient exhales.
- **Vesicular** breath sounds are heard in front of the chest, on both sides, and in back. They're longer and louder during inspiration than expiration.
- **Bronchovesicular** breath sounds can be auscultated over the mainstem bronchi and between the shoulder blades. They have a soft, medium pitched, breezy sound. They're lower-pitched than bronchial sounds, but higher-pitched than vesicular sounds.

Abnormal sounds

Abnormal breath sounds, also called **adventitious sounds,** help diagnose many respiratory disorders. These sounds are classified as:

- **Crackles** are crackling sounds, like hairs being rubbed together, usually heard first over the lung bases. Crackles are further classified by pitch as **high (fine), medium,** or **low (coarse).** Crackles are sometimes called **rales.**
- **Rhonchi** are loud, coarse, low-pitched bubbling sounds heard primarily when a patient exhales, although they may also be heard when the patient inhales. You'll auscultate rhonchi over the central airways.
- **Wheezes** are high-pitched, musical sounds that may occur during inspiration but occur predominantly during expiration. Wheezes are heard over the large bronchi.
- **Pleural friction rubs** are coarse, low-pitched abnormal breath sounds heard at the anterolateral chest wall (in front, near the ribs) during inspiration and expiration. A friction rub sounds like pieces of sandpaper being rubbed together.
- **Grunting** respirations refer to a grunting noise heard during expiration.
- **Stridor** is a crowing sound heard during inspiration that is caused by air whistling as it passes through swollen upper airways.
- **Decreased breath sounds** describes abnormally diminished sounds in areas of the lung.
- **Absent breath sounds** refers to a lack of sound over areas of the lungs that normally have breath sounds.

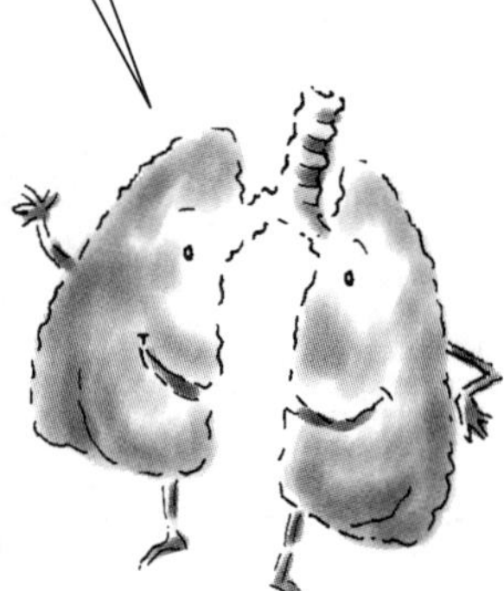
Abnormal breath sounds are also called **adventitious** sounds. It may help you to think of the word **adventure,** because these sounds are out of the ordinary.

heart disease and in older children and adults with long-standing pulmonary disease

- **cyanosis** — bluish discoloration of the skin and mucous membranes resulting from an excessive amount of deoxygenated hemoglobin in the blood
- **dyspnea** — shortness of breath, difficulty breathing, or labored breathing
- **expectoration** — ejection of mucus from the trachea and lungs by coughing and spitting
- **expiration** — act of exhaling air

- **hemoptysis** — coughing or spitting up blood
- **inspiration** — act of inhaling air
- **orthopnea** — discomfort in breathing except in an upright position (see *Three-pillow orthopnea*)
- **palpation** — assessment step; feeling the body surface with the hand
- **percussion** — assessment step; striking a part of the body with short, sharp blows of the fingers to detect changes in sound or mobilize lung secretions
- **respiratory rate** — number of breaths per minute
- **shunting** — condition in which blood moves from the venous circulation to the arterial circulation without participating in gas exchange, leading to hypoxemia
- **subcutaneous crepitus** — creaking sound produced by palpation or stroking of the skin; caused by bubbles of air or other gases such as CO_2 trapped in the subcutaneous tissue; may occur with pneumothorax
- **tactile fremitus** — vibration in the chest wall that may be felt when a hand is applied to the thorax while the patient is speaking.

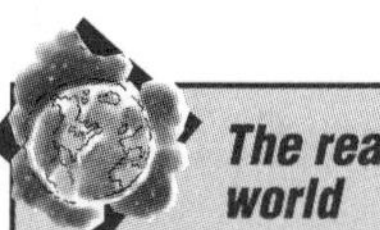

The real world

Three-pillow orthopnea

You may hear the term **three-pillow orthopnea** used to describe a patient's sleeping habits. This means the patient requires three pillows to breathe comfortably while sleeping.

Respiratory patterns

The following terms describe different respiratory patterns:

- **apnea** — absence of breathing (may be periodic)
- **apneustic breathing** — prolonged, gasping inspirations followed by extremely short, inefficient expirations
- **Biot's respirations** — irregular periods of apnea alternating with periods of four or five breaths having the same depth
- **bradypnea** — unusually slow, regular respirations
- **Cheyne-Stokes respirations** — alternating periods of apnea and deep, rapid breathing (see *Cheyne-Stokes*)
- **eupnea** — normal respiratory rate and rhythm
- **Kussmaul's respirations** — faster and deeper respirations than normal, without pauses
- **tachypnea** — abnormally rapid respiratory rate.

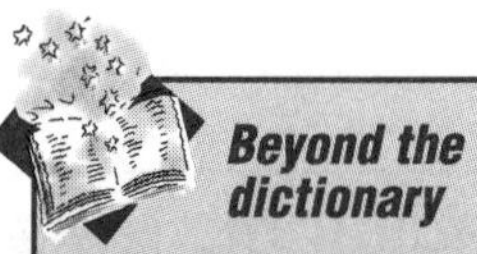

Beyond the dictionary

Cheyne-Stokes

Cheyne-Stokes respirations were named after John Cheyne, a Scottish doctor, and William Stokes, an Irish doctor.

Diagnostic tests

Below are the names of some diagnostic tests for respiratory disorders and classifications.

Ventilation tests

Ventilation tests, also called **pulmonary function tests,** include a series of measurements that evaluate the lungs' ventilatory function:

- **diffusing capacity for carbon monoxide (DLCO)** — amount of carbon monoxide diffused per minute across the alveolar membrane
- **expiratory reserve volume (ERV)** — volume of air that can be exhaled after normal expiration is completed
- **forced expiratory volume (FEV)** — volume of air expired in the 1st, 2nd, and 3rd seconds of the forced vital capacity test
- **forced vital capacity (FVC)** — volume of air that can be exhaled after maximum inspiration
- **functional residual capacity (FRC)** — volume of air remaining in the lungs after normal expiration
- **inspiratory capacity (IC)** — volume of air that can be inhaled after normal expiration
- **inspiratory reserve volume (IRV)** — volume of air that can be inspired after normal inspiration is complete
- **maximum voluntary ventilation (MVV)** — the greatest volume of air breathed per unit of time
- **minute volume (V_E)** — volume of air breathed per minute, calculated from the tidal volume
- **residual volume (RV)** — volume of air that is *always* in the lungs and can't be exhaled (must be measured indirectly)
- **tidal volume (V_T)** — volume of air inhaled or exhaled during normal breathing
- **total lung capacity (TLC)** — volume of the lungs at peak inspiration
- **vital capacity (VC)** — volume of air that can be exhaled after maximum inspiration.

Radiologic tests

Tests that use X-rays or electromagnetic waves to create images of interior structures are:

- **Chest radiography,** commonly known as **chest X-ray,** creates an image of the thorax to reveal abnormalities.
- **Magnetic resonance imaging (MRI)** is a procedure in which the patient is placed in a magnetic field into

which a radiofrequency beam is introduced. Resulting energy changes are measured and computed, generating images on a monitor. Cross-sectional images of the anatomy can be viewed in multiple planes.

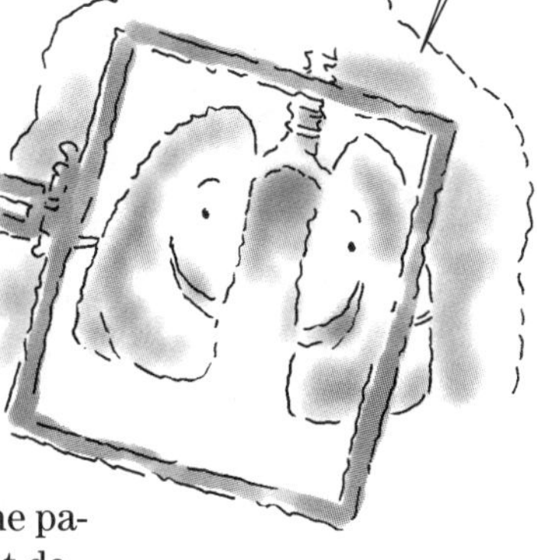

Radiologic tests help you get a good look at me.

- **Pulmonary angiography,** also called **pulmonary arteriography,** is the radiographic examination of the pulmonary circulation after injection of a radiopaque contrast dye into the pulmonary artery or one of its branches.
- **Thoracic computed tomography (CT) scan** provides cross-sectional views of the chest by passing an X-ray beam from a computerized scanner through the body at different angles. CT scanning may be done with or without an injected contrast dye.
- **Ventilation-perfusion scan** combines two procedures to evaluate the lungs' ventilation and perfusion. The ventilation scan is performed after the patient inhales a mixture of air and radioactive gas that delineates areas of the lung ventilated during respiration. The perfusion scan produces an image of pulmonary blood flow after I.V. injection of a radioactive dye.

Other tests

Here are other tests used to diagnose respiratory system disorders:

- **Arterial blood gas measurement** provides levels of O_2 and CO_2 in arterial blood to evaluate acid-base balance and to assess and monitor a patient's ventilation and oxygenation status. (See *What a gas!* and *What arterial blood gases reveal,* page 158.)
- **Bronchoscopy** is a visual inspection of the tracheobronchial tree using a bronchoscope to obtain a specimen for biopsy or culture, or to remove foreign bodies.
- **Culture and sensitivity tests** help identify the causative organism in bacterial, viral, or fungal infections.
- **Pulse oximetry** is a continuous noninvasive study of arterial blood oxygen saturation (Sao_2) using a probe or clip attached to a sensor site (usually earlobe or fingertip).
- **Sputum analysis** examines a sample of expectorated material from the patient's lungs.

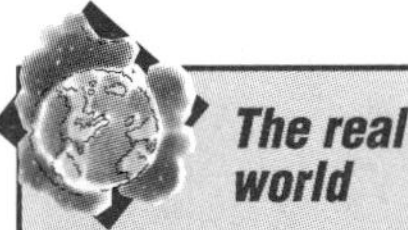

The real world

What a gas!

In practice, you'll commonly hear **arterial blood gases** referred to as *ABGs, blood gases,* or simply *gases*—as in "Let's draw some gases."

What arterial blood gases reveal

Arterial blood gases diagnose the following disorders:
- **respiratory acidosis,** or excess carbon dioxide (CO_2) retention, which is most often caused by hypoventilation
- **respiratory alkalosis,** which occurs when too much CO_2 is excreted (hyperventilation is the primary cause)
- **metabolic acidosis,** which reflects elevated acid levels and may be caused by loss of bicarbonate, excess acid production, or a combination of both
- **metabolic alkalosis,** which reflects elevated bicarbonate levels, decreased acid levels, or both (prolonged vomiting and loss of potassium can deplete the body's acid stores; overuse of alkaline medications, such as antacids, can produce elevated bicarbonate levels).

- **Thoracentesis** uses a needle to puncture the chest to aspirate fluid from the parietal cavity for diagnostic or therapeutic purposes.

Need some fluid? A **thoracentesis** uses a needle to aspirate the parietal cavity.

Respiratory disorders

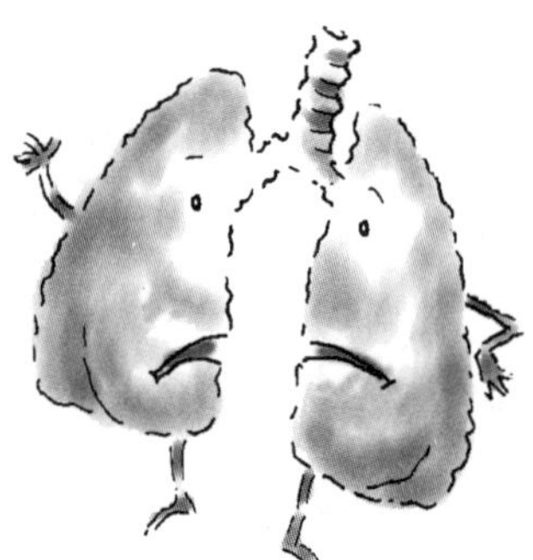

Here is a list of major respiratory disorders:
- **Acute bronchitis** is an inflammation of the bronchi accompanied by mucus production and subsequent obstruction of airflow. Infectious agents, such as influenza virus, streptococci, pneumococci, staphylococci, and *Haemophilus*, can cause acute bronchitis.
- **Acute respiratory failure (ARF)** is caused by the cardiac and pulmonary systems inadequately exchanging O_2 and CO_2 in the lungs.
- **Adult respiratory distress syndrome (ARDS)** is a form of pulmonary edema that can quickly lead to acute respiratory failure.
- **Asbestosis** is caused by prolonged inhalation of asbestos fibers, which become encased in the bronchioles and alveolar walls in a proteinlike sheath.
- **Atelectasis** is the collapse of lung tissue or incomplete expansion of a lung caused by the absence of air in a portion of the lung or the entire lung. (See *Atelectasis.*)

• **Bronchiectasis** is a condition marked by chronic abnormal dilation of bronchi and destruction of bronchial walls.
• **Chronic obstructive pulmonary disease (COPD)** refers to a group of long-term pulmonary disorders marked by resistance to air flow (hence the term **obstructive**). Types of COPD include:
–**asthma** — episodic airway obstruction caused by bronchospasm, increased mucus secretion, and mucosal edema; may be either **extrinsic (atopic),** a reaction to specific external allergens, or **intrinsic,** a reaction to internal, nonallergenic factors
–**chronic bronchitis** — characterized by excessive mucus production with productive cough lasting at least 3 months per year for 2 successive years; usually caused by prolonged exposure to bronchial irritants such as smoking, secondhand smoke, air pollution, dust, and toxic fumes
–**emphysema** — abnormal, permanent enlargement of the acini, accompanied by destruction of the alveolar walls.
• **Cor pulmonale** is a heart condition in which hypertension of the pulmonary circulation leads to enlargement of the right ventricle.
• **Croup** is a severe inflammation and obstruction of the upper airway that usually follows an upper respiratory tract infection. Croup is a childhood disease characterized by a sharp barklike cough.
• **Cystic fibrosis** is a multisystem genetic disorder, a defect of the exocrine glands, causing tenacious mucus in the lungs.
• **Empyema** is a form of pleural effusion in which the fluid in the pleural space contains pus.
• **Epiglottiditis** is an acute inflammation of the epiglottis that tends to cause airway obstruction.
• **Hemothorax** is a collection of blood in the pleural cavity.
• **Hypoxemia** is a deficiency of O_2 in the arterial blood, but isn't as severe as anoxia.
• **Hypoxia** is a deficiency of O_2 at a cellular level.
• **Legionnaires' disease** is an acute, noncommunicable bronchopneumonia caused by an airborne bacillus.
• **Lung abscess** is a lung infection accompanied by pus accumulation and tissue destruction.

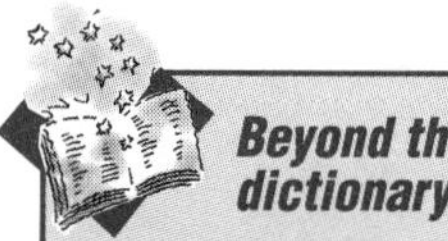
Beyond the dictionary

Atelectasis

Atelectasis derives from the Greek terms ***ateles,*** meaning *imperfect,* and ***ektasis,*** meaning *expansion.*

Beyond the dictionary

Pneuma: A breath of air

In English, the ***Pn-*** combination always indicates a word of Greek origin, and the ***p*** isn't pronounced. ***Pneuma,*** the Greek word for *breath, spirit,* or *wind,* has given rise to a number of words. In medical terminology it means *air* or *lung.* ***Thorax*** is a Greek word that means *chest.* It makes sense that a **pneumothorax** is a collection of air in the chest.

- **Pleural effusion** is accumulation of fluid in the interstitial and air spaces of the lung.
- **Pleurisy** is an inflammation of the pleurae characterized by dyspnea and stabbing pain, leading to restriction of breathing.
- **Pneumonia** is an acute infection of lung parenchyma often impairing gas exchange.
- **Pneumothorax** is a collection of air in the pleural cavity that leads to partial or complete lung collapse. (See *Pneuma: A breath of air.*) Different types of pneumothorax include:

–**closed pneumothorax** — condition in which air enters the pleural space from within the lungs
–**open pneumothorax** — condition in which atmospheric air flows directly into the pleural cavity
–**tension pneumothorax** — condition in which air in the pleural space compresses the thoracic organs, possibly causing **mediastinal shift** of organs and blood vessels, thus reducing blood flow to and from the heart.

- **Pulmonary edema** is a common complication of cardiac disorders in which extravascular fluid accumulates in the lung tissues and alveoli.
- **Pulmonary embolism** occurs when a clot or foreign substance lodges in a pulmonary artery.
- **Pulmonary fibrosis** is scar tissue formation in the connective tissue of the lungs.
- **Pulmonary hypertension** is any condition that increases resistance to blood flow in the pulmonary vessels. The most common cause is COPD.
- **Pulmonary infarction** occurs when lung tissue is denied blood flow and dies.

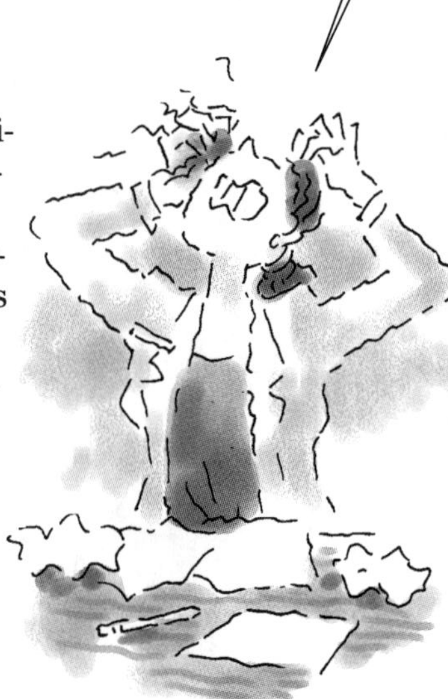
Don't let the name fool you. A **tension pneumothorax** doesn't result from stress. Instead, it occurs when air in the pleural space compresses the thoracic organs.

• **Respiratory distress syndrome,** also called **hyaline membrane disease,** is the most common cause of neonatal mortality. In respiratory distress syndrome, the premature infant develops widespread alveolar collapse.
• **Sarcoidosis** is a multisystem, granulomatous disorder that characteristically produces enlarged lymph nodes, pulmonary infiltration, and skeletal, liver, eye, or skin lesions.
• **Silicosis** is a progressive disease characterized by nodular lesions that commonly progress to fibrosis.
• **Sudden infant death syndrome** kills apparently healthy infants, usually between ages 4 weeks and 7 months, for reasons that remain unexplained even after an autopsy.
• **Tuberculosis** is an infectious disease in which pulmonary infiltrates accumulate in the lungs, cavities develop, and masses of granulated tissue form.

Treatments

Below are the devices, treatments, and surgical interventions used to improve oxygenation.

Tools of the trade

These are names of medical devices used to treat respiratory disorders:
• **bronchoscope** — used therapeutically to remove foreign bodies from the trachea and bronchi
• **chest tube** — a tube inserted through a thoracostomy into the pleural space and used to remove blood, fluid, or air in cases of hemothorax, pleural effusion, pneumothorax, or acute empyema

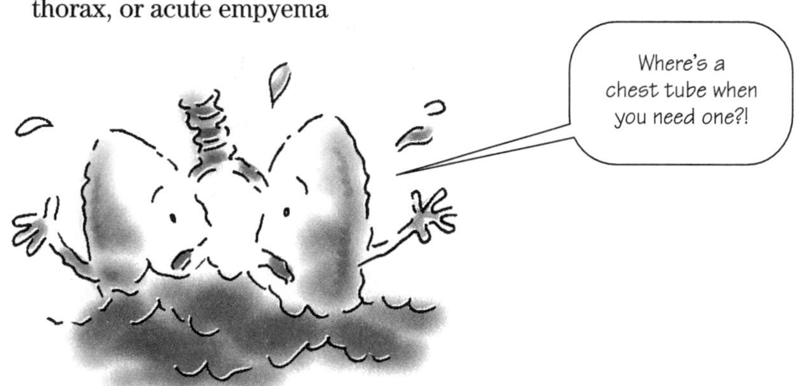

• **endotracheal tube** — a flexible catheter inserted into the trachea via the mouth or nose and used to deliver O_2 into the lungs
• **nasal cannula** — small tubes that deliver a variable, low-flow O_2 supply through the nasal passages
• **nebulizer** — a device that delivers a fine spray for inhalation of moisture or drug therapy
• **resuscitation bag** — an inflatable device that can be attached to a facemask or directly to an endotracheal or tracheostomy tube that is designed to pump O_2 or room air into the lungs
• **stethoscope** — an instrument used for auscultation of respiratory, cardiac, arterial, and venous sounds consisting of two earpieces connected by flexible tubing to a diaphragm, which is placed against the patient's chest or back
• **tracheostomy tube** — inserted into the surgical opening through the neck into the trachea, which is used to relieve upper airway obstruction and aid breathing; may be used with a mechanical ventilator
• **Venturi mask** — a device designed to deliver a high-flow, precise O_2 mixture.

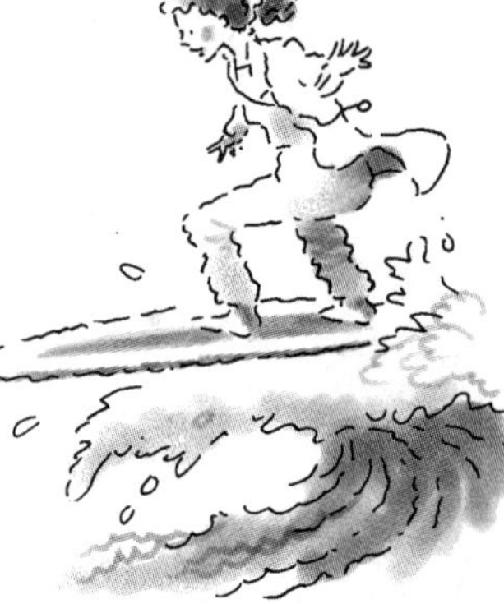
A nebulizer can be used to deliver moisture or drug therapy.

Surgery

Here are the names of surgical procedures used to treat respiratory disorders:
• **pneumonectomy** — surgical removal of the lung
• **thoracentesis** — a needle puncture of the chest performed to drain fluid from the parietal cavity
• **thoracostomy** — the surgical creation of an opening in the chest wall for the purpose of drainage.
• **thoracotomy** — a surgical incision in the chest wall made to excise a lung or portions of it. Thoracotomy can be further classified in three ways:
–**lobectomy** — the surgical excision of a lobe of a lung
–**segmental resection** — surgical removal of one or more of the lung's segments (removes more functional tissue than a lobectomy)
–**wedge resection** — the surgical removal of a triangular section of lung tissue

• **tracheotomy** — a surgical opening in the trachea, that provides an airway for intubated patients who need prolonged mechanical ventilation; also to help remove lung secretions and bypass upper airway obstruction.

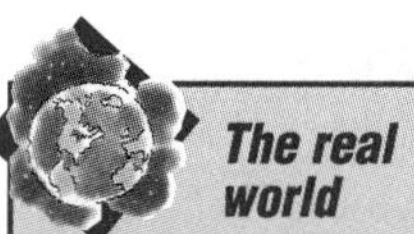

Vent 'em, bag 'em

The handheld resuscitation bag is commonly referred to as an **Ambu bag.** You may hear people refer to the process of using this device as *bagging the patient.* For example, "Disconnect him from the ventilator and bag him." If a patient requires a ventilator to assist with breathing, you may hear people say that the patient is *on a vent.*

Ventilation therapies

Ventilation therapy moves air in and out of a patient's lungs, but it doesn't ensure adequate gas exchange.

Manual ventilation

Manual ventilation uses a handheld resuscitation bag to deliver room air or O_2 to the lungs of a patient who can't breathe spontaneously. (See *Vent 'em, bag 'em.*)

Mechanical ventilation

Mechanical ventilators may supply negative or positive pressure. Negative pressure on the chest and lungs expands them during inspiration and is used to treat neuromuscular disorders. Positive pressure, the most commonly used mechanical ventilation system, is used to treat respiratory disorders.

Be positive

The **positive-pressure system** exerts positive pressure on the airway to inflate alveoli during inspiration. The inspiratory cycles of these ventilators may vary in volume, pressure, or time. There are three inspiratory cycle types:
• **Pressure-cycled** ventilation provides a continuous flow of O_2 until a preset pressure is reached.
• **Time-cycled** ventilation provides flow for a preset amount of time.
• **Volume-cycled** ventilation delivers a preset volume of air.

In the mode

Ventilation is provided through several ventilator modes:
• **Control mode** completely controls the patient's respiration, delivering a set tidal volume at a prescribed rate.
• **Assist mode** allows the patient to initiate a breath and receive a tidal volume from the machine.
• **Assist-control mode** allows the patient to initiate breathing, but a backup control delivers a preset number of breaths at a set volume.

• **Continuous positive-airway pressure (CPAP)** maintains positive pressure in the airways throughout the entire respiratory cycle.
• **Positive end-expiratory pressure (PEEP)** applies positive pressure during expiration.
• **Pressure support ventilation** augments the patient's spontaneous breath with a preset pressure. It doesn't provide the entire volume. The rate is set not by the machine but by the patient's spontaneous efforts.
• In **synchronized intermittent mandatory ventilation (SIMV),** a machine delivers a set number of specific-volume breaths. The patient can breathe on his own between SIMV breaths at volumes that differ from those on the machine. SIMV is commonly used as a weaning tool, conditioning the patient's respiratory muscles.

Drug therapy

Drug therapy for respiratory disorders includes:
• **antitussives** to suppress cough
• **decongestants** to relieve swelling in nasal passages
• **expectorants,** which liquefy secretions to help remove mucus
• **methylxanthine agents** to relax bronchial smooth muscle in patients with asthma and stimulate respiratory drive in patients with bronchitis, emphysema, and apnea
• **mucolytics** to enhance mucus removal.

Other therapies

Here are other therapies to treat respiratory disorders:
• **Aerosol treatments** deliver drugs by way of a nebulizer, which turns liquid into a spray the patient breathes.
• **Deep breathing** loosens secretions and opens airways.
• **Oxygen therapy** is delivered by a nasal cannula, catheter, mask, or transtracheal catheter; it prevents hypoxemia and eases the patient's breathing.
• **Postural drainage** uses gravity to help move secretions from the lungs and bronchi into the trachea to be coughed up.
• **Percussion** involves cupping hands and fingers together and clapping them alternately over the patient's lung fields to loosen secretions for expectoration.
• An **ultrasonic nebulizer** mobilizes thick secretions and promotes a productive cough.

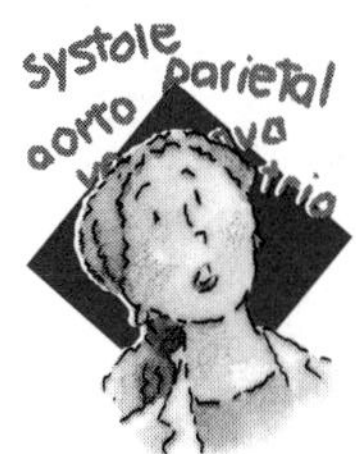

Vocabulary builders

At a crossroads

Completing this crossword puzzle will help you breathe more easily about respiratory system terms. Good luck!

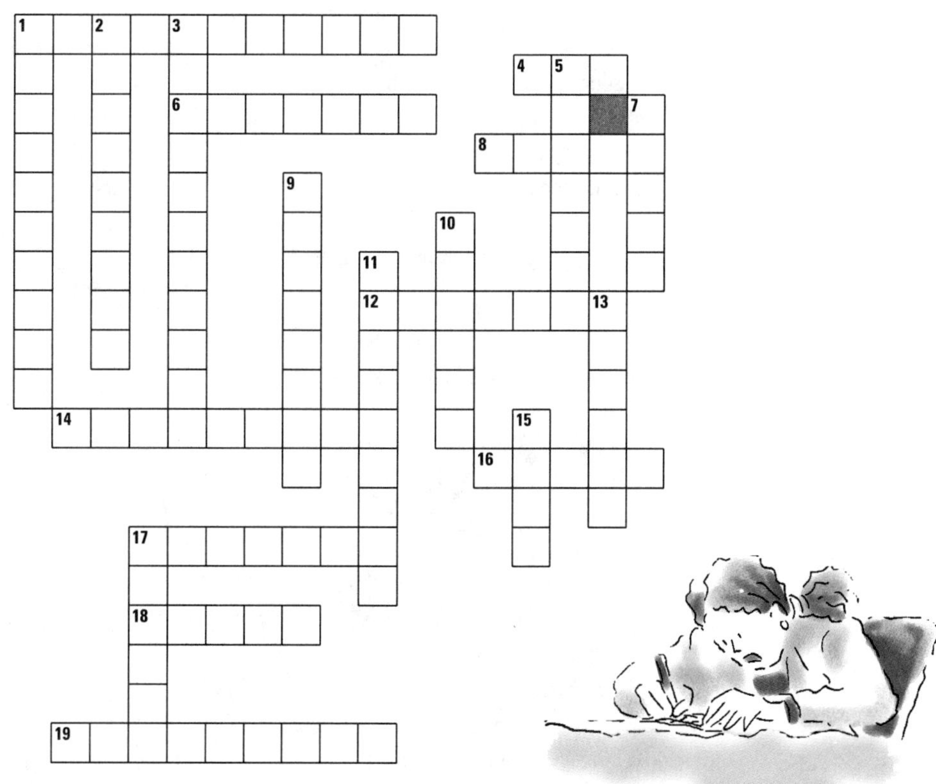

Across

1. Space between the lungs
4. Acronym for volume of air that can be exhaled after maximum inspiration
6. Another word for windpipe
8. Absence of breathing
12. Deficiency of O_2 at a cellular level
14. Surgical excision of a lung lobe
16. Slit on the lungs' medial surface
17. Bony structures that form the posterior walls of the nasal passages
18. Lung that is shorter, broader, and larger than the other
19. Unusually slow, regular respirations

Down

1. Type of ventilation that uses a positive-pressure system
2. Most important muscle for respiration
3. Drug type that acts to suppress cough
5. Eponym for mask designed to deliver a high-flow, precise O_2 mixture
7. Another word for nostrils
9. Another word for larynx
10. What separates the nasal passages
11. Plural form of pharynx
13. Chief respiratory unit for gas exchange
15. Eponym for respirations characterized by irregular periods of apnea alternating with four or five breaths of the same depth
17. Another word for tracheal bifurcation

Answers are on page 168.

Match game

It's important to know the the terms for different breath sounds. Match the description of each breath sound below to its name.

Clues

Normal sounds

1. Loud, high-pitched sounds that are heard next to the trachea and are loudest on expiration ____
2. Sounds heard in front of the chest, on both sides, and in back that are longer and louder during inspiration than expiration ____
3. Soft, medium-pitched, breezy sounds that are lower pitched than bronchial sounds but higher pitched than vesicular sounds ____

Abnormal sounds

4. Sounds like hairs being rubbed together, usually heard first over the lung bases ____
5. Loud, coarse, low-pitched bubbling sounds heard primarily during expiration ____
6. High-pitched, musical sounds that may occur during both inspiration and expiration but predominantly during expiration ____
7. Coarse, low-pitched sounds heard at the anterolateral chest wall (in front, near the ribs) during inspiration and expiration that sound like pieces of sandpaper being rubbed together ____
8. Crowing sound heard during inspiration, caused by air whistling as it passes through swollen upper airways ____
9. Abnormally diminished breath sounds in areas of the lung ____
10. Lack of sound over areas of the lungs that normally have breath sounds ____

Choices

A. Absent
B. Bronchial
C. Bronchovesicular
D. Crackles
E. Decreased
F. Pleural friction rubs
G. Rhonchi
H. Stridor
I. Vesicular
J. Wheezes

Answers are on page 168.

Scrambled or overeasy

Fill in the answers for the following questions, then unscramble the circled letters to find the answer to the puzzle.

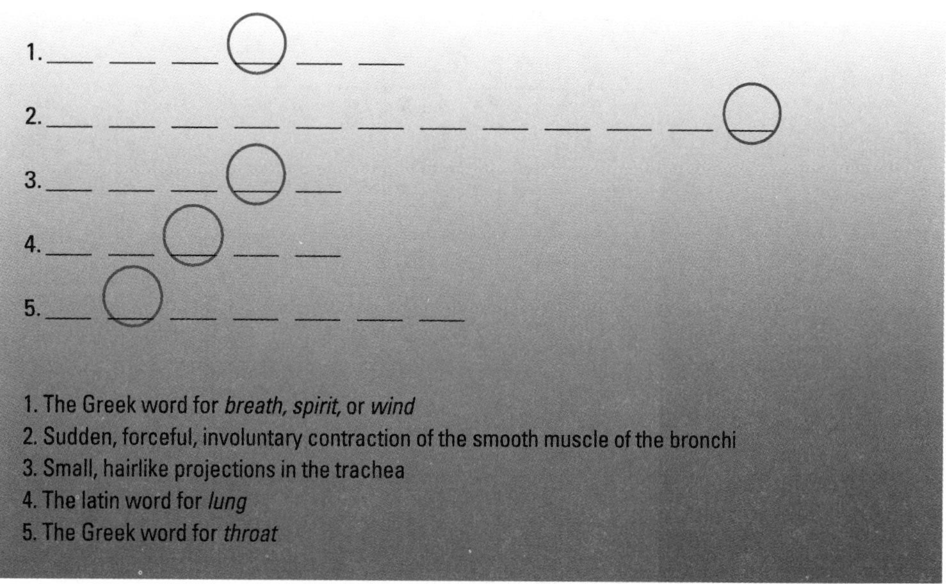

1. The Greek word for *breath, spirit,* or *wind*
2. Sudden, forceful, involuntary contraction of the smooth muscle of the bronchi
3. Small, hairlike projections in the trachea
4. The latin word for *lung*
5. The Greek word for *throat*

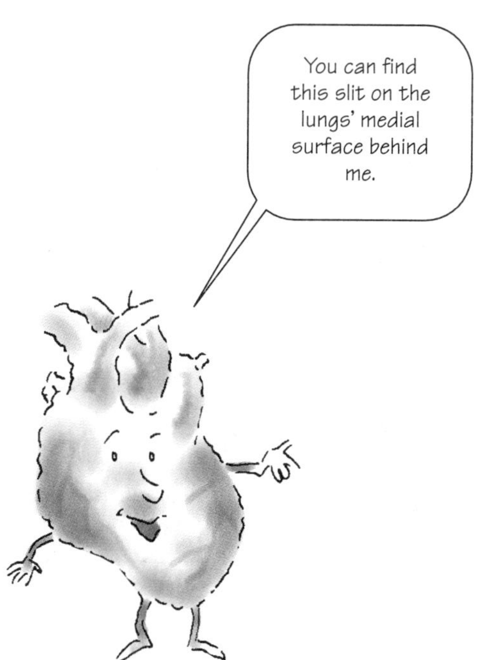

You can find this slit on the lungs' medial surface behind me.

Answers are on page 168.

Answers

At a crossroads

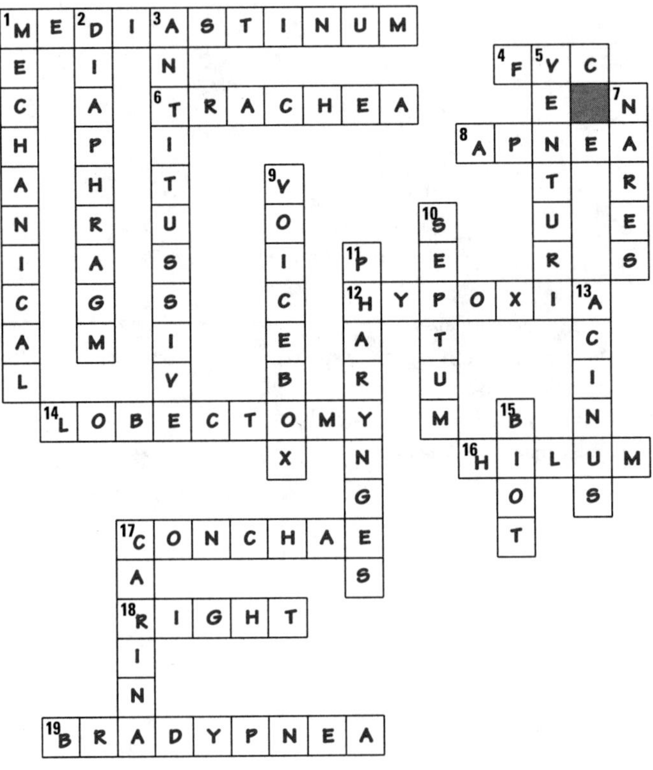

Match game

1. B; 2. I; 3. C; 4. D; 5. G; 6. J; 7. F; 8. H; 9. E; 10. A.

Scrambled or overeasy

1. Pneuma; 2. Bronchospasm; 3. Cilia; 4. Pulmo; 5. Pharynx.
Answer to puzzle — Hilum

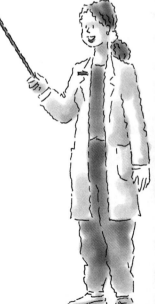

Gastrointestinal system

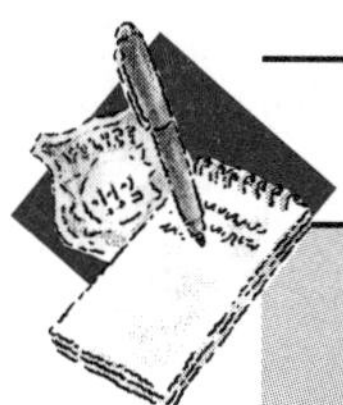

Just the facts

In this chapter, you'll review:

- terminology related to the structure and function of the GI system
- terminology needed for physical examination
- tests that help diagnose GI disorders
- common GI disorders and their treatments.

GI structure and function

This chapter introduces terms associated with the GI system, the system responsible for digestion and elimination. The first part of the word **gastrointestinal, *gastro-*,** is a Greek word that means *stomach;* it's used in many medical terms. The second part of the word refers, of course, to the intestines. But the GI system includes more than just the stomach and the intestines. (See *Pronouncing key GI system terms*, page 170.)

Let's see. **Gastro** means stomach; **entero** means intestine; and **-ology** means study. Seems simple — **gastroenterology** is the study of the stomach and intestines.

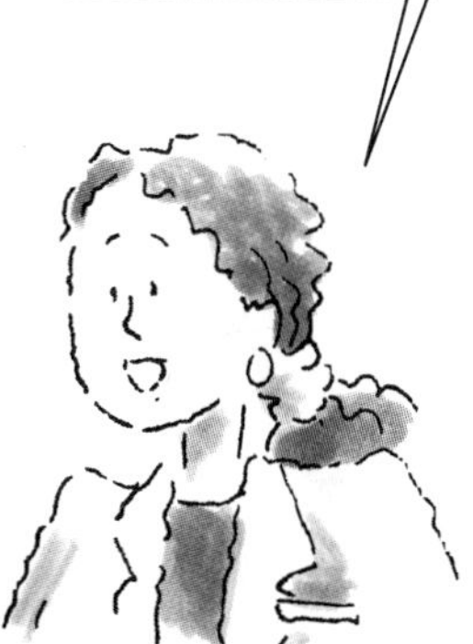

Two parts

The GI system has two major components:
- **alimentary canal** (also called the **GI tract**) — the mouth, pharynx, esophagus, stomach, and intestines
- **accessory GI organs** — the liver, gallbladder, biliary duct system, and pancreas.

Two functions

Together, the alimentary canal and the accessory organs serve two major functions:
- **digestion** — the breakdown of food and fluid into simple chemicals that can be absorbed into the bloodstream and transported throughout the body

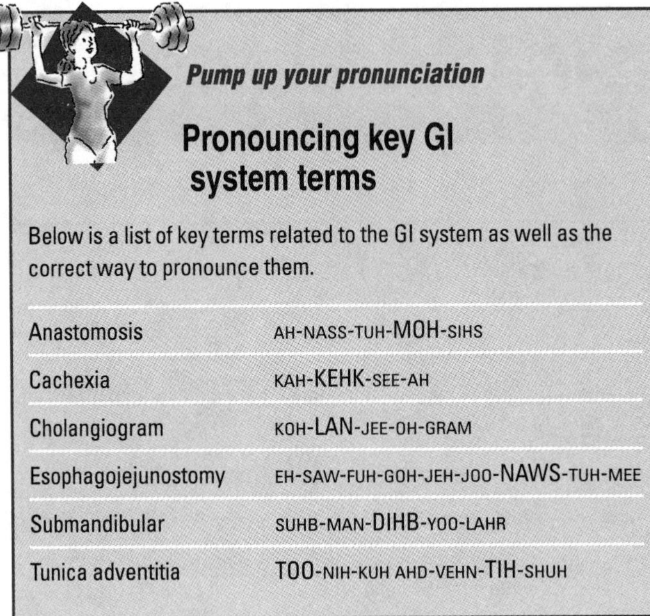

Pump up your pronunciation

Pronouncing key GI system terms

Below is a list of key terms related to the GI system as well as the correct way to pronounce them.

Term	Pronunciation
Anastomosis	AH-NASS-TUH-MOH-SIHS
Cachexia	KAH-KEHK-SEE-AH
Cholangiogram	KOH-LAN-JEE-OH-GRAM
Esophagojejunostomy	EH-SAW-FUH-GOH-JEH-JOO-NAWS-TUH-MEE
Submandibular	SUHB-MAN-DIHB-YOO-LAHR
Tunica adventitia	TOO-NIH-KUH AHD-VEHN-TIH-SHUH

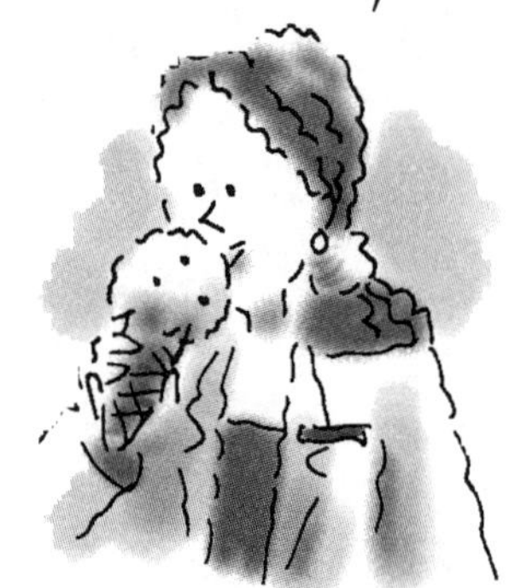

Digesting this ice cream begins in the **oral cavity** — that's the mouth.

• **elimination** — the expulsion of waste products from the body through excretion of feces.

Alimentary canal

Here are the terms and descriptions of structures of the alimentary canal.

Mouth

Also called the **buccal cavity** or **oral cavity,** the mouth is bounded by the lips, cheeks, **palate** (the roof of the mouth), and tongue. It also contains the teeth. The mouth initiates the mechanical breakdown of food. Ducts connect the mouth with three major pairs of **salivary glands,** which secrete **saliva** to moisten food during chewing. The three pairs are:

• **parotid** — located at the side of the face in front of and below the external ear

• **submandibular** — located, as the name indicates, beneath the **mandible,** or lower jaw

• **sublingual**—located, as the name indicates, under the tongue. (See *Structures of the GI system.*)

Structures of the GI system

The GI system includes the alimentary canal (the pharynx, esophagus, stomach, and small and large intestines) and the accessory organs (the liver, biliary duct system, and pancreas).

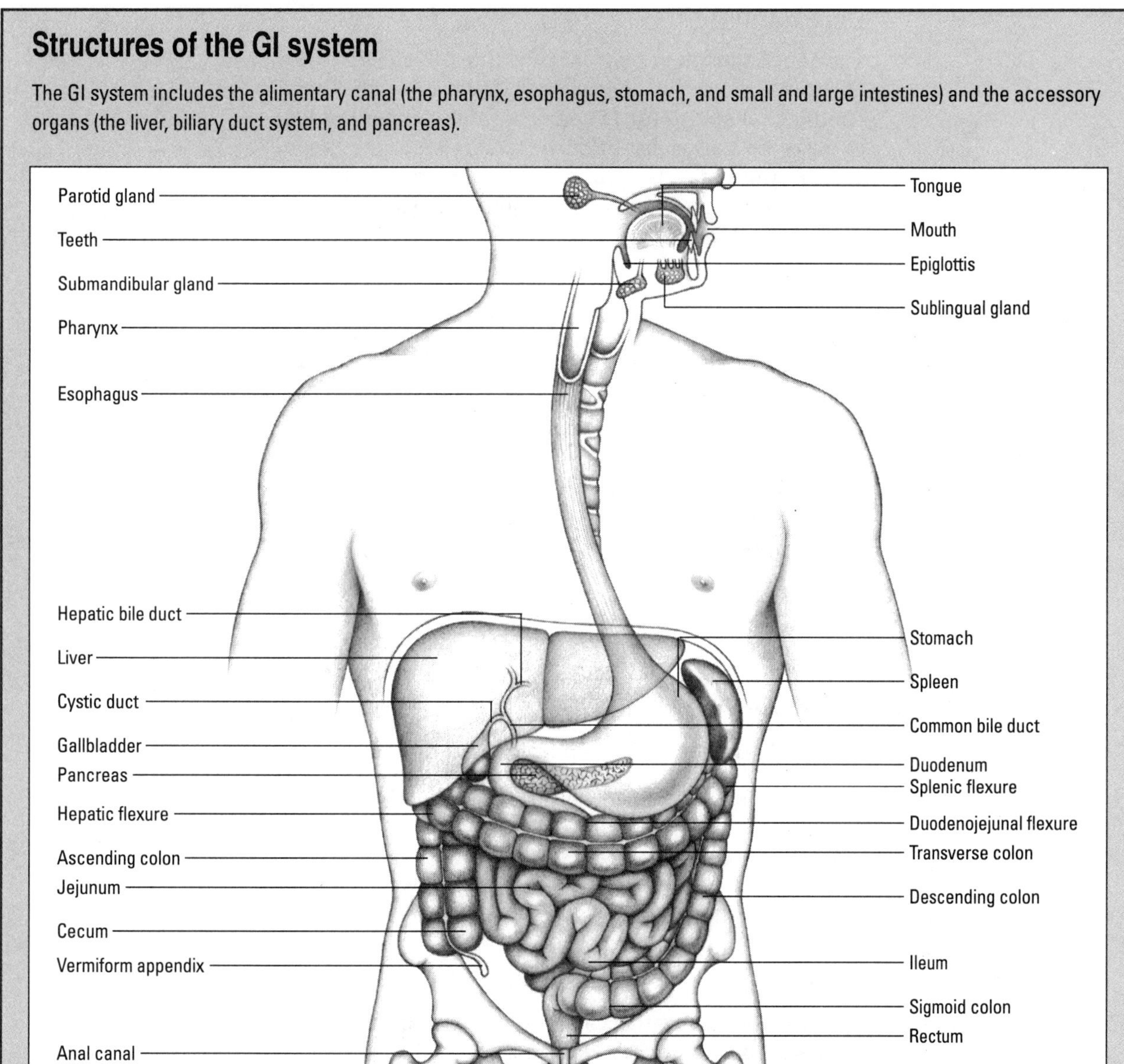

Pharynx

The **pharynx,** or throat, a cavity extending from the base of the skull to the esophagus, aids swallowing by grasping food and propelling it toward the esophagus.

Esophagus

The **esophagus** is a muscular tube that extends from the pharynx through the mediastinum to the stomach. The **esophageal sphincter** (a sphincter at the upper border of the esophagus) must relax for food to enter the esophagus. **Peristalsis** (the rhythmic contraction and relaxation of smooth muscle) propels liquids and solids through the esophagus into the stomach.

Stomach

The **stomach** is a collapsible, pouchlike structure in the upper left part of the abdominal cavity, just below the diaphragm. Its upper border attaches to the lower end of the esophagus. The **cardiac sphincter** guards the opening to the stomach and opens as food approaches. The lateral surface of the stomach is called the **greater curvature;** the medial surface, the **lesser curvature.**

The stomach has four main regions:

The **cardia** lies near the junction of the stomach and esophagus.

The **fundus** is the enlarged portion above and to the left of the esophageal opening into the stomach.

The **body** is the middle portion of the stomach.

The **pylorus** is the lower portion, lying near the junction of the stomach and the duodenum. (See *A close-up of the stomach.*)

The stomach serves as a temporary storage space for food and also begins digestion.

Intestines

After mixing food with gastric secretions, the stomach breaks it down into **chyme,** a semifluid substance, and then moves the gastric contents into the intestines, which consist of the small intestine and the large intestine.

Small but really lo-o-o-o-n-n-g

Although it's called "small," the narrow tube called the **small intestine** is actually about 20′ (6.1 m) long and is composed of three major divisions:

- The **duodenum** is the most superior division.
- The **jejunum** is the middle portion.

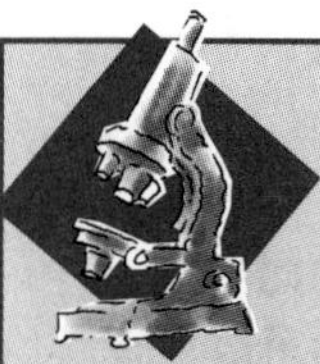

Zoom in

A close-up of the stomach

The body of the stomach lies between the **lower esophageal,** or **cardiac, sphincter** and the **pyloric sphincter.** Between these sphincters lie the fundus, body, antrum, and pylorus. These areas have a rich variety of mucosal cells that help the stomach carry out its tasks.

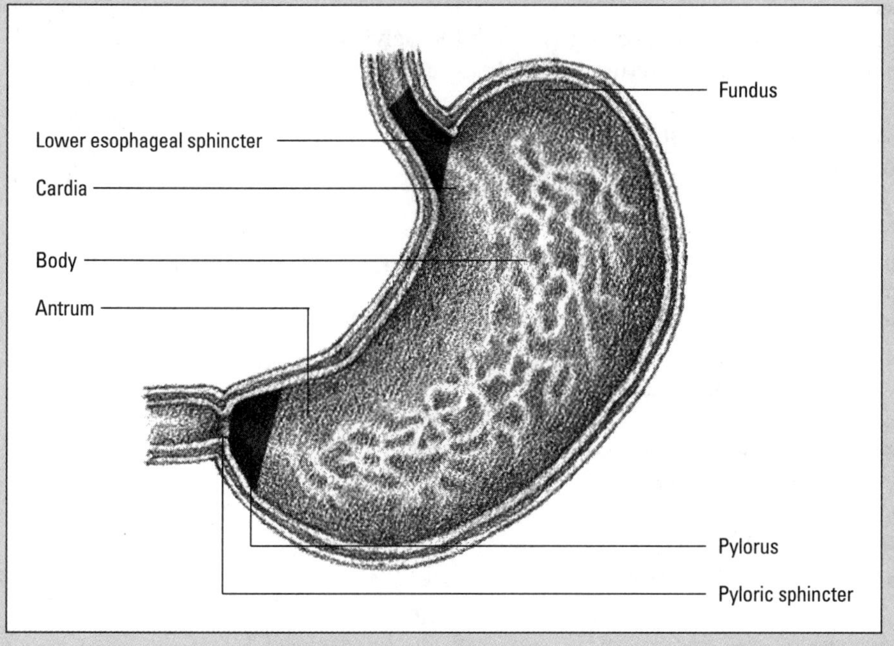

- The **ileum** is the most inferior portion.

The small intestine completes food digestion. Food molecules are absorbed through its wall into the circulatory system, from which they're delivered to body cells.

Now LARGE

The **large intestine** extends from the **ileocecal valve** (the valve between the ileum of the small intestine and the first segment of the large intestine) to the **anus.** The large intestine absorbs water, secretes mucus, and eliminates digestive wastes. It has five segments:

- The **cecum,** a saclike structure, makes up the first few inches of the large intestine beginning just below the ileocecal valve.

- The **ascending colon** rises on the right posterior abdominal wall, then turns sharply under the liver at the hepatic flexure.
- The **transverse colon,** situated above the small intestine, passes horizontally across the abdomen and below the liver, stomach, and spleen. At the left splenic flexure it turns downward.
- The **descending colon** starts near the spleen and extends down the left side of the abdomen into the pelvic cavity.
- The **sigmoid colon** descends through the pelvic cavity, where it becomes the rectum. (See *Sigmoid has an "S" shape.*)
- The **rectum,** the last few inches of the large intestine, terminates at the **anus.**

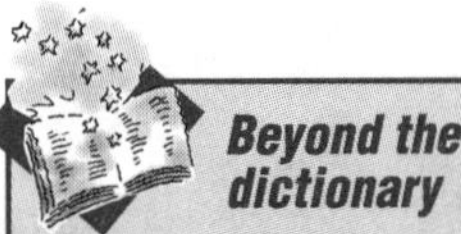

Beyond the dictionary

Sigmoid has an "S" shape

The term **sigmoid** derives from the Greek word ***sigma,*** the name of the eighteenth letter of the Greek alphabet. In Greek, the letter is represented like this: ς, a kind of truncated **s,** which pretty closely resembles the shape of the sigmoid colon.

Inner lining

The wall of the GI tract consists of several layers. The innermost layer, the **mucosa** (also called the **tunica mucosa**), consists of epithelial and surface cells and loose connective tissue.

The **submucosa** (also called the **tunica submucosa**) encircles the mucosa. It's composed of loose connective tissue, blood and lymphatic vessels, and a nerve network.

Around the submucosa lies the **tunica muscularis,** which is composed of skeletal muscle in the mouth, pharynx, and upper esophagus and longitudinal and circular smooth muscle fibers elsewhere in the tract.

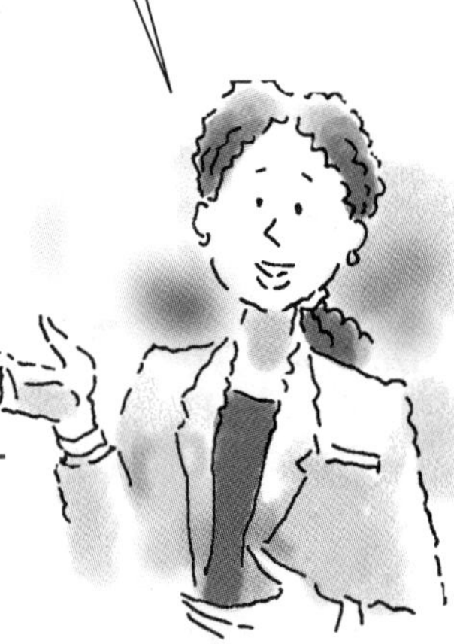

Many of these words share a common term, tunica, which comes from Latin and means sheath.

Outer covering

The **visceral peritoneum** is the GI tract's outer covering. In the esophagus and rectum, it's also called the **tunica adventitia;** elsewhere in the GI tract, it's called the **tunica serosa.**

The visceral peritoneum covers most of the abdominal organs and lays next to an identical layer, the **parietal peritoneum,** that lines the abdominal cavity.

Vital accessories

Accessory organs — the liver, the biliary duct system, and pancreas — contribute hormones, enzymes, and bile, which are vital to digestion. They deliver their secretions to the duodenum through the **hepatopancreatic ampul-**

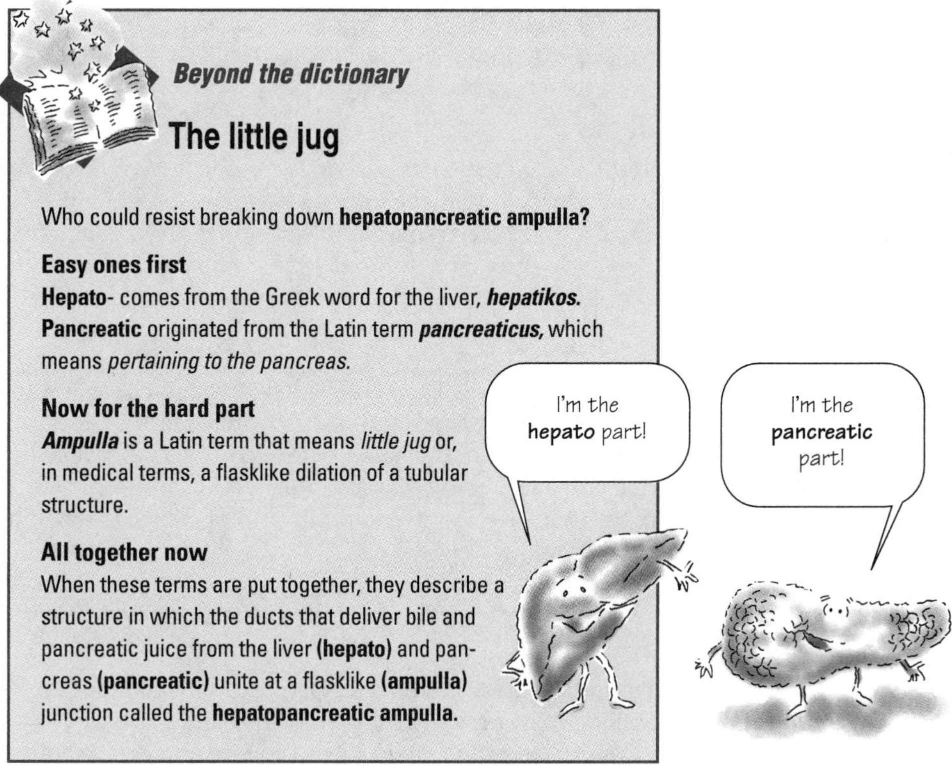

Beyond the dictionary

The little jug

Who could resist breaking down **hepatopancreatic ampulla?**

Easy ones first

Hepato- comes from the Greek word for the liver, ***hepatikos.*** **Pancreatic** originated from the Latin term ***pancreaticus,*** which means *pertaining to the pancreas.*

Now for the hard part

Ampulla is a Latin term that means *little jug* or, in medical terms, a flasklike dilation of a tubular structure.

All together now

When these terms are put together, they describe a structure in which the ducts that deliver bile and pancreatic juice from the liver **(hepato)** and pancreas **(pancreatic)** unite at a flasklike **(ampulla)** junction called the **hepatopancreatic ampulla.**

la, also called the **ampulla of Vater** (named after Abraham Vater, a German anatomist). (See *The little jug.*)

The entry of bile and pancreatic juice is controlled by a muscular valve called the **hepatopancreatic sphincter,** or **Oddi's sphincter** (named after Ruggero Oddi, an Italian doctor).

Liver and lobule

The **liver's** digestive function is to produce bile for export to the duodenum. The **liver's** functional unit, the **lobule,** consists of a plate of hepatic cells, or **hepatocytes,** that encircle a central vein and radiate outward.

Sinusoids

Separating the hepatocyte plates from each other are **sinusoids,** the liver's capillary system.

Toxic clean up

Kupffer's cells, which line the sinusoids, remove bacteria and toxins that have entered the blood through the intestinal capillaries. (Kupffer's cells are named after Karl Wilhelm von Kupffer, a German anatomist.)

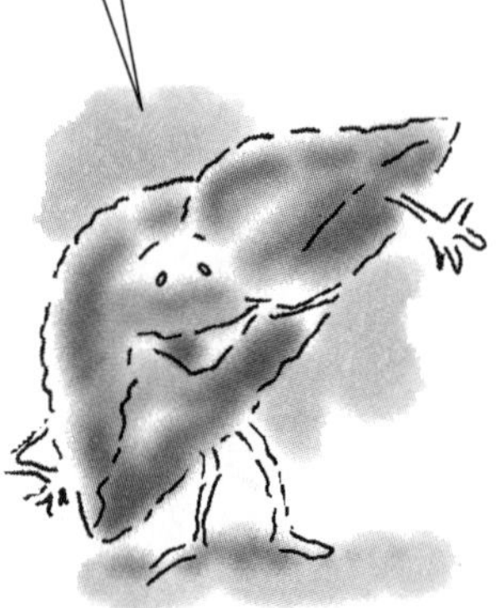
My three ducts are the common hepatic duct, cystic duct, and common bile duct.

Ducts

Bile, recycled from bile salts in the blood, leaves through biliary ducts that merge into the right and left hepatic ducts to form the **common hepatic duct.** This duct joins the **cystic duct** from the gallbladder to form the **common bile duct,** which leads to the duodenum.

Bully for bile

A yellow-greenish liquid composed of water, cholesterol, bile salts, electrolytes, and phospholipids, **bile** breaks down fats and neutralizes gastric secretions in chyme. Bile prevents jaundice by assisting with excretion of **conjugated bilirubin,** an end product of normal hemoglobin breakdown.

Gallbladder

The **gallbladder** is a pear-shaped organ that is nestled under the liver and joined to the larger organ by the cystic duct. The gallbladder's job is to store and concentrate bile produced by the liver. (See *Why not bilebladder?*)

Of all the gall!

When stimulated by a hormone called **cholecystokinin,** the gallbladder contracts, the hepatopancreatic ampulla relaxes, and bile is released into the common bile duct for delivery to the duodenum. (See *Bile, bladder, and protein.*)

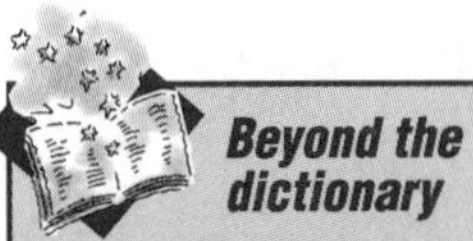

Bile, bladder, and protein

Cholecystokinin is easy to dissect:
Chole- is Greek for bile.
Cysto- comes from the Greek word ***kystis,*** meaning *bladder.*
Kinin is a general term for plasma proteins — like this hormone.

Pancreas

The **pancreas** lies behind the stomach, with its head and neck extending into the curve of the duodenum and its tail lying against the spleen. The pancreas contains two cell types:

- **endocrine cells,** from which hormones are secreted into the blood
- **exocrine cells,** from which enzymes are secreted through ducts to the digestive system.

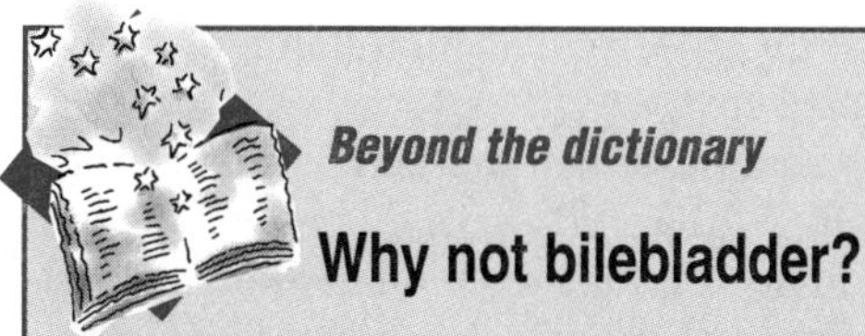

Beyond the dictionary

Why not bilebladder?

We might just as well call the gallbladder a **bilebladder** because the two words, **gall** and **bile,** refer to the same thing. **Gall** appears in Old English as early as the year 825 in a translation of the Psalms. The word **gall** actually refers to the yellowish color of bile. The word **bile,** on the other hand, is a relatively recent borrowing from Latin by way of French; this word doesn't show up in English until the 17th century.

In the islets of Langerhans

The pancreas's endocrine function involves the **islets of Langerhans,** named for Paul Langerhans (1847-1888), the German doctor who discovered them. These microscopic structures — over 1 million of them — are scattered throughout the pancreas and house two cell types:

- **alpha cells,** which secrete **glucagon,** a hormone that stimulates the breakdown of glycogen to glucose in the liver — a process referred to as **glycogenolysis**
- **beta cells,** which secrete **insulin** to promote carbohydrate metabolism.

Physical examination terms

Before you can perform a complete examination of the GI tract, you need to understand the associated terminology:

- **Aaron's sign** refers to pain in the chest or abdominal area that is elicited by applying gentle but steadily increasing pressure over McBurney's point (2″ [5.1 cm] below the right anterior superior spine of the ilium, on a line between that spine and the umbilicus). A positive sign indicates appendicitis.
- **Abdominal distention** refers to increased abdominal girth — the result of increased intra-abdominal pressure forcing the abdominal wall outward.
- **Anorexia** is a loss of appetite.

- **Ascites** refers to the abnormal accumulation of serous fluid in the peritoneal cavity.
- **Auscultation** is an assessment method; it means to listen carefully, usually with a stethoscope.
- **Ballottement,** lightly tapping or bouncing fingertips against the abdominal wall, elicits abdominal muscle resistance or guarding.
- **Bowel sounds** are auscultated with a stethoscope and provide information about **bowel motility** (movement) and the underlying vessels and organs. Normally, air and fluid moving through the bowel create soft, bubbling sounds that are often mixed with soft clicks and gurgles, that occur every 5 to 15 seconds. Bowel sounds are described using the following terms:
  –**absent bowel sounds,** when no bowel sounds are heard
  –**borborygmi,** the familiar "growling stomach" of a hungry patient
  –**hyperactive,** which describes rapid, high-pitched, loud gurgling sounds
  –**hypoactive,** which occur at a rate no greater than one per minute.
- **Cachexia** is a profound state of overall ill health and malnutrition characterized by weakness and emaciation.
- **Colic** is acute abdominal pain.
- **Constipation** refers to a decreased passage of stools. Stools are characteristically hard and dry.
- **Cullen's sign** refers to irregular, bluish hemorrhagic patches on the skin around the umbilicus and occasionally around abdominal scars. Cullen's sign indicates massive hemorrhage.
- **Diarrhea** is rapid movement of fecal material through the intestines that causes poor absorption of water and nutrients. Stools are watery and frequent.
- **Dyspepsia** is gastric discomfort, such as fullness, heartburn, bloating, and nausea, that occurs after eating.
- **Dysphagia** is difficult or painful swallowing.
- **Emesis,** from Greek, is an expulsion of the stomach contents by vomiting.
- **Epigastrium** refers to the upper and middle regions of the abdomen.
- **Fecal impaction** is an accumulation of hardened feces in the rectum or sigmoid colon that can't be evacuated.
- **Fecal incontinence** refers to an inability to prevent the discharge of feces.

Colic is acute abdominal pain.

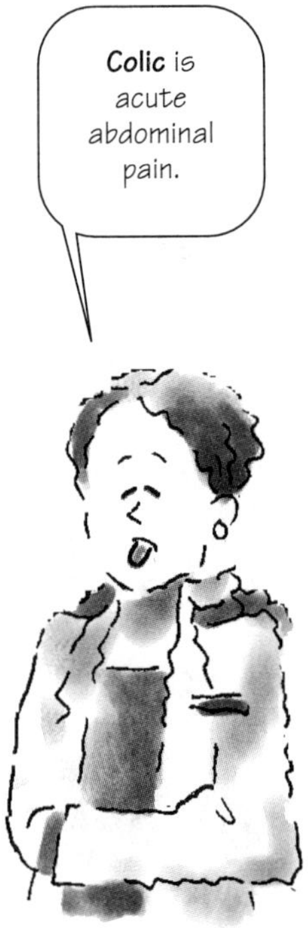

- **Flatulence** refers to a sensation of gaseous abdominal fullness.
- **Grey Turner's sign** is characterized by a bruiselike discoloration of the skin of the flanks that appears 6 to 24 hours after the onset of retroperitoneal hemorrhage in acute pancreatitis.
- **Guarding** is moving away or flinching when a tender area of the abdomen is touched.
- **Heartburn,** also referred to as **pyrosis,** is a burning sensation in the esophagus or below the sternum in the region of the heart.
- **Hematemesis** is vomiting blood.
- **Hemoperitoneum** refers to a leakage of blood into the peritoneal cavity.
- **Hepatomegaly** is an enlarged liver.
- **Hypogastrium** is the lowest, middle abdominal region.
- **Ileus** is a mechanical intestinal obstruction.
- **Jaundice** is a yellow appearance of the skin, mucous membranes, and sclerae of the eyes, resulting from elevated serum bilirubin levels.
- **Melena** is the passage of black, tarry stools — a common sign of upper GI bleeding.
- **Murphy's sign** is the arrest of inspiratory effort when gentle finger pressure beneath the right subcostal arch and below the margin of the liver causes pain during deep inspiration. This classic (but not always present) sign of acute cholecystitis may also occur in hepatitis.
- **Nausea** is an unpleasant feeling that typically precedes vomiting.
- **Occult blood** is an amount of blood so small that it can be seen or detected only by a chemical test or microscopic examination.
- **Pica** refers to the craving and ingestion of normally inedible substances, such as plaster, charcoal, clay, wool, ashes, paint, and dirt.
- **Polyphagia** is consuming abnormally large amounts of food.
- **Polydipsia** is chronic, excessive thirst.
- **Rebound tenderness,** also referred to as **Blumberg's sign,** is pain that occurs when a hand pressing on the abdomen is suddenly released.
- **Rectal tenesmus** is a spasmodic contraction of the anal sphincter with a persistent urge to defecate and involuntary, ineffective straining. This occurs in inflamma-

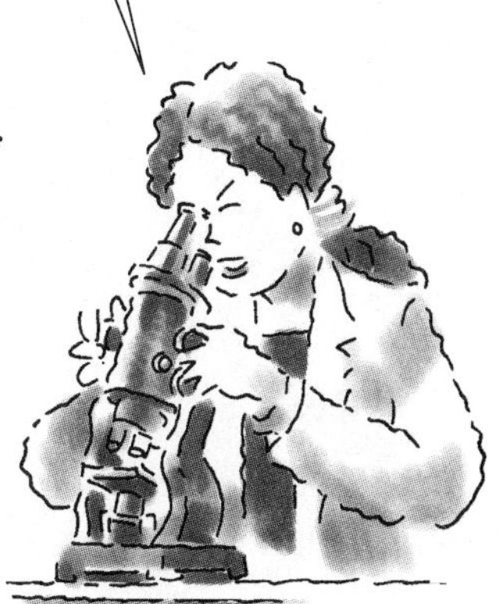
Occult blood refers to minute amounts of blood that can be seen or detected only by a chemical test or microscopic examination.

tory bowel disorders, such as ulcerative colitis and Crohn's disease, and in rectal tumors.

- **Rigidity** describes a stiff abdominal wall, sometimes called a "boardlike abdomen."
- **Rovsing's sign,** named after the Copenhagen surgeon Niels Rovsing (1862-1927), who first described this symptom, occurs in acute appendicitis. Pressure on the left lower quadrant of the abdomen will cause pain in the right lower quadrant.
- **Steatorrhea** is excessive fat in the feces that floats and is frothy and foul-smelling.
- **Tympany** is a clear, hollow, drumlike sound heard when palpating the abdomen.
- **Vomiting** is forcibly expelling the contents of the stomach through the mouth. Vomiting can be described as:

–**cyclic** (recurring attacks of vomiting)
–**dry** (attempt to vomit without emesis)
–**projectile** (ejected with great force).

Diagnostic tests

Below are diagnostic tests used to identify GI disorders.

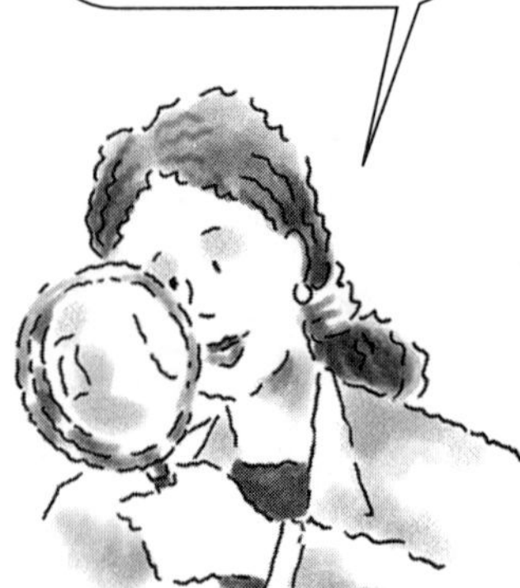
The different serum tests look at the levels of substances in the blood. For example, a serum bilirubin test measures bilirubin level.

Blood tests

Serum studies of enzymes, proteins, and formed elements are used to investigate disorders involving the liver, pancreas, gallbladder, and intestinal tract. You'll see the following tests ordered most often:

- The **alkaline phosphatase test** measures the enzyme activity of several alkaline phosphatase isoenzymes found in the liver, bone, kidneys, intestines, and biliary system.
- The ***Helicobacter pylori*** **antibodies test** checks for the presence of *H. pylori,* which is associated with chronic gastritis and idiopathic chronic duodenal ulceration.
- The **serum amylase test** measures the level of the pancreatic enzyme alpha-amylase, which is active in the digestion of starch and glycogen. Amylase is released with pancreatic damage.

- The **serum bilirubin test** measures serum levels of bilirubin, the main pigment in bile and the major product of hemoglobin breakdown.
- The **serum lipase test** measures the amount of lipase in the blood; large amounts indicate pancreatic damage.
- The **total cholesterol test** measures the circulating levels of free cholesterol and cholesterol esters.

Radiologic and imaging tests

Tests that use X-rays, electromagnetic waves, and sound waves to create images of internal structures of the GI system and its function include:

- **Abdominal X-ray,** also called a **flat plate of the abdomen,** helps detect and evaluate tumors and other abdominal disorders.
- **Barium enema** is the radiographic examination of the large intestine after rectal instillation of barium, a radiopaque contrast medium.
- **Barium swallow** is the radiographic examination of the throat and esophagus after ingestion of a radiopaque contrast medium.
- **Cholangiogram** is an X-ray of the gallbladder and biliary duct system that is obtained by injecting a radiopaque contrast medium.
- **Computerized tomography (CT) scan** translates the action of multiple X-ray beams into three-dimensional images.
- **Contrast radiography** is a general term that describes several procedures that use a radiopaque contrast medium to accentuate differences among densities of fat, air, soft tissue, and bone.
- **Endoscopic retrograde cholangiopancreatography** is a radiographic examination of the pancreatic ducts and hepatobiliary tree after injection of a contrast medium into the **duodenal papilla** (small nipplelike elevation). This is done by use of a endoscope guided by use of fluoroscopy. (See *I'd rather say ERCP,* page 182.)
- **Liver-spleen scan** uses a gamma-ray camera to record the distribution of radioactivity within the liver and spleen after injection of a radioactive colloid.
- **Magnetic resonance imaging (MRI)** creates images by computer analysis of electromagnetic waves directed into the tissues.

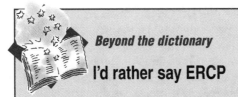

Beyond the dictionary

I'd rather say ERCP

Endoscopic retrograde cholangiopancreatography (ERCP) is a real mouthful, but this word is easy to dissect: **Endoscopic** refers to the optical instrument used in the procedure. **Retrograde** means *moving against the usual flow* and refers to dye injected the wrong way in the ampulla of Vater. **Cholangio-** refers to the biliary tract, **pancrea** means *pancreas*, and **-graphy** is a recording. Therefore, ERCP is a recording of the function of the biliary tract and pancreas.

- **Percutaneous transhepatic cholangiography** examines the biliary system in which a radiopaque contrast medium is introduced through a catheter inserted through the skin into the liver.
- **Ultrasonography** creates images of deep structures of the body by computer analysis of ultrasonic (sound) waves directed into the tissues.
- **Upper GI and small bowel series** involves the fluoroscopic examination of the esophagus, stomach, and small intestine after the patient ingests a contrast medium.

Other tests

Other tests used to diagnose abnormalities of the GI system include:

- **Basal gastric secretion test** measures basal acid secretion during fasting by aspirating stomach contents through a nasogastric tube.
- **Breath hydrogen analysis** is a simple method of detecting lactose intolerance.
- **Colonoscopy** is an endoscopic examination of the colon.
- **Endoscopy** is a visual inspection of a body cavity using an optical instrument called an **endoscope.**
- **Esophageal acidity test** evaluates the competence of the lower esophageal sphincter — the major barrier to reflux — by measuring the pH within the esophagus with an electrode that is attached to a special catheter.

• **Fecal lipids test** is used to detect excessive excretion of lipids in patients with signs of malabsorption.
• **Gastric acid stimulation test** measures the secretion of gastric acid for 1 hour after subcutaneous injection of a drug that stimulates gastric acid output.
• **Laparoscopy** is an endoscopic examination of the interior of the peritoneal cavity.
• **Percutaneous liver biopsy** involves aspiration of a core of liver tissue for analysis.
• **Peritoneal fluid analysis** examines a specimen of peritoneal fluid obtained by paracentesis for appearance, red blood cell and white blood cell counts, cytologic studies, microbiologic studies for bacteria and fungi, and determinations of protein, glucose, amylase, ammonia, and alkaline phosphatase levels.
• **Sigmoidoscopy** is an endoscopic examination of the sigmoid colon.
• **Stool culture** is a bacteriologic examination of the feces.
• **Urine bilirubin test** detects abnormally high urine concentrations of direct bilirubin, possibly indicating liver disease.
• **Urine urobilinogen test** detects impaired liver function by measuring urine levels of urobilinogen, which results from the reduction of bilirubin by intestinal bacteria.

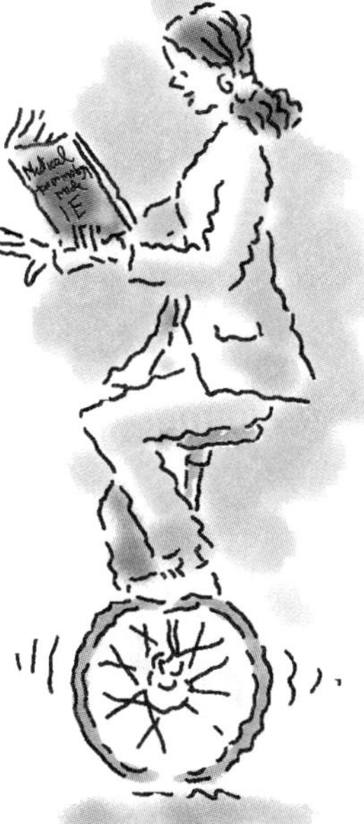
Sigmoidoscopy is an endoscopic examination of the sigmoid colon.

GI disorders

Here are descriptions of disorders of the organs of the GI system.

Mouth and esophagus

The following are important terms used to describe disorders of the upper alimentary canal:
• **Esophageal atresia** refers to a closed esophagus.
• **Esophageal diverticula** are hollowed outpouchings in the esophageal wall.
• **Esophageal stricture** is a narrowing of the esophagus.
• **Esophageal varices** are enlarged, torturous veins in the lower esophagus that are caused by portal hypertension.

- **Esophagitis** is the inflammation of the mucous membrane that lines the esophagus.
- **Gastroesophageal reflux** refers to the backflow of gastric or duodenal contents into the esophagus.
- **Gingivitis** is an inflammation of the gums.
- **Glossitis** is an inflammation of the tongue.
- **Hiatal hernia** is the protrusion of the stomach through a structural defect in the diaphragm at the esophageal opening.
- **Mallory-Weiss syndrome** refers to lacerations in the mucous membrane at the esophagogastric junction that result in massive bleeding. The syndrome is typically preceded by vomiting.
- **Periodontitis** refers to progression of gingivitis involving an inflammation of the oral mucosa.
- **Stomatitis** is an inflammation of the mouth.
- **Tracheoesophageal fistula** is an abnormal connection between the trachea and the esophagus.
- **Vincent's angina,** also known as **trench mouth,** causes necrosis and ulceration of the gums.

Stomatitis looks like it may be related to **stomach** — and it is. The root shared by both words, ***stoma,*** means *mouth, or opening.*

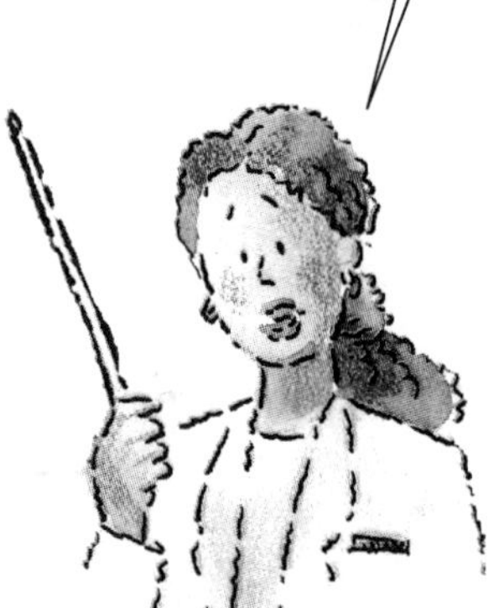

Stomach and intestines

Here are terms that relate to diseases and abnormalities of the stomach and intestines:

- **Celiac disease** is a chronic disease in which an individual can't tolerate foods containing gluten or wheat protein.
- **Crohn's disease** is a chronic inflammatory bowel disease that usually involves the proximal portion of the colon and, less commonly, the terminal ileum. It's named after the American surgeon Burrill Crohn (1884-1983), who first described it in 1932.
- **Diverticular disease** refers to bulging pouches **(diverticula)** in the GI wall — most often in the sigmoid colon — that push the mucosal lining through the surrounding muscle. (See *A diversion on diverticulum.*) Diverticular disease has two clinical forms:

–**Diverticulitis** is the inflammation of one or more diverticula.

–**Diverticulosis** is the presence of diverticula without accompanying inflammation.

- **Gastritis** refers to inflammation of the stomach and stomach lining.

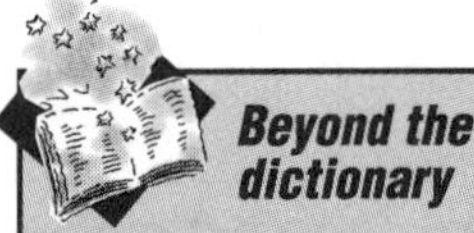

A diversion on diverticulum

A **diverticulum** is, in fact, a *diversion.* The small pouches divert contents of the GI tract; this action gives the structures their name.

• **Gastroenteritis** is inflammation of the lining of the stomach and intestines that accompanies numerous GI disorders.
• **Hirschsprung's disease,** also called **congenital megacolon,** is a congenital disorder of the large intestine characterized by the absence or marked reduction of nerve cells in the colorectal wall, which results in impaired intestinal motility and constipation.
• **Inactive colon** is a state of chronic constipation that, if left untreated, may lead to fecal impaction.
• **Inguinal hernia** is protrusion of the large or small intestine, omentum, or bladder into the inguinal canal resulting from weakened abdominal muscles, traumatic injury, or aging. The hernia is:
–**reducible** if it can be moved back into place easily
–**incarcerated** if it can't be reduced
–**strangulated** if a portion of the herniated intestine becomes twisted or swollen so that blood flow is stopped.

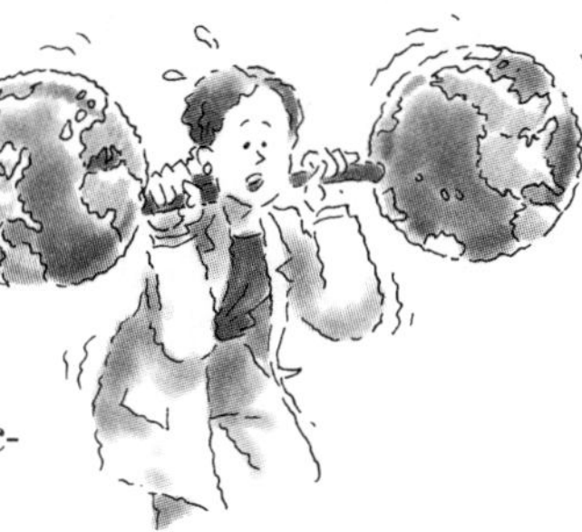
I hope this hernia is reducible!

• **Intestinal obstruction** occurs when the **lumen** (opening) of the bowel is partly or fully blocked. Obstruction is classified as mechanical or nonmechanical:
–**Mechanical obstruction** results from foreign bodies or compression of the bowel wall.
–**Nonmechanical obstruction** results from physiologic disturbances, such as paralytic ileus, electrolyte imbalance, and blood clots in the mesenteric vessels.
• **Intussusception** refers to a telescoping of a portion of bowel into an adjacent distal portion.
• **Irritable bowel syndrome** is a condition characterized by diarrhea resulting from increased bowel motility alternating with constipation.
• **Necrotizing enterocolitis** is characterized by diffuse or patchy intestinal necrosis and is accompanied by infection in about one-third of cases.
• **Paralytic ileus** is a physiologic form of intestinal obstruction that usually develops in the small bowel after abdominal surgery.
• **Peptic ulcer** is a disruption in the gastric or duodenal lining that occurs when normal defense mechanisms are overwhelmed or impaired by acid or pepsin.
• **Peritonitis** is an acute or chronic inflammation of the **peritoneum** (the membrane that lines the abdominal cavity and covers visceral organs).

• **Pseudomembranous enterocolitis** is an acute inflammation and **necrosis** (tissue death) of the small and large intestines, usually affecting only the mucosa.
• **Ulcerative colitis** is a chronic, inflammatory disease that affects the mucosa of the colon and produces edema and ulcerations. It typically begins in the rectum and sigmoid colon and commonly extends upward into the entire colon. It rarely affects the small intestine.
• **Volvulus** is a twisting of intestine at least 180 degrees on its mesentery, resulting in blood vessel compression and ischemia.

Anus and rectum

Disorders of the anus and rectum include:
• **Anal fissure** is a laceration or crack in the lining of the anus.
• **Anorectal abscess** is a localized collection of pus due to inflammation of the soft tissue near the rectum or anus.
• **Anorectal fistula** is an abnormal opening in the anal skin that may communicate with the rectum. Inflammation caused by an anorectal abscess may cause the fistula to form.
• **Anorectal stenosis** is narrowing of the anorectal sphincter.
• **Anorectal stricture** occurs when the anorectal lumen size decreases.
• **Hemorrhoids** are varicosities in the veins of the rectum or anus that result in swelling and pain.
• **Pilonidal cyst** is a hair-containing dermoid cyst that forms in the midline gluteal fold.
• **Proctitis** is an acute or chronic inflammation of the rectal mucosa.
• **Pruritus ani** is perianal itching, irritation, or superficial burning.
• **Rectal polyps** are masses of tissue that rise above the mucosal membrane and protrude into the GI tract.
• **Rectal prolapse** is the circumferential protrusion of one or more layers of the mucous membrane through the anus.

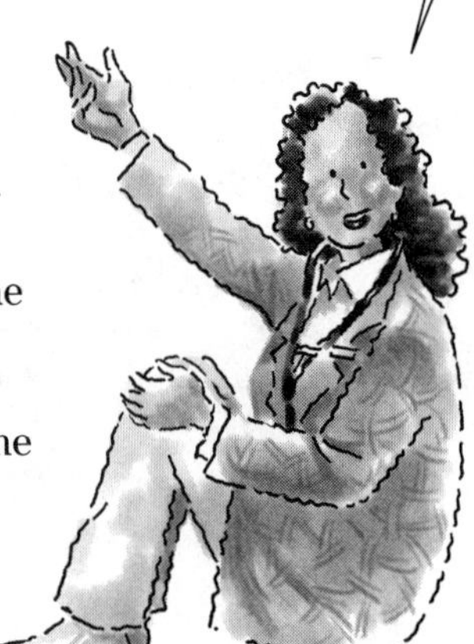
Proctitis is an acute or chronic inflammation of the rectal mucosa.

Accessory organs

Disorders of the appendix, liver, gallbladder, and pancreas include:

- **Appendicitis** is an inflammation of the vermiform appendix due to an obstruction.
- **Cholecystitis** is acute or chronic inflammation of the gallbladder, typically caused by gallstones.
- **Cholelithiasis** is the presence of gallstones in the gallbladder. (See *Lithos = stone.*)
- **Choledocholithiasis** occurs when gallstones pass from the gallbladder and lodge in the common bile duct, causing complete or partial obstruction.
- **Cirrhosis** refers to a chronic, degenerative liver disease in which the lobes are covered with fibrous tissue, the liver parenchyma degenerates, and the lobules are infiltrated with fat.
- **Fatty liver,** also known as **steatosis,** is the accumulation of triglycerides and other fats in liver cells.
- **Hepatic coma** is a neurologic syndrome that develops as a complication of hepatic encephalopathy.
- **Hepatic encephalopathy** is a degenerative brain condition caused by advanced liver disease.
- **Hepatitis** occurs in two forms, nonviral and viral:

–**Nonviral hepatitis** is usually caused by exposure to toxins or drugs.

–**Viral hepatitis** is an acute inflammation of the liver marked by liver-cell destruction, necrosis, and **autolysis** (destruction of tissue by enzymes).

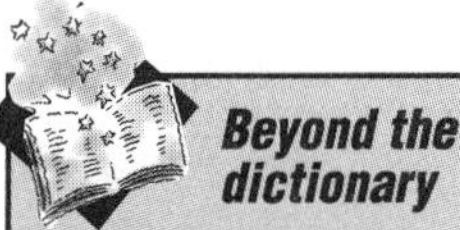

Beyond the dictionary

Lithos = stone

Cholecystitis is a combination of Greek terms: ***chole*** means *bile*; ***cyst*** means *bladder*, and ***-itis*** means *inflammation*. So it makes sense that cholecystitis is *inflammation of the gallbladder*.

Now take it one step further. ***Lithos*** is the Greek term for *stone*, so it makes sense that **cholelithiasis** is the term for *gallstones*.

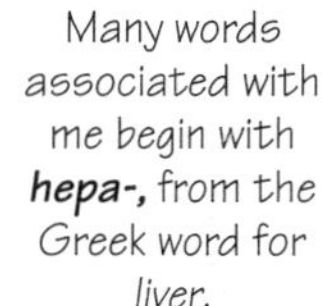

Many words associated with me begin with **hepa-,** from the Greek word for *liver*.

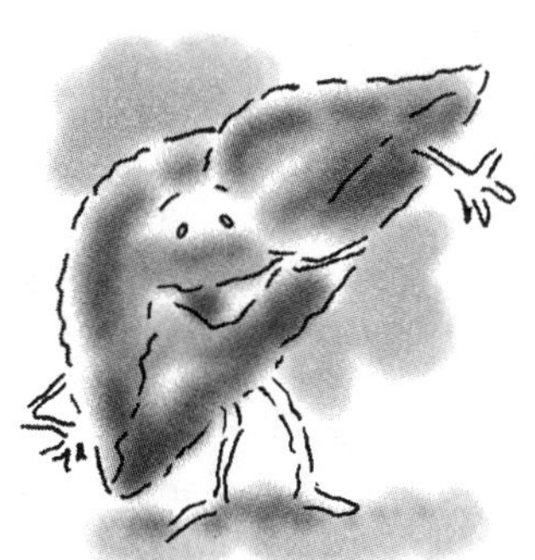

Assessment findings are similar for the different types of hepatitis. The five forms of viral hepatitis are:
–**type A,** which is spread by direct contact through the oral-fecal route
–**type B,** which is transmitted by contaminated serum through blood transfusion, needles, I.V. drug use, and direct contact with body fluids
–**type C,** which is spread through needle sticks, blood transfusion, and I.V. drug use
–**type D,** which is found only in patients with acute or chronic episodes of hepatitis B and requires the presence of hepatitis B surface antigen (hepatitis D is rare, except among I.V. drug users)
–**type E,** which is transmitted by the oral-fecal and waterborne routes, much like type A (because this virus is inconsistently shed in the feces, detection is difficult).

- **Pancreatitis** is an acute or chronic inflammation of the pancreas.
- **Portal hypertension** is increased pressure in the portal vein as a result of obstruction of blood flow through the liver.
- **Wilson's disease** is a rare inherited metabolic disorder characterized by excessive copper retention in the liver, brain, kidneys, and corneas. These deposits of copper eventually lead to hepatic failure.

Lavage and **gavage** are two similar sounding words that can be easily confused. Just remember, **lavage** means the stomach is being *laundered;* **gavage** means you're *giving* food to the stomach.

Treatments

Here are terms identifying surgical procedures and other treatments to correct GI disorders.

GI tubes

Here are terms related to GI tubes used to treat patients with GI disorders:

- **Gastric lavage** is irrigation or washing of the stomach with sterile water or saline solution using a nasogastric tube.
- **Gavage** is feeding a patient through a stomach tube.
- **Intestinal decompression** removes fluids and gas from the intestine by the insertion of one of several types of tubes:

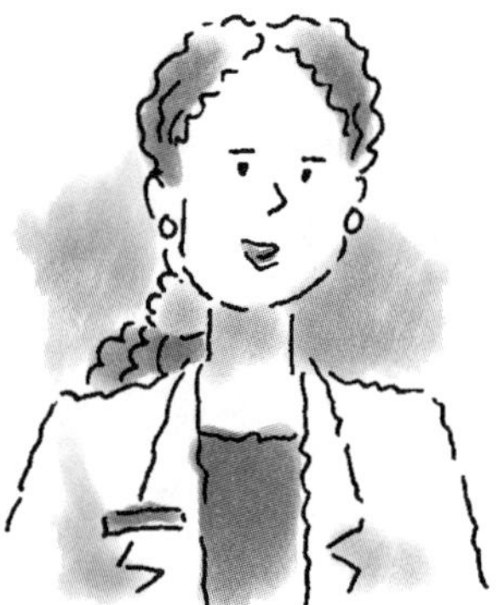

–The **Miller-Abbott tube** is a double-lumen tube in which one lumen contains a weighted balloon to ease passage and the other lumen facilitates drainage.
–The **Harris tube,** used for gastric and intestinal decompression, is a mercury-weighted single-lumen tube that is inserted through the nose and carried through the digestive tract by gravity.
–The **Cantor tube,** used to relieve obstruction in the small intestine, is a double-lumen nasoenteric tube. One lumen is used to inflate the distal balloon with air; the other, to instill mercury to weight the tube. The tube also allows for aspiration of intestinal contents.

- **Nasogastric intubation** is insertion of a tube into the stomach through the nose.
- **Sengstaken-Blakemore intubation** is insertion of a triple-lumen catheter used to stop hemorrhaging from esophageal varices. Two lumens end in balloons; one is inflated in the stomach to hold the catheter in place and compress the vessels around the cardia, and the other is inflated in the esophagus to exert pressure against varices in the wall of the esophagus. The third lumen is used to **aspirate** (withdraw) stomach contents.

Pharyngeal and esophageal surgeries

Surgical procedures performed on the esophagus include:

- **cricopharyngeal myotomy** — a partial or total incision of the cricopharyngeal muscle that relieves diverticula or severe cricopharyngeal muscle spasm
- **esophagectomy** — removal of part of the esophagus.
- **esophagogastrectomy** — removal of all or part of the stomach and esophagus
- **esophagogastrostomy** — removal of a portion of the esophagus then connecting the remaining healthy portion to the stomach
- **esophagojejunostomy** — attachment of the jejunum to the esophagus to provide a bypass for food for patients with esophageal stricture.

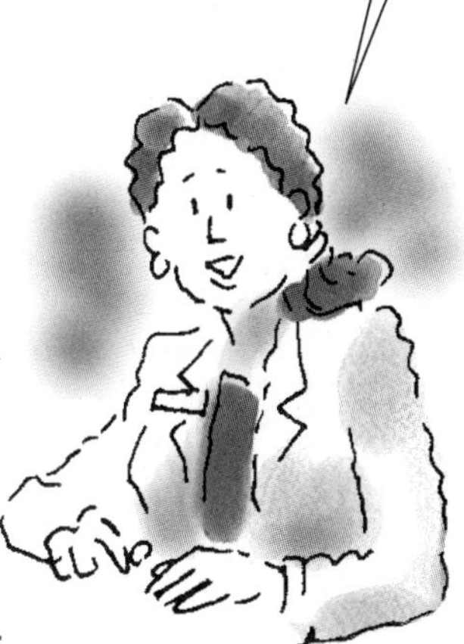

Remember, the suffix ***-ectomy*** means *removal of,* and the suffix ***-ostomy*** means *creation of an opening.*

Gastric and abdominal surgeries

Surgical procedures on the stomach are explained below:

- **Antrectomy** is the removal of the **antrum,** the lower part of the stomach, which produces gastric acid.

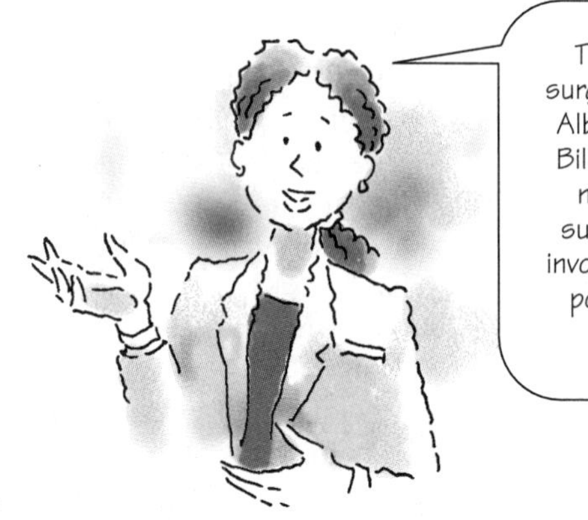

The Austrian surgeon Christian Albert Theodore Billroth gave his name to two surgeries. Both involve removing a portion of the stomach.

- **Billroth I** is a partial removal of the distal portion of the stomach; the remaining stomach is connected to the duodenum.
- **Billroth II** is a surgical excision of a portion of the stomach with connection of the remaining portion to the jejunum.
- **Gastrostomy** is the creation of a hole into the stomach through the abdominal wall to insert an feeding tube.
- **Laparotomy** is a surgical opening of the abdomen. (See *Gastric lingo*.)
- **Pyloroplasty** is surgical enlargement of the pylorus to improve drainage of gastric contents into the small bowel.
- **Total gastrectomy** is removal of the entire stomach.
- **Vagotomy with gastroenterostomy** is removal of the vagus nerves and creation of a **stoma** (artificial opening) for gastric drainage.

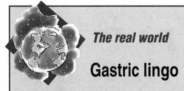

The real world

Gastric lingo

Let's run another lap

In practice, people commonly refer to an **exploratory laparotomy** as an *exploratory lap.* So you might hear someone say, "We need to take this patient for an exploratory lap."

NG tube

Rarely will you hear someone refer to a **nasogastric tube** by its full name. In practice, it's simply referred to as an *NG tube.*

Bowel surgery

Listed below are important surgical terms concerning the small intestine, large intestine, and colon:

- **Abdominal perineal resection** is a procedure in which a colostomy is created and the distal sigmoid colon, rectum, and anus are removed.
- **Anastomosis** is a surgical procedure in which two blood vessels, ducts, or other tubelike structures are joined to allow flow of substances between them.
- **Colectomy** is excision of a portion of the colon.
- **Hemicolectomy** is the removal of one-half or less of the colon.
- **Hemorrhoidectomy** is the surgical excision of a hemorrhoid.
- **Ileostomy** is the creation of an opening between the ileum and the abdominal wall through which fecal matter is expelled.

Colostomy

A **colostomy,** bowel surgery that creates an opening between the colon and the abdominal wall through which feces are expelled, may be created in different portions of the intestine and structured several ways.

Different locations

Named according to their location in the colon, the four types of colostomy are:

- **ascending**
- **transverse**
- **descending**
- **sigmoid.**

Different structures

These are the main types of colostomy construction:

- A **double-barrel colostomy** creates two separate stomas — usually temporarily — on the abdominal wall. The proximal stoma is the functioning end and is continuous with the upper GI tract. The distal stoma, also referred to as a **mucous fistula,** opens into the nonfunctioning section of the colon that is continuous with the rectum.

• An **end colostomy** creates a single stoma on the abdomen created from the end of the colon, which is brought out through an opening in the abdominal wall.
• A **loop colostomy** involves bringing a loop of bowel through an incision in the abdominal wall.

Liver surgery

Important terms concerning liver surgery are listed below:
• **Hepatic lobectomy** is removal of a lobe of the liver.
• **LeVeen shunt** is a plastic tube implanted to shunt ascites fluid from the peritoneal cavity through the jugular vein to the superior vena cava.
• **Liver resection** is removal of a portion of the diseased or damaged liver tissue.
• **Liver transplant** is reserved for patients with a life-threatening liver disorder that doesn't respond to other treatment.
• **Partial hepatectomy** is excision of a portion of the liver.
• **Transjugular intrahepatic portosystemic shunt** is a nonsurgical procedure in which the right internal jugular vein is accessed and a metallic, flexible stent is inserted into a new pathway created by balloon dilation of the tissue between the hepatic and portal veins in the liver. This artificial shunt creates a new pathway for blood flow and reduces portal hypertension.

Let me help with **transjugular intrahepatic portosystemic shunt. Transjugular** means the catheter is inserted through the jugular; **intrahepatic** means it goes through the hepatic vein; **porto** means it then goes through the portal vein; **systemic** means it then shunts blood into systemic circulation.

Gallbladder and appendix surgery

Surgical procedures performed on the gallbladder and appendix are explained below:
• **Appendectomy** is the removal of the vermiform appendix.
• **Cholecystectomy** is removal of the gallbladder. (See *Open chole.*)
• **Cholecystoduodenostomy** is anastomosis of the gallbladder and duodenum.
• **Choledochojejunostomy** is anastomosis of the common bile duct to the jejunum of the small intestine.

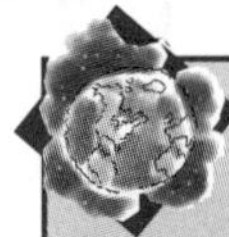

The real world

Open chole

You may hear a conventional **cholecystectomy** be referred to as an *open chole,* pronounced KOHLEE. This means an open abdominal incision was required to remove the gallbladder, as opposed to **laparoscopic surgery,** which doesn't require an abdominal incision.

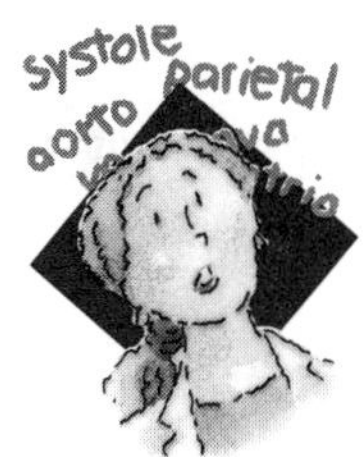

Vocabulary builders

At a crossroads

Completing this crossword puzzle will help you digest GI system terms. Good luck!

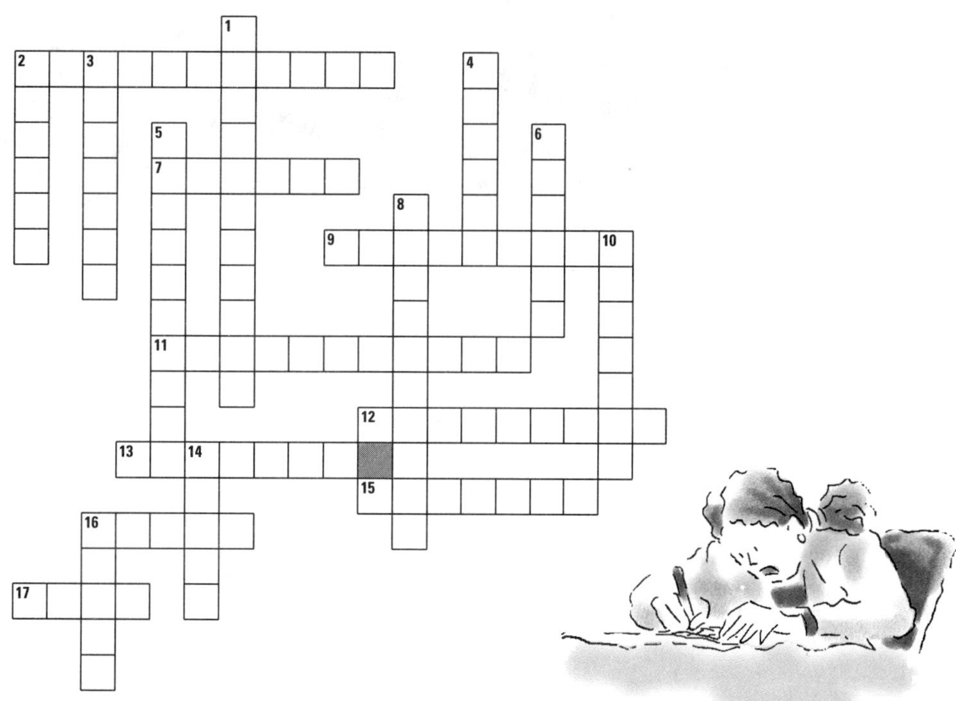

Across

2. Rhythmic contraction and relaxation of smooth muscle in the alimentary canal
7. Liver's functional unit
9. Inflammation of the tongue
11. Another name for Vincent's angina (two words)
12. Difficult or painful swallowing
13. Clear, hollow, drumlike sound heard on abdominal palpation
15. Greek word that means *little jug*
16. Saclike structure that makes up the first few inches of the large intestine
17. Yellow-green liquid that breaks down fats and neutralizes gastric secretions

Down

1. Pear-shaped organ nestled under the liver
2. Roof of the mouth
3. Eponym for diagnostic sign of appendicitis
4. Enlarged portion of the stomach above and to the left of the esophageal opening
5. Canal also called the GI tract
6. Root from Greek that means *stomach*
8. Growling sound in the stomach that indicates hunger
10. Part of the colon named after a Greek letter
14. Also called the buccal cavity
16. Acute abdominal pain

Answers are on page 196.

Match game

Eponyms can be confusing. There are lots of eponyms for GI structures, disorders, and tests. See if you can match each person to their discovery.

Clues	Choices
1. ________ Sphincter	A. Karl Wilhelm von Kupffer, German anatomist
2. Ampulla of _______	B. Paul Langerhans, German doctor
3. _______ cells	C. Ruggero Oddi, Italian doctor
4. Islets of _______	D. Burrill Crohn, American surgeon
5. _______'s disease	E. Abraham Vater, German anatomist

Maybe we should call this Joy's confusion.

Answers are on page 196.

Scrambled or overeasy

Fill in the answers for the following questions, then unscramble the circled letters to find the answer to the puzzle.

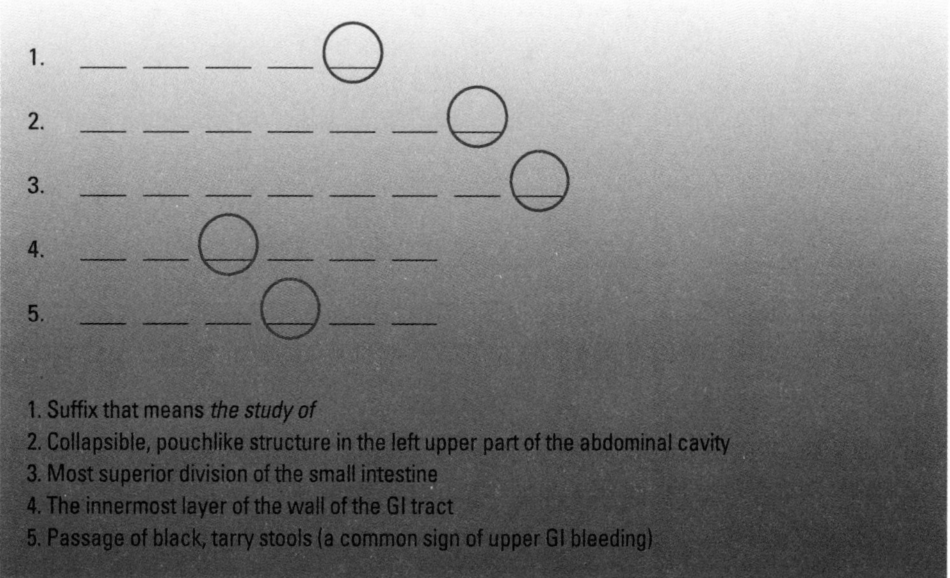

1. Suffix that means *the study of*
2. Collapsible, pouchlike structure in the left upper part of the abdominal cavity
3. Most superior division of the small intestine
4. The innermost layer of the wall of the GI tract
5. Passage of black, tarry stools (a common sign of upper GI bleeding)

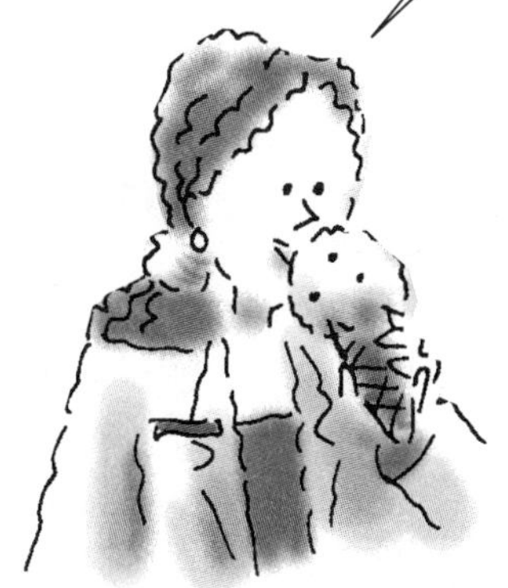

Sure, it looks and tastes like ice cream now, but my stomach will soon break it down into this semifluid substance.

Answers are on page 196.

Answers

At a crossroads

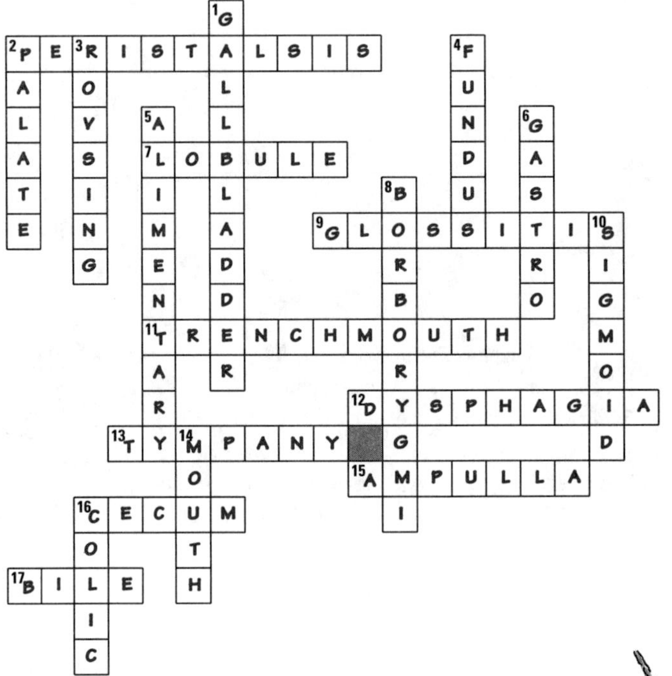

Match game

1. C; 2. E; 3. A; 4. B; 5. D.

Scrambled or overeasy

1. Ology; 2. Stomach; 3. Duodenum; 4. Mucosa; 5. Melena.
Answer to puzzle — Chyme

Urinary system

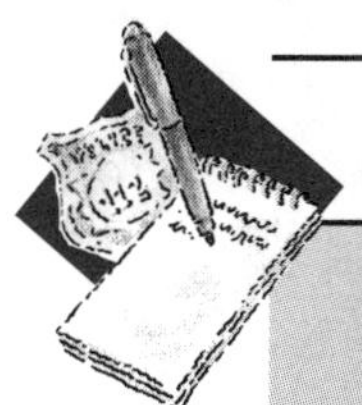

Just the facts

In this chapter, you'll review:

- terminology related to the structure and function of the urinary system
- terminology needed for physical examination
- tests that help diagnose urinary disorders
- common urinary disorders and their treatments.

Urinary structure and function

The **urinary tract** is the body's water treatment plant. It filters the blood and collects and expels the resulting liquid waste products as urine. To help you understand many of the terms relating to this waste control system, three key root words deserve special attention.

In the key of pee

The first key root is the syllable ***ur-*** or its other forms, ***urin-*** or ***uro-***. This term derives from the Greek verb ***ourein,*** which means *to urinate.* Appropriately, the study of the urinary system is called **urology.**

Two keys to the kidneys

The second and third key terms refer to the kidneys. The second is the adjective **renal.** This word derives from ***ren,*** the Latin word for *kidney.* The kidneys are the filter of our bodies' water treatment plant and perform a number of other vital functions, including:

- regulating acid-base balance
- regulating electrolyte balance

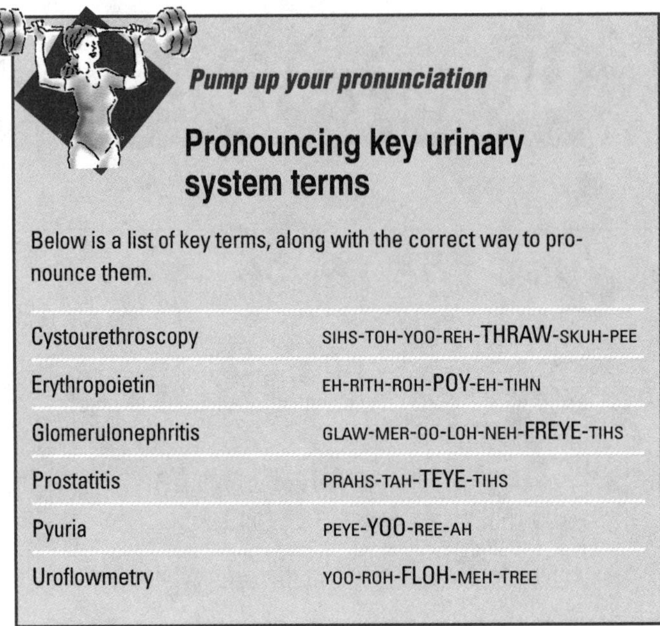

Pump up your pronunciation

Pronouncing key urinary system terms

Below is a list of key terms, along with the correct way to pronounce them.

Cystourethroscopy	SIHS-TOH-YOO-REH-THRAW-SKUH-PEE
Erythropoietin	EH-RITH-ROH-POY-EH-TIHN
Glomerulonephritis	GLAW-MER-OO-LOH-NEH-FREYE-TIHS
Prostatitis	PRAHS-TAH-TEYE-TIHS
Pyuria	PEYE-YOO-REE-AH
Uroflowmetry	YOO-ROH-FLOH-MEH-TREE

- regulating blood pressure
- aiding in red blood cell (RBC) formation.

The word **renal** can show up in a variety of medical contexts.

A medical subspecialization within urology focuses on just the renal system. The name of this specialization, **nephrology,** employs the Greek word for *kidney*, ***nephros,*** instead of the Latin ***ren. Nephro-,*** or ***nephr-,*** our third key term, is identical in meaning with ***ren,*** and you'll find many words containing these two roots side by side. (See *Pronouncing key urinary system terms.*)

Kidneys

The **kidneys** are bean-shaped, highly vascular organs located at the small of the back on either side of the vertebral column between the 12th thoracic and 3rd lumbar vertebrae. The right kidney, crowded by the liver, is positioned slightly lower than the left. Although each kidney is only about 4″ (10.2 cm) long, these organs are complicated structures with many functioning units. They receive about 20% of the blood pumped by the heart each minute.

Adrenal gland influence

Atop each kidney lies an **adrenal gland.** These glands affect the renal system by influencing blood pressure and sodium and water retention by the kidneys.

Checking in and checking out

The kidneys receive waste-filled blood from the **renal artery,** a large branch of the abdominal **aorta.** After passing through a complicated network of smaller blood vessels and filtering structures within the kidneys, the filtered blood returns to the circulation by way of the **renal vein,** which empties into the **inferior vena cava,** the major ascending vein of the lower body. (See *Major structures of the kidney,* page 200.)

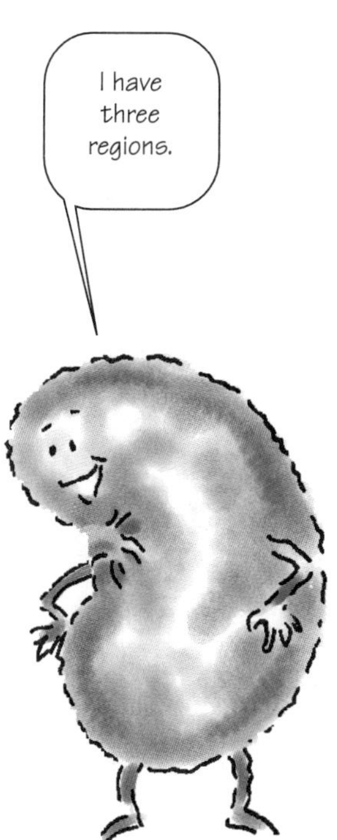

A tri-umph of organ-ization

Each kidney has three regions. The **renal cortex,** or outer region, contains blood-filtering mechanisms. The **renal medulla,** or middle region, contains 8 to 12 **renal pyramids,** which are striated wedges composed of tubular structures.

The tapered portion of each pyramid, called the **apex,** empties into a cuplike **calyx** (plural: **calyces**). The calyces channel urine from the renal pyramids into the **renal pelvis,** which is an expansion of the upper end of the ureters.

Getting to know the nephron

The **nephron** is the functional and structural unit of the kidney; each kidney contains about 1.25 million nephrons. The nephron has two main activities:

- selective resorption and secretion of ions
- mechanical filtration of fluids, wastes, electrolytes, and acids and bases.

Glom on the glomerulus

Three processes — **glomerular filtration, tubular reabsorption,** and **tubular secretion** — take place in the nephrons, ultimately leading to urine formation.

Each nephron consists of a long tubular system with a closed, bulbous end called the **glomerular capsule,** or **Bowman's capsule.** Within the capsule are a cluster of

Zoom in

Major structures of the kidney

The illustration below shows the structures of the kidney, which plays a major role in the elimination of wastes and excess ions (in urine); blood filtration; acid-base, electrolyte, and blood pressure regulation; and blood cell formation.

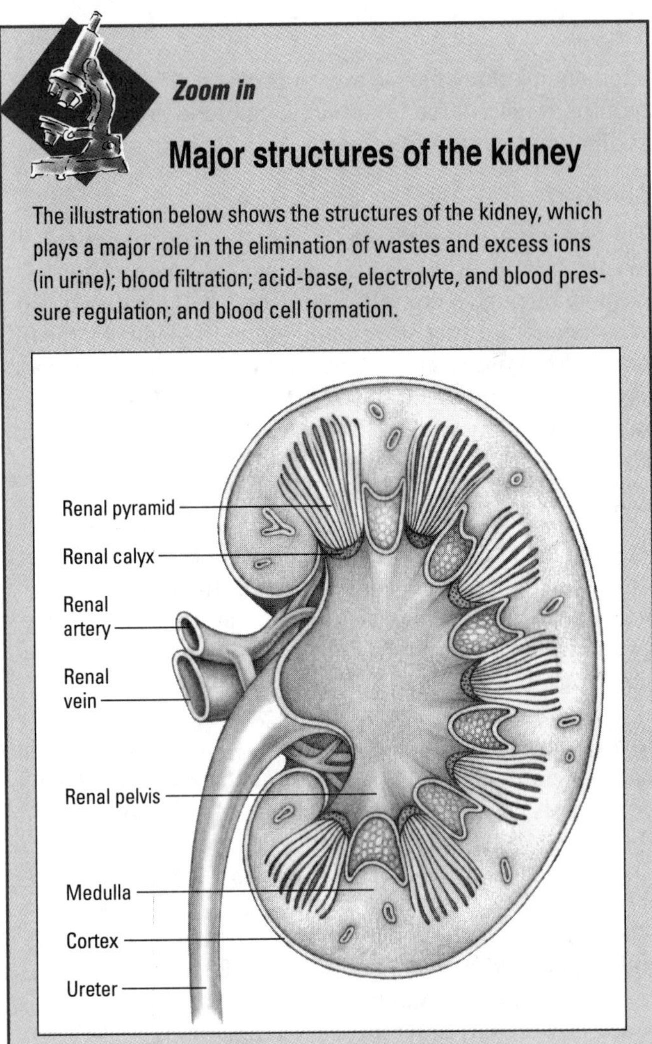

capillaries called the **glomerulus** (plural: **glomeruli**). The glomerulus acts as a bulk filter and passes protein-free and RBC-free filtrate into the tubular system of the nephron. (See *The nephron.*)

A tireless inner tube

This tubular system has three parts through which the filtrate passes in succession:

- The **proximal convoluted tubules,** along with glomeruli, are located in the cortex of the kidney. This part of the nephron has freely permeable cell membranes

Zoom in

The nephron

The illustration below shows the structures of the nephron, which performs resorption and secretion of ions and mechanical filtration.

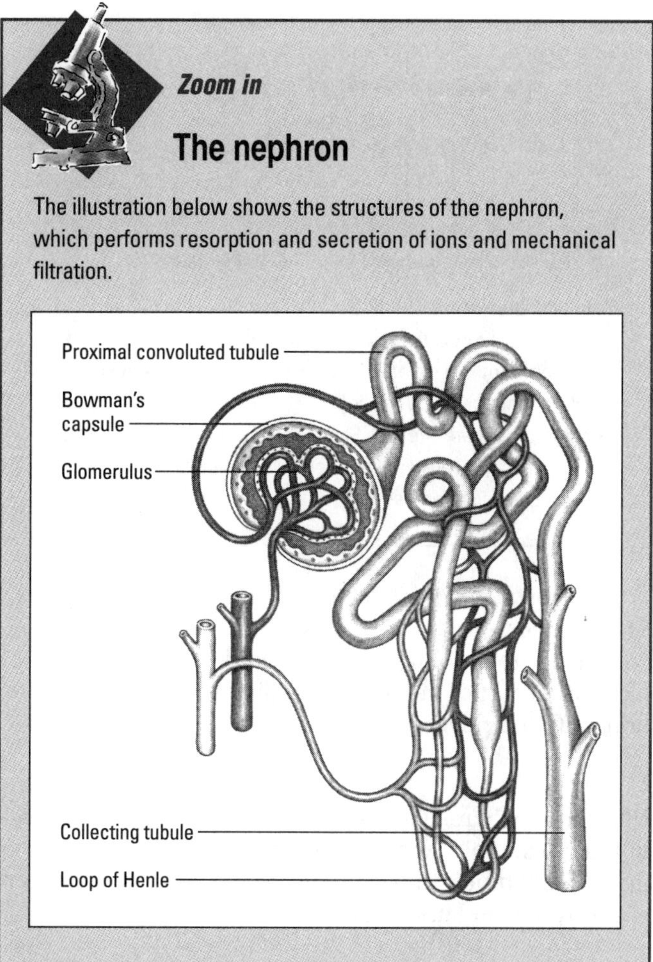

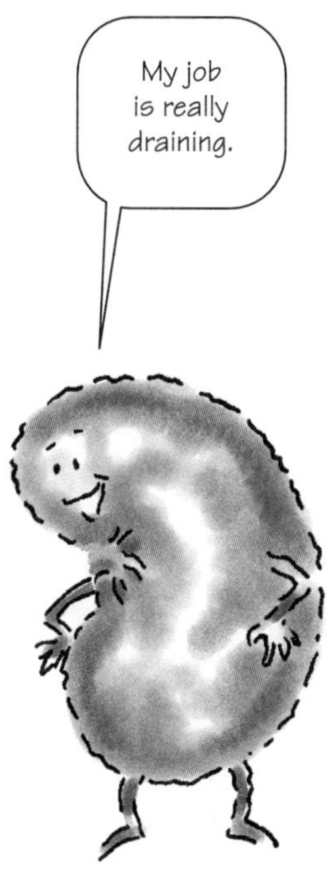

that allow glucose, amino acids, metabolites, and electrolytes from the filtrate to pass into nearby capillaries and back into the circulatory system.

- The **loop of Henle,** which forms the renal pyramid in the medulla, is a U-shaped continuation of the renal tubule. In the descending loop more water is removed from the filtrate; in the ascending part, sodium and chloride are removed to maintain osmolality.
- The **distal convoluted tubule,** like the proximal tubule, is located in the cortex. In the distal tubule, more sodium and water are removed as potassium and hydrogen ions and ammonia are introduced.

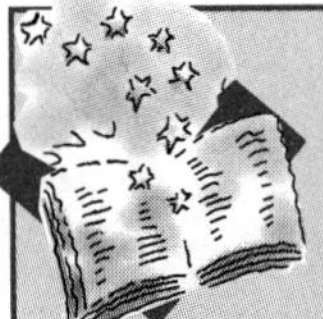

Beyond the dictionary

Two *-in* words

The words **renin** and **angiotensin** both end with the suffix ***-in,*** which derives from Latin and means *of* or *belonging to.*

Ren-* and *angiotens-

As in the word **renal,** the ***ren-*** in **renin** indicates the kidneys; the word literally means *related to the kidneys.* ***Angio-*** derives from Greek and means *blood vessel;* **tens** comes from Latin ***tensum,*** meaning *stretched.* The word **angiotensin** thus means *relating to the stretching (or tension) imposed on blood vessels,* which is measured as blood pressure.

The distal end joins the distal end of other nephrons. Their concentrated filtrate, now urine, flows into larger collecting tubules. These tubules arch back into in the medulla as part of the renal pyramids and empty the urine into the calyces.

It's a hormone thing

Hormones help regulate tubular reabsorption and secretion. For example, **antidiuretic hormone (ADH)** acts in the distal tubule and collecting ducts to increase water reabsorption and urine concentration.

Remember renin

By secreting the enzyme **renin,** the kidneys play a crucial role in regulating sodium retention and, therefore, blood pressure and fluid volume. This regulation takes place mostly through a complicated cascade of events in the **renin-angiotensin system.** (See *Two* **-in** *words.*)

In the liver, renin converts the substance **angiotensinogen** to **angiotensin I.**

Traveling to the lungs, angiotensin I is converted to **angiotensin II,** a potent vasoconstrictor that acts on the adrenal cortex to stimulate the production of the hormone aldosterone.

Retention regulation

Aldosterone affects tubular reabsorption by regulating sodium retention and helping control potassium secretion in the tubules. When serum potassium levels rise, the adrenal cortex responds by increasing aldosterone secretion. Increased aldosterone levels increase sodium and water retention and depress the formation of more renin.

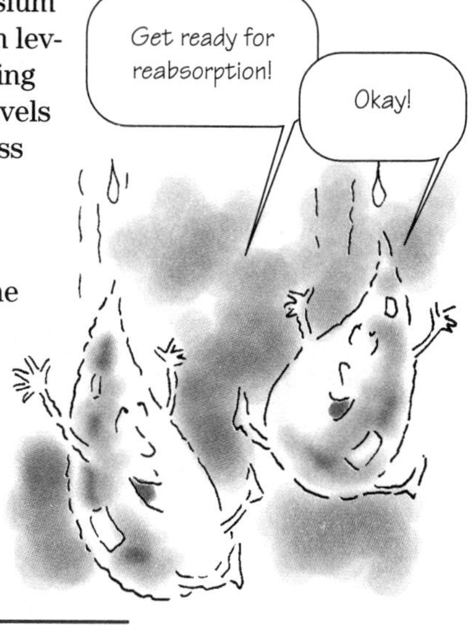
Get ready for reabsorption!
Okay!

RBC production

Low levels of oxygen in the arterial blood tell the kidneys that the body needs more RBCs to deliver oxygen to the tissues. In response, the kidneys secrete a hormone called **erythropoietin,** which travels to the bone marrow and stimulates increased RBC production. Each kidney has a **ureter,** a tube that carries urine by peristalsis from the kidney to the bladder.

Bladder

A hollow, sphere-shaped, muscular organ in the pelvis, the **bladder** stores urine. Urination results from **involuntary** (reflex) and **voluntary** (learned or intentional) processes. When urine fills the bladder, parasympathetic nerve fibers in the bladder wall cause the bladder to contract and the **internal sphincter** to relax.

You can relax now

This parasympathetic response is called the **micturition reflex.** Then the cerebrum stimulates voluntary relaxation and contraction of the **external sphincter** of the bladder, causing urine to pass into the urethra for elimination from the body.

Urethra

The **urethra** is a small duct that channels urine outside the body from the bladder. (See *The urinary tract,* page 204.)

Females

In the female, the urethra is embedded in the anterior wall of the vagina behind the **symphysis pubis** (the bony

Zoom in

The urinary tract

The illustration below shows the structures of the urinary tract.

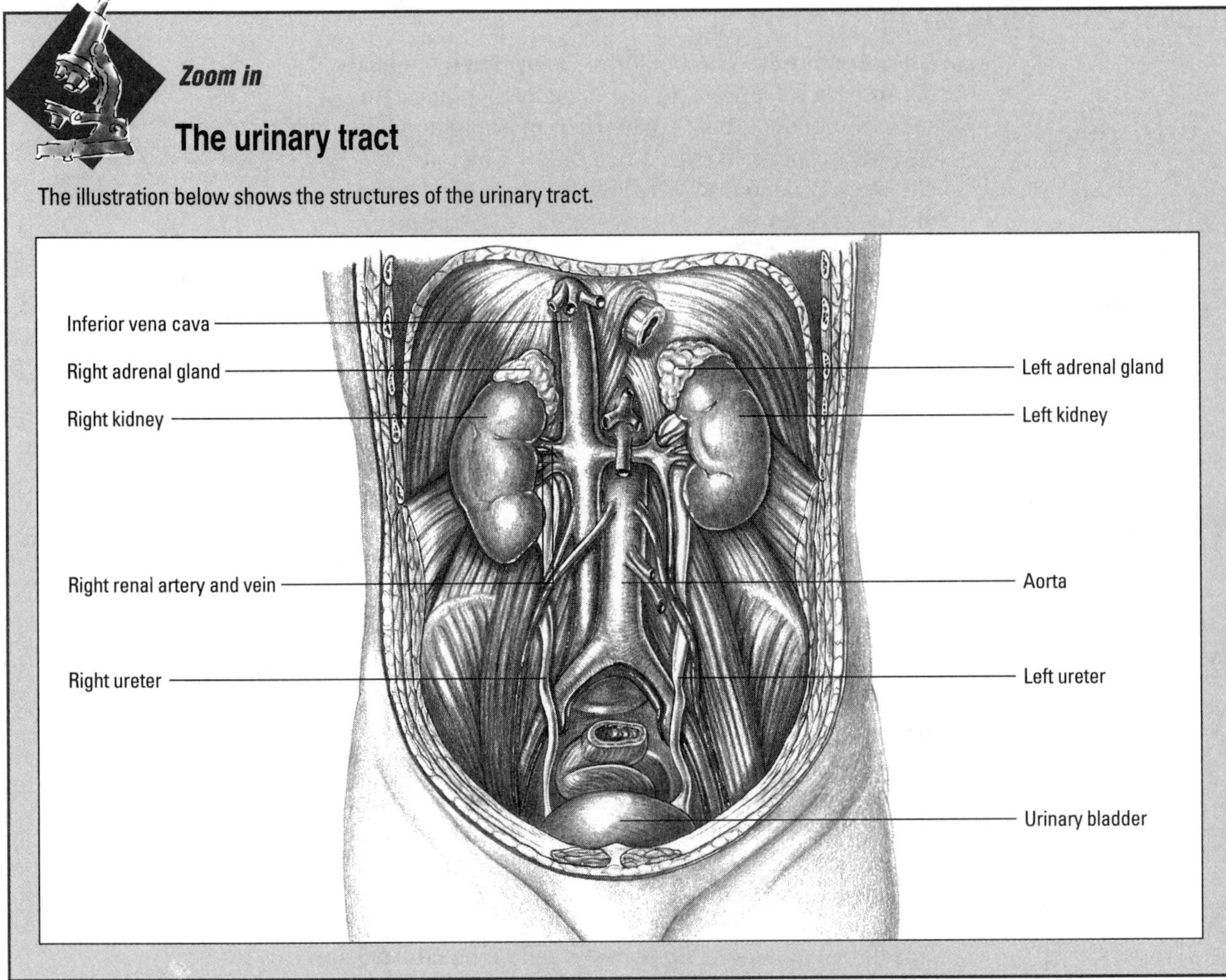

prominence under the pubic hair). The urethra connects the bladder with an external opening called the **urethral meatus,** located anterior to the vaginal opening.

Males

In the male, the urethra passes vertically through the **prostate gland,** then extends through the **urogenital diaphragm** (a triangular ligament) and the **penis.** The male urethra serves as a passageway for semen as well as urine.

Physical examination terms

Examining a patient's urinary system requires observation, palpation, and keen interviewing skills. Before you can perform a complete physical examination, you must know these essential urinary system terms:

- **Anuria** is the absence of urine production.
- **Azotemia,** or **uremia,** refers to accumulation of excess amounts of nitrogenous bodies, particularly **urea,** in the blood.
- **Dysuria** is painful or difficult urination.
- **Enuresis** refers to nighttime urinary incontinence in a girl over age 5 or boy over age 6.
- **Glycosuria** is the abnormal presence of glucose in the urine.
- **Hematuria** is the presence of blood in the urine.
- **Nocturia** refers to excessive urination at night.
- **Oliguria** is diminished urine production in relation to fluid intake, usually less than 400 ml in 24 hours.
- **Polyuria** is excessive production of urine.
- **Proteinuria** refers to the presence of protein in the urine.
- **Pyuria** is pus in the urine.
- **Renal colic** is sharp, severe pain occurring in the lower back, radiating forward into the area of the groin caused by kidney stones.
- **Thornton's sign** is severe flank pain resulting from kidney stones.
- **Urinary hesitancy** is difficulty beginning urination and subsequent decreased urine flow.
- **Urinary incontinence** refers to a loss of control over bladder and urethral sphincters, resulting in involuntary leakage of urine.
- **Urinary tenesmus** is persistent, ineffective, painful straining to empty the bladder.
- **Urine retention** is retaining urine in the bladder.

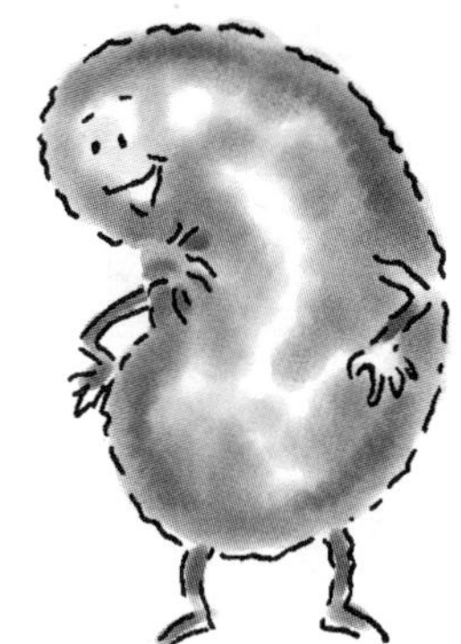

Look! Many of these words have a common root — ***uria.*** It comes from the Greek word ***ouron,*** which means urine.

Diagnostic tests

Here are common diagnostic tests for patients with urinary system disorders.

Urine and bladder tests

The following urine and bladder tests provide the most direct assessment of urinary function:

• **Cystometry** assesses the bladder's neuromuscular function, including bladder sensation, capacity, and the presence or absence of detrusor muscle contractions. A **cystometer** is the instrument used to measure the amount, flow, and time of voiding.

• **External sphincter electromyography** evaluates urinary incontinence by measuring electrical activity of the urinary sphincter muscle.

• **24-hour urine specimen** collects urine over a 24-hour period to determine levels of the following:
–**creatinine,** a nitrogenous waste product produced by working muscle tissue and normally excreted in the urine
–**protein,** normally absent from urine
–**uric acid,** an end product of protein metabolism normally excreted in the urine.

• **Urea clearance** measures urine levels of **urea,** the chief end product of protein metabolism. This test measures **glomerular filtration rate (GFR),** but is less reliable than the creatinine clearance.

• **Urinalysis** tests the urine for color, turbidity, specific gravity, pH, protein, glucose, and ketone bodies. This test also examines sediment for blood cells, casts, and crystals.

• **Urine culture** checks for bacterial growth in the urine, which is normally sterile.

• **Urine myoglobin** detects the presence of **myoglobin,** a red pigment found in the cytoplasm of cardiac and skeletal muscle in the urine.

• **Urine osmolality** is the concentration or osmotic pressure of urine expressed in milliosmols per kilogram of water.

• **Uroflowmetry** measures the volume of urine expelled from the urethra in milliliters per second **(urine flow rate)** and also determines the urine flow pattern. Abnormal results can indicate obstruction of the urethra.

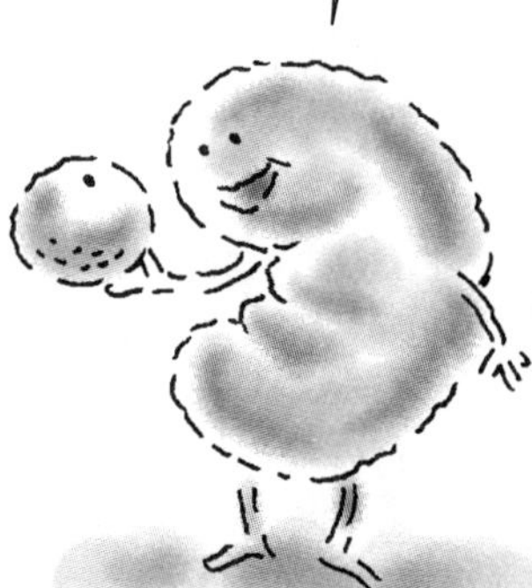

The ***glom-*** of **glomerular** derives from the Latin word ***glomus,*** meaning *ball,* and is akin to the Latin ***globus,*** meaning *globe.*

Blood studies

Here are several blood tests used to diagnose urinary disease and evaluate kidney function:

- **Anion gap** is the measurement of the total concentrations of anions and cations in the blood. An increased anion gap is present with renal failure.
- **Blood urea nitrogen (BUN)** level measures the amount of serum nitrogenous urea. Levels are elevated with kidney failure and dehydration.
- **Calcium and phosphorus levels** indicate the kidney's efficient conversion of vitamin D to a metabolite essential for calcium absorption in the intestines.
- **Chloride tests** measure serum levels of chloride, which helps regulate blood pressure and acid-base balance, and is excreted by the kidneys.
- **Complete blood count (CBC)** includes the evaluation of white blood cells, RBCs, hemoglobin, and hematocrit. Abnormal levels may indicate urinary tract infection or disease.
- **Creatinine clearance** assesses the GFR by measuring how well the kidneys remove creatinine from the blood over a 24-hour period. This test is an excellent indicator of renal function because it requires blood and urine specimens.
- **Serum creatinine** measures blood levels of creatinine. Creatinine levels are elevated with renal damage.
- **Serum osmolality** tests the concentration of serum expressed in milliosmols per kilogram of water.
- **Serum potassium levels** measure blood potassium, essential for proper renal functioning.
- **Serum sodium levels** are evaluated in relation to the amount of water in the body. Abnormal ratios may indicate renal disease.
- **Serum uric acid levels** measure uric acid, a normal by-product of metabolism that is excreted by the kidneys. Levels may be abnormally high with gout or impaired renal function. Below-normal levels may indicate problems with renal tubular absorption.

Radiologic and imaging tests

Here are the names of radiologic, tomographic, sonographic, and endoscopic diagnostic procedures:

- **Computerized tomography (CT) scan** generates a three-dimensional, computerized image of the kidneys.
- **Cystourethroscopy** uses an endoscopic instrument to examine the bladder, bladder neck, and urethra.

- **Excretory urography,** also known as **I.V. pyelography,** injects a radiopaque contrast medium to visualize renal structures, ureter, bladder, and the urethra. (See *IVP in action.*)
- **Kidney-ureter-bladder (KUB) X-ray** is just that, an X-ray of the kidneys, ureter, and bladder.
- **Magnetic resonance imaging (MRI)** creates precise three-dimensional (tomographic) images of tissue by passing magnetic energy through the body.
- **Nephrotomography** creates a tomogram of the kidneys after I.V. injection of a contrast medium.
- **Radionuclide renal scan** requires injecting a **radionuclide** (radioactive material) before **scintigraphy,** which records the relative distribution of radioactivity in the tissues and, therefore, proper functioning of those tissues.
- **Renal angiography** creates X-ray images of renal arterial circulation by injecting a contrast medium into the femoral artery.
- **Renal venography** creates X-ray images of the kidneys by injecting a contrast medium into a vein.
- **Retrograde cystography** instills a contrast medium into the bladder, followed by radiographic examination.
- **Ultrasonography** visualizes the urinary system by measuring and recording the reflection of pulses of ultrasonic waves directed into the tissue.
- **Voiding cystourethrography** demonstrates the efficiency of bladder filling and excretion by instilling a contrast medium into the patient's bladder through a urinary catheter. Radiographs are then taken before, during, and after voiding. (See *Cystourethrography.*)

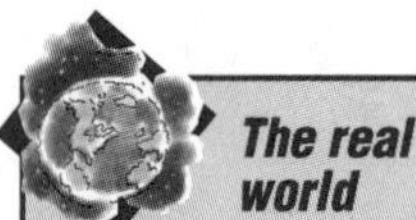

The real world

IVP in action

In practice, you'll hear **excretory urography** referred to as an **IVP,** an abbreviation for an older name of the test, intravenous pyelography. For example, you might hear someone say, "We need to take the patient for an IVP to check for an obstruction in the ureter."

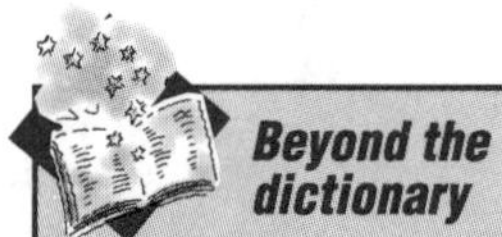

Beyond the dictionary

Cystourethrography

In **cystourethrography** the prefix ***cysto-*** is the Greek word element for *bladder.* ***Urethro*** refers to the urethra and ***-graphy*** is a method of recording. Thus, *cystourethrography* is a procedure that records (through radiography) bladder and urethra function.

Urinary system disorders

Terms naming disorders of the urinary system are presented here.

Acute renal failure

Acute renal failure is the sudden interruption of renal function, caused by obstruction, poor circulation, or kidney disease. Types of this potentially life-threatening condition are classified by the cause of onset:

- **Intrarenal failure,** also called **intrinsic** or **parenchymal renal failure,** results from damage to the kidneys' filtering structures.
- **Postrenal failure** results from obstruction of urine outflow.
- **Prerenal failure** is caused by any condition that reduces blood flow to the kidneys **(hypoperfusion).**

Stages of acute renal failure

Each type of acute renal failure has three distinct phases:

- The **oliguric phase** is marked by decreased urine output (less than 400 ml in 24 hours).
- The **diuretic phase** occurs when the kidneys produce a high volume of urine.
- The **recovery phase** occurs when the cause of diuresis is corrected, azotemia gradually disappears, and the patient begins to improve.

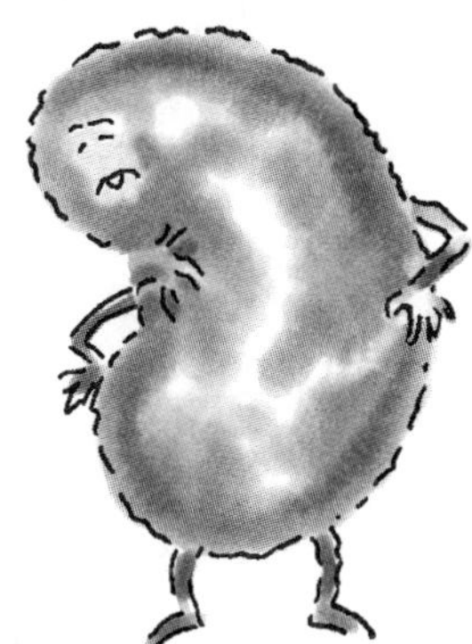
I can't work without a blood supply.

Other disorders

- **Acute poststreptococcal glomerulonephritis** is a relatively common inflammation of the glomeruli after a streptococcal infection of the respiratory tract.
- **Acute pyelonephritis** is a sudden inflammation of the kidney and its pelvis caused by bacteria.
- **Acute tubular necrosis (ATN),** also called **acute tubulointerstitial nephritis,** destroys the tubular segment of the nephron, leading to renal failure and uremia.
- **Alport's syndrome** is a hereditary kidney inflammation in which the patient may have recurrent gross or microscopic hematuria.
- **Benign prostatic hyperplasia** occurs when the prostate gland enlarges enough to compress the urethra, causing urinary obstruction.
- **Chronic glomerulonephritis** is an inflammation of the glomerulus of the kidney characterized by decreased urine production, blood and protein in the urine, and edema.

• **Chronic renal failure** is the typically slow, progressive loss of kidney function and glomerular filtration.
• **Cystitis** refers to inflammation of the bladder, usually caused by an ascending infection.
• **Cystocele** is a herniation of the urinary bladder through the vaginal wall. (See *Cystocele is all Greek.*)
• **Fanconi's syndrome** is a kidney disorder that produces malfunctions of the proximal renal tubules, leading to elevated potassium levels, elevated sodium levels, glucose in the urine and, eventually, rickets and retarded growth and development.
• **Hydronephrosis** refers to a distention of the kidneys by urine that is caused by obstruction of the ureter.
• **Hypospadias** is a condition in which the urethra opening is on the ventral surface of the penis. This condition rarely occurs in females, where the opening occurs within the vagina.
• **Nephrotic syndrome** is a condition marked by proteinuria, low blood albumin levels, and edema.
• **Neurogenic bladder** refers to any dysfunction of the nerves that control the bladder. The patient's bladder becomes spastic or flaccid, and urinary incontinence results.
• **Polycystic kidney disease** is characterized by multiple cysts of the kidney.
• **Prostatitis,** an inflammation of the prostate gland, may be acute or chronic.
• **Renal calculi** are **kidney stones** that form from minerals normally dissolved in the urine, such as calcium or magnesium.
• **Renal hypertension** is hypertension that occurs as a consequence of kidney disease and excessive release of the enzyme renin, which ultimately produces vasoconstriction and hypertension.
• **Renal infarction** occurs when a thrombus or embolus causes ischemia of a kidney.
• **Renal vein thrombosis** is clotting in the renal vein that results in renal congestion, engorgement and, possibly, infarction.
• **Ureterostenosis** is a ureteral stricture.
• **Urethritis** is inflammation of the urethra.
• **Vesicoureteral reflux** is a condition in which urine flows from the bladder back into the ureters and eventually into the renal pelvis or the parenchyma.

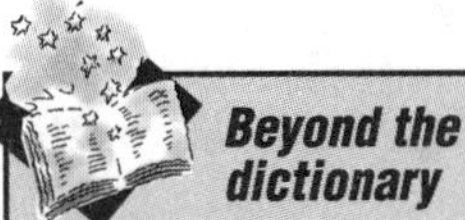

Beyond the dictionary

Cystocele is all Greek

Cystocele is an easy word. **Cysto-** comes from Greek ***kystis,*** which means *bladder* or *pouch.* **Cele-** is also derived from a Greek word, ***kele,*** which means *hernia.*

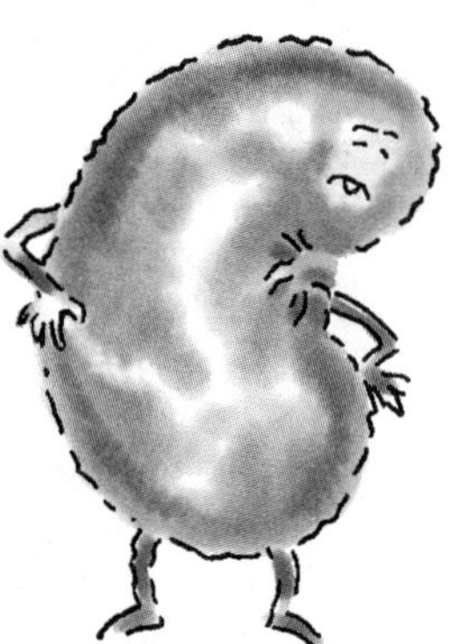
Ouch! These stones really hurt!

Treatments

Noninvasive procedures, dialysis, and surgeries that treat disorders of the urinary and renal systems are presented here.

Lithotripsy

There are two procedures that use a process called **lithotripsy** to reduce the size of renal calculi:
- **Extracorporeal shock-wave lithotripsy (ESWL)** is a noninvasive treatment that breaks up calculi with high-energy shock waves to allow their passage out of the body.
- **Percutaneous ultrasonic lithotripsy** uses an ultrasonic probe inserted through a nephrostomy tube into the renal pelvis. The probe generates ultrahigh-frequency sound waves that shatter calculi and continuous suctioning removes the fragments.

Catheters

Catheters are used in several way to treat urinary system disorders:
- An **external catheter,** also called a **Texas** or **condom catheter,** is a urine collection device that fits over the penis and resembles a condom.
- An **indwelling urinary catheter** is a urinary catheter with a balloon end designed to remain in the urinary bladder for a prolonged time. (See *Don't fool with my Foley.*)
- An **intermittent catheterization** is a procedure that drains urine remaining in the bladder after each voiding.

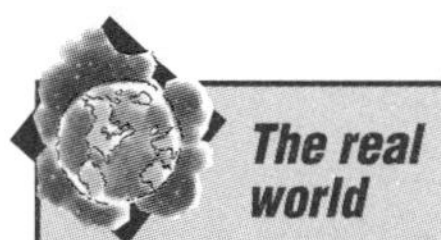

The real world

Don't fool with my Foley

You may hear an indwelling urinary catheter referred to as a *Foley,* named after Dr. Frederick Foley, the American doctor who designed the device.

Dialysis

Dialysis is a technique for removing waste products from the body when the kidneys fail. Several types of dialysis are explained here:
- **Continuous ambulatory peritoneal dialysis (CAPD)** is a form of peritoneal dialysis that allows the patient to continue daily activities.

• **Continuous arteriovenous hemofiltration (CAVH)** filters toxic wastes from the patient's blood and infuses a replacement solution such as lactated Ringer's solution.
• **Continuous arteriovenous ultrafiltration (CAVU)** uses equipment similar to that in CAVH but removes fluid from the patient's blood at a slower rate.
• **Continuous-cycling peritoneal dialysis (CCPD)** uses a machine to perform dialysis at night while the patient sleeps, and the patient performs CAPD in the daytime.
• **Hemodialysis** removes toxic wastes and other impurities directly from the blood of a patient with renal failure. Blood is pumped through a **dialyzing unit** to remove toxins and is then returned to the body.
• **Peritoneal dialysis** removes toxins from the patient's blood by using the peritoneal membrane surrounding the abdominal cavity as a **semipermeable dialyzing membrane.** In this technique, a dialyzing solution **(dialysate)** is instilled through a catheter inserted into the peritoneal cavity. By diffusion, the dialysate draws excessive concentrations of electrolytes and toxins through the peritoneal membrane. Next, excess water is drawn through the membrane. After an appropriate dwelling time, the dialysate is drained, taking toxins and wastes with it.

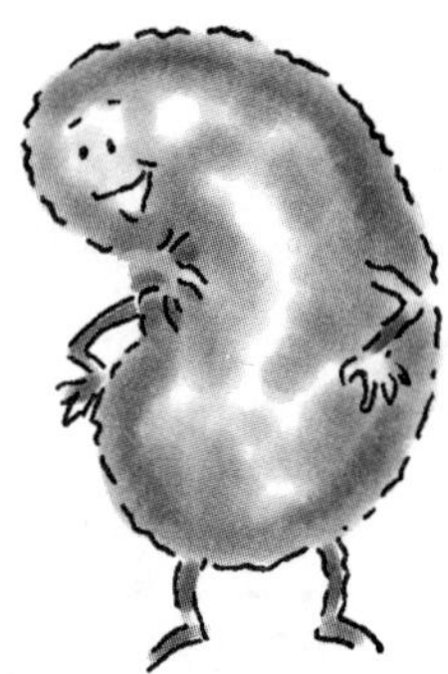

Surgery

Common surgical procedures to correct urinary system disorders include:
• **Cystectomy** is the partial or total removal of the urinary bladder and surrounding structures. Cystectomy may be partial, simple, or radical:
–A **partial cystectomy,** also called **segmental cystectomy,** involves **resection** (removal) of only cancerous tissue within the bladder. The patient's bladder function is usually preserved.
–A **simple,** or **total, cystectomy** involves resection of the entire bladder, but surrounding structures aren't removed.
–A **radical cystectomy** removes the bladder, prostate, and seminal vesicles in men. The bladder, urethra, uterus, fallopian tubes, ovaries, and a segment of the vaginal wall are removed in women.

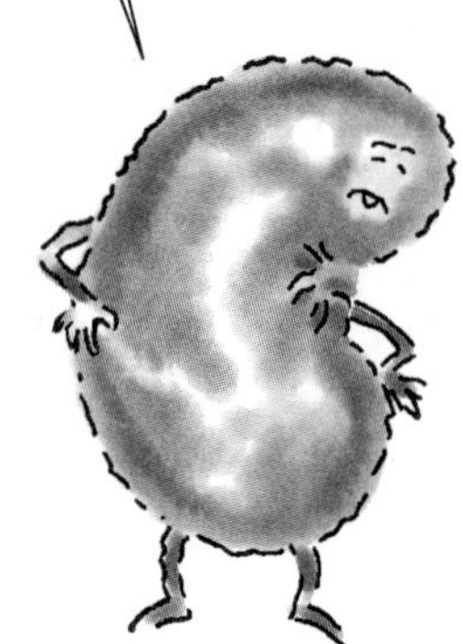

Now that you've got dialysis, I guess you don't need me any more.

• **Cystotomy** uses a catheter, which is inserted through the patient's suprapubic area into the bladder to temporarily divert urine away from the urethra and into a closed collection chamber.
• **Kidney transplantation** is one of the most common and successful organ transplant surgeries. This treatment is an alternative to dialysis for patients with end-stage renal disease.
• **Marshall-Marchetti-Krantz operation** helps correct urinary incontinence in female patients by restoring a weakened urinary sphincter.
• **Prostatectomy** is surgical removal of the prostate gland to remove diseased or obstructive tissue and restore urine flow through the urethra. One of four approaches is used:
–**Radical perineal prostatectomy** approaches the prostate through an incision in the perineum between the scrotum and the rectum.
–**Retropubic prostatectomy** uses a low abdominal incision to approach the prostate without opening the patient's bladder.
–**Suprapubic prostatectomy** uses an abdominal approach to open the bladder and remove the prostate gland.
–**Transurethral prostatectomy** approaches the prostate gland through the penis and bladder, using a surgical instrument called a **resectoscope.** The scope has an electric cutting wire to remove tissue.
• **Transurethral resection of the bladder (TURB)** is a relatively simple procedure that uses a cystoscope to remove small lesions from the bladder.
• **Urinary diversion** is a procedure that provides an alternative route for urine excretion when the normal channels are damaged or defective. Several types of urinary diversion surgery are performed.
–The **ileal conduit** diverts urine through a segment of the small bowel **(ileum),** which is removed for this purpose. A stoma formed on the abdominal wall continually empties urine into a collection bag.
–A **continent vesicostomy** allows urine to be diverted to a reservoir constructed from a portion of the bladder wall. A stoma is formed, and accumulated urine can be drained by inserting a catheter into the stoma.
–In a **ureterostomy,** one or both ureters are dissected from the bladder and brought to the skin surface to form one or two stomas that continuously drain urine.

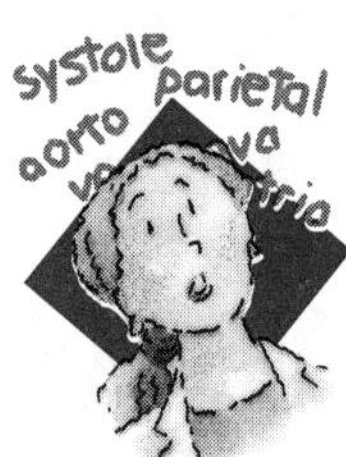

Vocabulary builders

At a crossroads

Completing this crossword puzzle will help you filter through urinary system terms. Good luck!

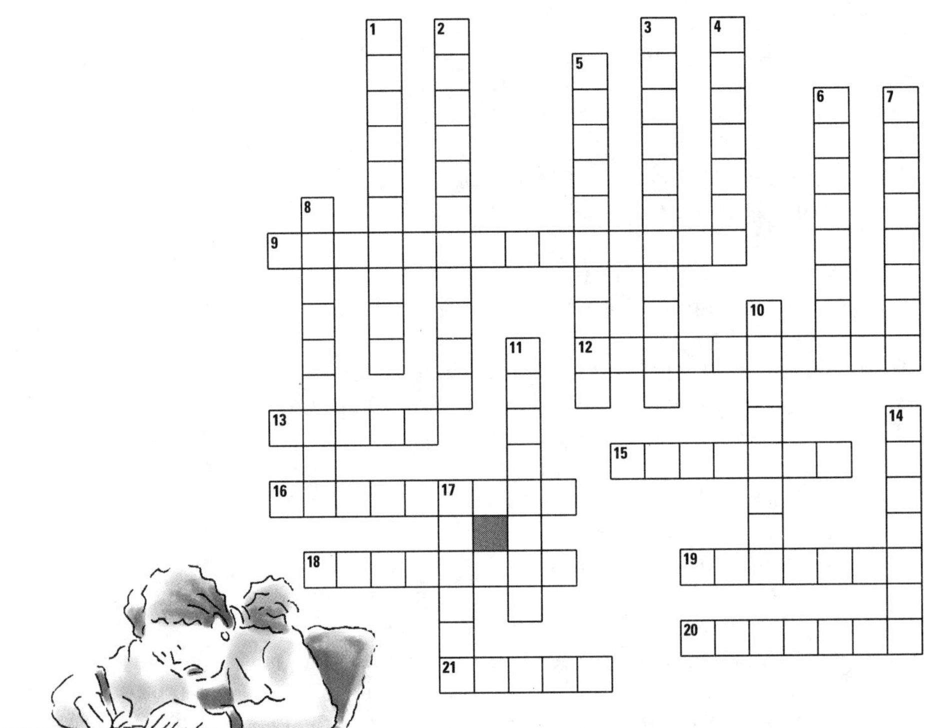

Across

9. Bacterial kidney infection
12. Analysis of urine
13. Artery that brings blood to the kidney
15. Kidney stones
16. Blood in the urine
18. Phase of renal failure when kidneys produce high volume of urine
19. Structure that collects and holds urine
20. Structure through which urine exits the body
21. Hormone involved with blood pressure

Down

1. Study of the renal system
2. Protein in the urine
3. Inflammation of the prostate gland
4. Syndrome resulting from a hereditary kidney inflammation
5. Network of capillaries
6. Striated wedges in the renal medulla
7. Technique for removing waste products when kidneys fail
8. Herniation of the bladder
10. Scant urine output
11. Bladder infection
14. Difficult urination
17. Structure that carries urine from kidney to bladder

Answers are on page 216.

Match game

Match the correct GI system term with its definition.

Clues	Choices
1. Catheter that is left in place ____	A. Dialysate
2. External catheter ____	B. Ureterostomy
3. Used for bladder training ____	C. Peritoneal dialysis
4. Uses the peritoneal membrane ____	D. Cystectomy
5. Uses blood ____	E. Indwelling catheter
6. Dialyzing solution ____	F. Strengthening exercises
7. Surgical removal of the prostate gland ____	G. Ileal conduit
8. Bladder surgery ____	H. Condom catheter
9. Ureters brought to the skin surface ____	I. Prostatectomy
10. Diverts urine through small bowel ____	J. Hemodialysis

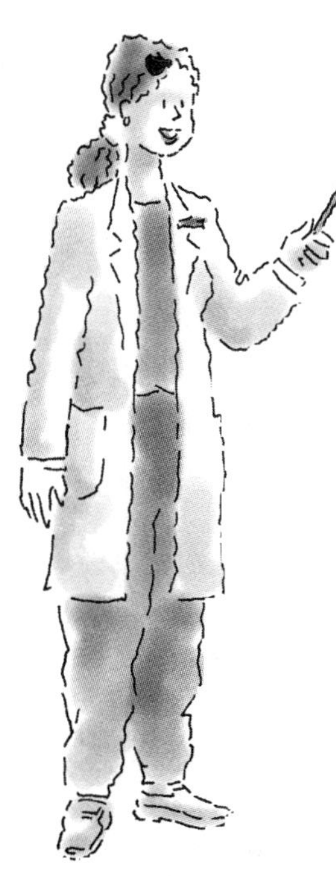
Match the answers to the questions up top and fill in the blanks down below.

Finish line

Fill in the blanks to complete the definition for each GI disorder, treatment, or test.

1. Inflammation of the bladder is called ________.
2. Inflammation of the renal glomeruli without infection is called ______.
3. The severe pain caused by kidney stones is called _______.
4. Kidney stones are also called _______.
5. A coagulated, necrotic area in the kidney caused by occlusion of blood vessels is called renal ________.
6. The phase of acute renal failure marked by decreased urine output is the _______ phase.
7. The phase of acute renal failure marked by excess urine output is called the _______ phase.
8. The initials IVP stand for ________.

Answers are on page 216.

Answers

At a crossroads

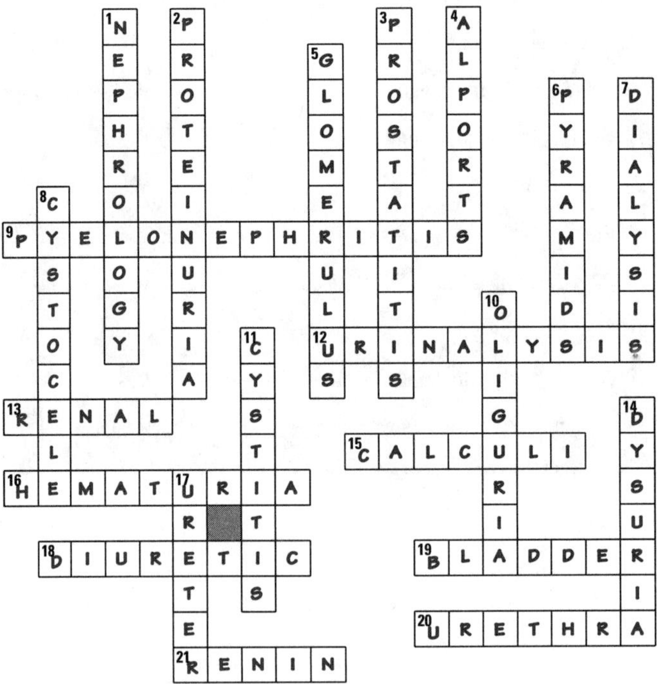

Match game

1. E; 2. H; 3. F; 4. C; 5. J; 6. A; 7. I; 8. D; 9. B; 10. G.

Finish line

1. Cystitis; 2. Glomerulonephritis; 3. Renal colic; 4. Calculi; 5. Infarction; 6. Oliguric; 7. Diuretic; 8. Intravenous pyelography.

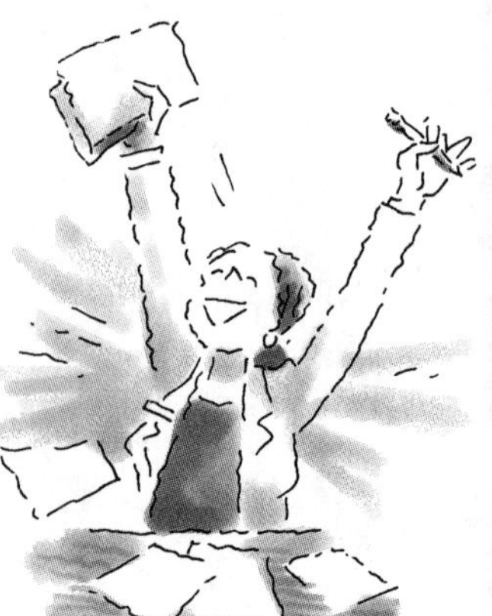

10 Reproductive system

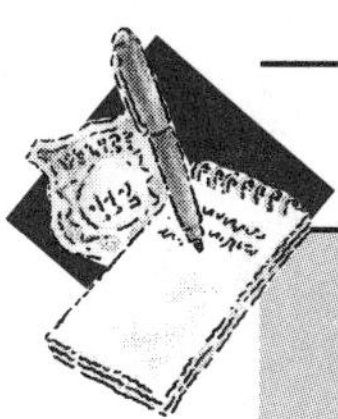

Just the facts

In this chapter, you'll review:

- terminology related to the structure and function of the reproductive system
- terminology needed for physical examination
- tests that help diagnose common reproductive disorders
- reproductive system disorders and their treatments.

Reproductive structure and function

Essential terminology related to the structure and normal function of the male and female reproductive systems and associated organs is presented here. A clear understanding of these systems will help you remember the terminology. (See *Pronouncing key reproductive system terms*, page 218.)

The male reproductive system produces sperm and some male sex hormones.

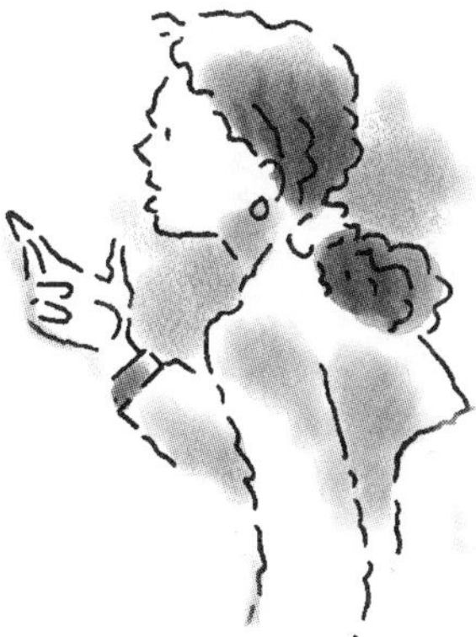

Male reproductive system

The male reproductive system consists of the organs that produce, transfer, and introduce mature sperm into the female reproductive tract, where fertilization occurs. In addition to producing male sex cells, the male reproductive system secretes some of the male sex hormones. The male reproductive organs include the penis, scrotum, testes, duct system, and accessory reproductive glands.

Pump up your pronunciation

Pronouncing key reproductive system terms

Below is a list of key terms, along with the correct way to pronounce them.

Abruptio placentae	AHB-RUP-SHEE-OH PLAH-SEN-TAY
Ballottement	BAH-LAWT-MEHNT
Epididymis	EHP-IH-DID-IH-MISS
Leydig's cells	LEYE-DIGZ SELLS
Oophorectomy	OH-AWF-UH-REK-TUH-MEE
Symphysis pubis	SIM-FIH-SISS PYOO-BISS

Penis

The **penis** deposits **sperm** (mature male germ cells) in the female reproductive tract through copulation and acts as the terminal duct for the urinary tract.

3 columns

The cylindrical penile shaft contains three columns of spongy vascular tissue that respond to sexual stimulation by becoming engorged with blood. Two of the three columns of this erectile tissue are bound together by heavy fibrous tissue and form the **corpora cavernosa,** the major part of the penis. The third column, on the underside of the shaft, is called the **corpus spongiosum.** The corpus spongiosum encases the urethra. (See *Caves and sponges.*)

So sensitive

The **glans penis,** at the distal end of the shaft, is a cone-shaped structure formed from the corpus spongiosum. Its lateral margin forms a ridge of tissue known as the **corona.** The glans is highly sensitive to sexual stimulation.

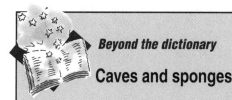

Beyond the dictionary

Caves and sponges

The terms **corpora cavernosa** and **corpus spongiosum** describe the columns of spongy vascular tissue in the penile shaft that respond to sexual stimulation.

Latin roots

Corpora is simply the plural of ***corpus,*** a Latin word for the main part of a bodily structure. ***Cavernosa*** relates to a cave or cavity. ***Spongiosum*** relates to a sponge, which is made up of little cavities.

Get outta here

Thin, loose skin covers the penile shaft. The **urethral meatus** opens through the glans to allow urination and ejaculation. (See *Structures of the male reproductive system,* page 220.)

Scrotum

The **scrotum,** meaning *pouch,* contains the primary male sex organs and joins with the penis at the **penoscrotal junction.** A thin layer of skin covers the scrotum, overlying a tighter, muscular layer. Within the scrotum are two sacs that each contain a testis, an epididymis, and a spermatic cord. The seam where the two sacs join is called the **median raphe** and is visible on the exterior of the scrotum. (See *The rap on the median raphe,* page 221.)

Eggs?

The **testes,** also called **testicles,** are two egg-shaped glands within the scrotum. Enclosed in a fibrous white capsule, each testicle is divided into numerous compartments, or **lobules.** The lobules contain **seminiferous tubules,** where **spermatogenesis** (sperm formation) takes place when a male reaches puberty and throughout life. Stimulated by male sex hormones, sperm continuously form within these tubules.

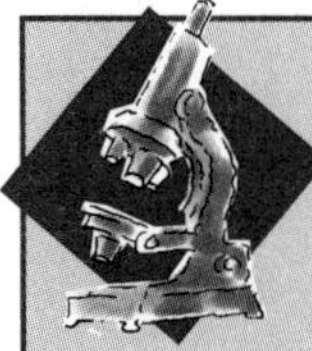

Zoom in

Structures of the male reproductive system

The male reproductive system, pictured here, consists of the penis and the scrotum and its contents—the prostate gland and the inguinal structures.

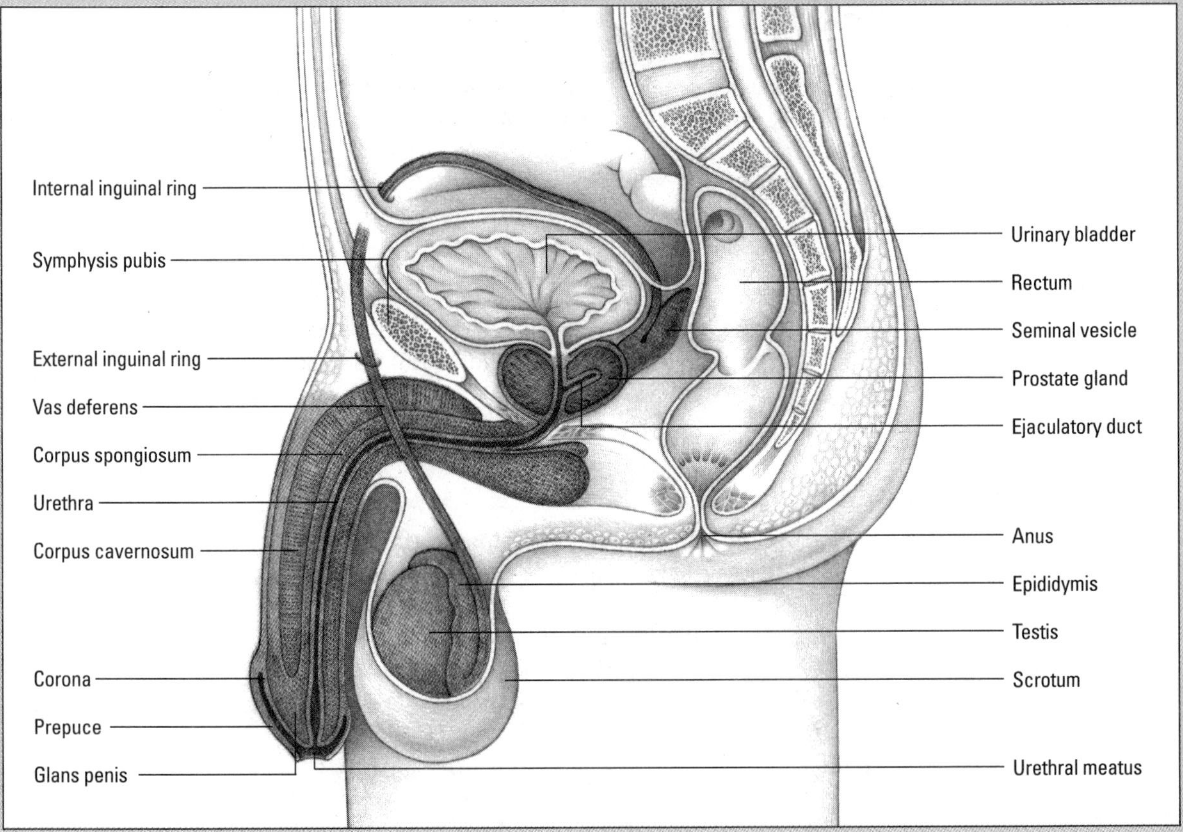

Epie? — did he miss what?

The **epididymis** is a complicated duct system that delivers sperm from the testes to the ejaculatory ducts near the bladder. This system is composed of two **epididymides** — a pair of coiled, tubular reservoirs located along the border of each testicle. These structures store sperm before ejaculation, secrete part of the seminal fluid, and serve as a passage for sperm.

Vas is da differens?

Mature sperm travels from the epididymis to the **vas deferens,** or **ductus deferens.** These two tubes begin at the epididymis, pass through the **inguinal canal** formed by the pelvic girdle, and enter the ejaculatory duct inside the prostate gland. Each vas deferens is enclosed by a **spermatic cord,** a compact bundle of vessels, nerves, and muscle fibers.

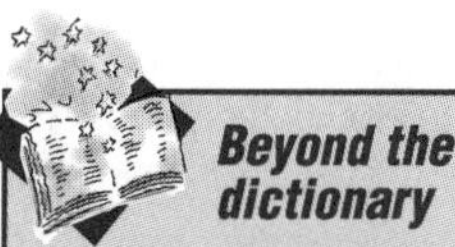

Beyond the dictionary

The rap on the median raphe

The seam where the two scrotal sacs join is called the **median raphe** and is visible on the exterior of the scrotum. Median comes from the Latin term ***medianus,*** meaning *in the midline of a structure;* ***raphe*** is the Greek word for *seam.*

Duct work

The **ejaculatory ducts** are two short tubes formed by the vas deferens and the ducts of the seminal vesicles. They pass through the prostate gland and enter the urethra. The **seminal vesicles,** two pouches located along the bladder's lower edge, produce most of the liquid part of semen, the thick whitish secretion that is discharged during ejaculation. The seminal vesicles also produce **prostaglandins,** potent hormonelike fatty acids.

Prostate gland

The walnut sized **prostate gland** is located under the bladder and surrounds the urethra. The three lobules of this gland are the left and right lateral lobes and the **median** (middle) lobe. They continuously secrete **prostatic fluid** — a thin, milky substance that comprises about one-third of the semen volume and activates the sperm.

Hormones

Male sex hormones, called **androgens,** are produced in the testes and the adrenal glands.

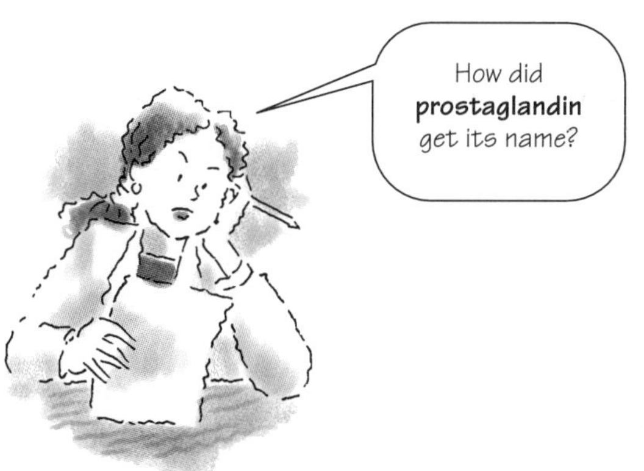

How did **prostaglandin** get its name?
Doctors used to think it was produced in the **prostate gland.** Think ***prosta + gland + in.***

It takes testosterone

Interstitial cells, called **Leydig cells,** are found in tissue between the seminiferous tubules (the tubules that produce and conduct sperm). Leydig cells secrete **testosterone,** the most important male sex hormone. A man's body needs testosterone for development of the sexual organs, secondary sex characteristics (such as a beard), and the formation of sperm.

Two other hormones — **luteinizing hormone (LH),** also known as **interstitial cell–stimulating hormone,** and **follicle-stimulating hormone (FSH)** — directly affect testosterone secretion.

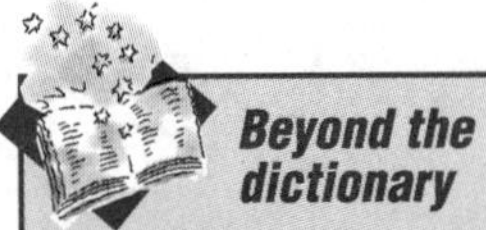

Beyond the dictionary

Addendum on the pudendum

The term **pudendum** derives from the Latin ***pudendus.*** This means, literally, *that of which one is to be ashamed.* In late classical and Latin and early Christian writings, the word came to refer to the external genitalia of both sexes. Now, it more commonly refers to female genitalia.

Female reproductive system

The ovaries are the basic female reproductive organs. Internal and external female reproductive organs include the fallopian tubes, the uterus, the vagina, and mammary glands.

External structures

As in males, the female **mons pubis** is a triangular pad of tissue, covered by skin and pubic hair, located over the **symphysis pubis,** the joint formed by the union of the pubic bones.

Just for her

The external female genitals, sometimes referred to as the **pudendum,** are contained in the region called the **vulva.** (See *Addendum on the pudendum.*)

Two **labia majora** form the sides of the vulva. The **labia minora,** two moist mucosal folds, lie within and alongside the labia majora.

The **perineum** consists of muscles, fascia, and ligaments between the anus and vulva. (See *External structures of the female reproductive system.*)

Small but important

The **clitoris** is a small, erectile organ located at the anterior of the vulva. Less visible are the multiple openings of **Skene's glands,** mucus-producing glands found on both sides of the **urethral meatus,** or opening. **Bartholin's glands,** other mucus-producing glands, are located on each side of and behind the vaginal opening. The **hymen,**

Zoom in

External structures of the female reproductive system

This illustration shows the external structures of the female reproductive system.

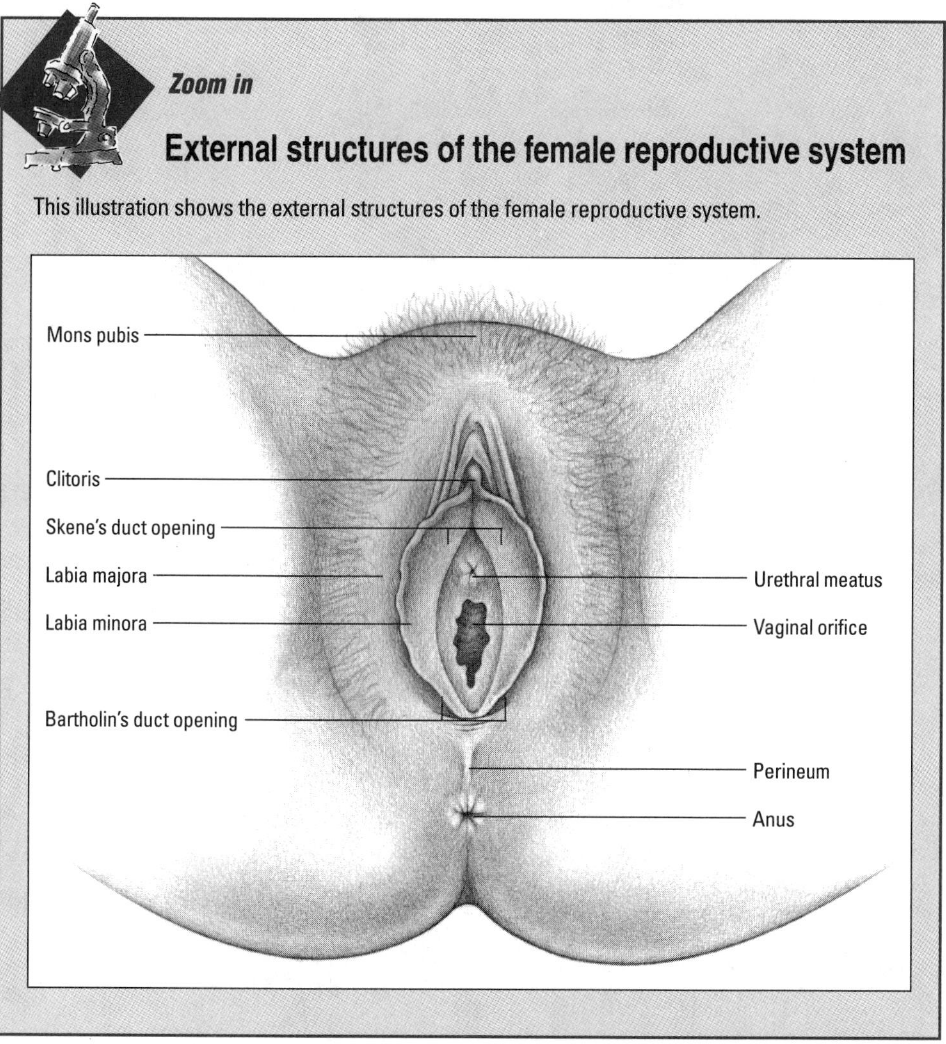

a tissue membrane varying in size and thickness, may completely cover the vaginal opening.

Internal organs

The **vagina** is a highly elastic muscular tube located between the urethra and the rectum. It's lined with a mucous membrane that lubricates the vagina during sexual activity. **Rugae,** folds of tissue in the vaginal walls, allow the vagina to stretch. (See *Internal structures of the female reproductive system*, page 224.)

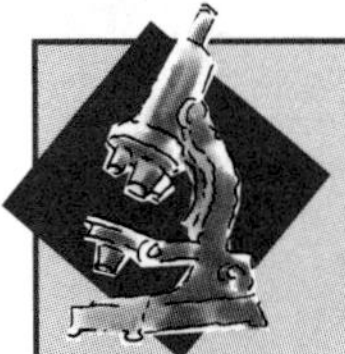

Zoom in

Internal structures of the female reproductive system

These illustrations show the internal structures of the female reproductive system.

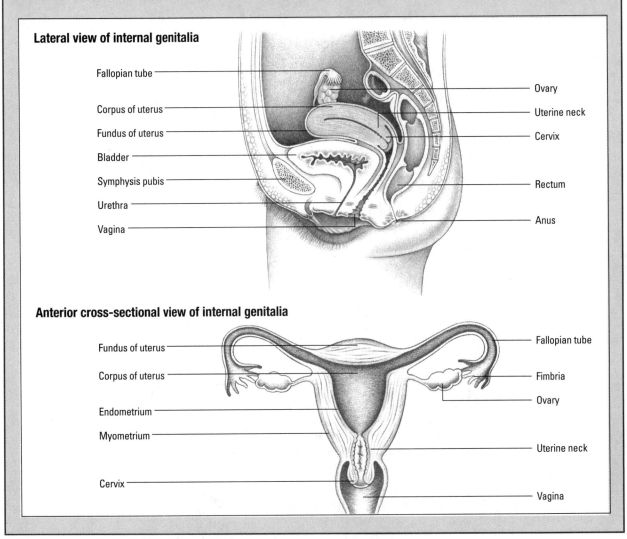

Lateral view of internal genitalia

Anterior cross-sectional view of internal genitalia

The pear-fect uterus

The vagina leads to the **uterus,** a small, firm, pear-shaped muscular organ resting between the bladder and rectum. The uterus usually lies at a 90-degree angle to the vagina.

The mucous membrane that lines the uterus is called the **endometrium.** The muscular layer is called the **myometrium.** (See *Metrium matters.*)

The uterine neck, or **isthmus,** joins the upper uterus or **fundus,** to the **cervix,** the part of the uterus that extends into the vagina. The fundus and isthmus make up the **corpus,** or main body of the uterus.

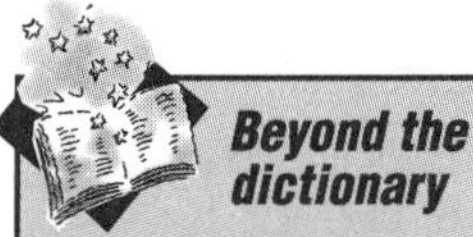

Beyond the dictionary

Metrium matters

The mucous membrane lining the uterus is called the **endometrium.** The muscular layer is called the **myometrium.** The root of these words, ***metrium,*** comes from the Greek word ***meter,*** which is related to and means the same thing as the English word **mother.** ***Metrium*** also refers to the uterus.

Certainly the cervix

The mouth of the cervix is called the **os,** a Latin term for a body orifice. The **internal os** opens from the cervix into the cervical canal, and the **external os** leads from the cervical canal to the vagina. A mucous membrane called the **endocervix** lines the cervical canal.

Fundamentally fallopian

The **fallopian tubes** are a pair of ducts attached to the uterus at the upper angles of the fundus. These long, narrow, muscular tubes have fingerlike projections, called **fimbriae,** on the free ends that partially surround the ovaries. (See *Fallopian facts.*)

Fertilization of the **ovum** (egg), or female sex cell, usually occurs in the outer third of the fallopian tube.

The ovaries

The **ovaries** are two almond-shaped organs that are located on each side of the pelvis and connected to the uterus by a ligament. The main function of the ovaries is to produce mature ova.

At birth, each ovary contains approximately 50,000 **graafian follicles,** mature ovarian vesicles that each

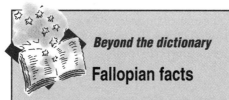

Beyond the dictionary

Fallopian facts

Although the correct function of the fallopian tubes had been known for more than 2,000 years, these structures received their name from Gabrielle Fallopio, a 16th-century Italian surgeon. He described and named the tubes in his book *Observationes anatomicae* (published in 1562), which corrected a number of widely held false ideas about anatomy.

contain an ovum. During childbearing years, one of these graafian follicles produces a mature ovum during the first half of each menstrual cycle.

Her hormones

The ovaries release **progesterone** and the female sex hormone **estrogen** at puberty. They also release a mature egg during the menstrual cycle. When expelled from the ovary, ova are caught by the fimbriated ends of the fallopian tubes.

The ovarian cycle

The Latin word ***menstrualis*** means monthly. The average **menstrual cycle** occurs over 28 days, roughly a month. Regulated by fluctuating, reciprocating hormones, this monthly cycle is divided into three phases: menstrual, proliferative, and luteal.

Phase I — menstrual

The **menstrual** or **preovulatory** phase begins the 1st day of menstruation. As the cycle begins, low estrogen and progesterone levels in the bloodstream stimulate the hypothalamus to secrete **gonadotropin-releasing hormone.** In turn, this substance stimulates the anterior pituitary to secrete FSH and LH. When the FSH level rises, LH output increases.

Phase II — proliferative

The **proliferative** or **follicular** phase lasts from day 6 to day 14. During this time, LH and FSH act on the ovarian follicle containing the ovum and stimulate estrogen secretion. After 14 days, estrogen production decreases, the follicle matures, and ovulation occurs. Normally, one follicle matures and is released from the ovary during each cycle.

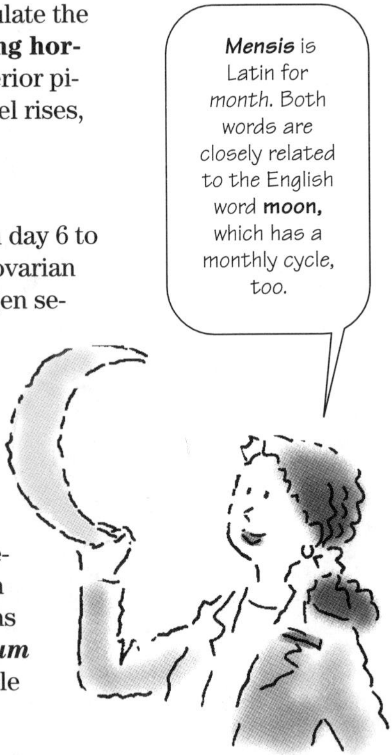

Phase III — luteal

During the **luteal phase,** which lasts about 14 days, FSH and LH levels drop. Estrogen levels decline at first. Then estrogen increases, along with progesterone levels, as the **corpus luteum** begins functioning. This yellow structure (***corpus luteum*** is Latin for *yellow body)* develops after the follicle ruptures and produces progesterone.

Mensis is Latin for *month.* Both words are closely related to the English word **moon,** which has a monthly cycle, too.

During this phase, the endometrium responds to progesterone by becoming thicker and preparing to nourish a fertilized ovum. About 10 to 12 days after ovulation, the corpus luteum diminishes as progesterone and estrogen levels drop. When a fertilized ovum isn't present and hormone levels can't sustain the thickened endometrium, the lining is shed. The process of shedding the lining is known as **menses.**

Breasts

The **mammary glands,** or **breasts,** are milk-producing structures. Breast development is controlled by estrogen and progesterone, hormones secreted by the ovaries. Each breast contains ducts surrounded by **acini** (milk-secreting cells). Individual ducts join with others to form larger ducts, which circle the **nipple** and end in tiny openings on the nipple surface. The anterior lobe of the pituitary gland produces a lactogenic hormone called **prolactin** to stimulate milk production.

The **areola** is a pigmented area (in Latin, the word means *a little open space*) around the breast nipple. (See *The female breast,* page 228.)

Menopause

Most women cease menstruation between ages 40 and 55. The term **menopause** applies if menses are absent for 1 year. **Climacteric** refers to a woman's transition from reproductive fertility to infertility. This change occurs over a period of several years.

At the onset of menopause, estrogen and progesterone levels decrease and testosterone secretion increases. The body compensates for estrogen deficiency by producing **estrone,** a weaker form of estrogen.

Pregnancy

Pregnancy occurs with **conception,** when an ovum in the fallopian tube is penetrated by one sperm cell. The fertilized ovum, or **zygote,** immediately forms a rounded mass of cells and travels from the tube to the uterus. In the uterus, it attaches to the endometrial lining and begins growing.

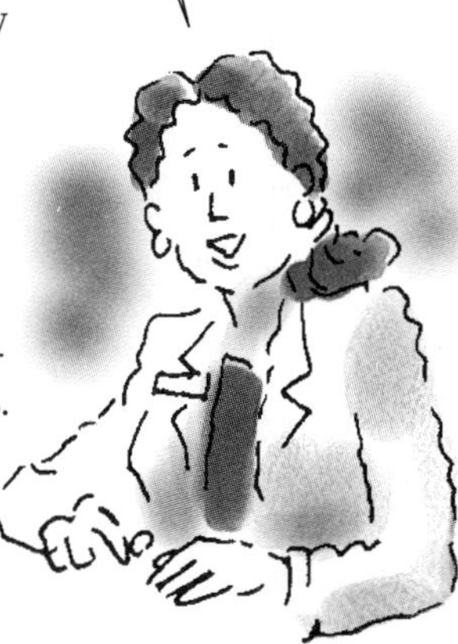
Lactos is Latin for *milk.* ***Genesis*** is Greek, meaning *creation.* **Lactogenesis** means *milk production.*

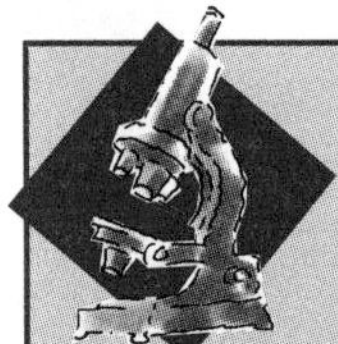

Zoom in

The female breast

Here is a closer look at terms related to the female breast.

Structures of the breast

The **areola** — the pigmented area in the center of the breast — contains the **nipple**. Pigmented erectile tissue in the nipple responds to cold, friction, and sexual stimulation. The interior of each breast is composed of glandular and fibrous tissue. Glandular tissue contains 15 to 20 lobes made up of clustered **acini,** tiny saclike duct terminals that secrete milk. Fibrous **Cooper's ligaments** support the breasts.

Milk production and drainage

Acini draw the ingredients to make milk from the blood in surrounding capillaries. **Lactiferous ducts** and **sinuses** store milk during lactation, conveying it to and through the nipples.

Glands on the areolar surface, called **Montgomery's tubercles,** produce sebum that lubricates the areola and nipple during breast-feeding.

Lateral cross section

Clavicle

Adipose tissue

Acini of lobule

Glandular lobe

Collecting and main ducts

Areola

Montgomery's tubercle

Nipple

Lactiferous duct orifice

Lactiferous sinus

Lactiferous duct

Take a closer look at the body's milk-producing system.

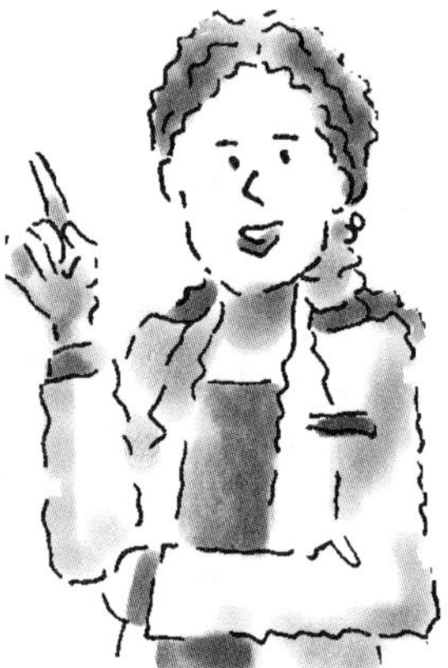

Embryonic stage

During the 2nd through the 8th week of pregnancy, the **embryonic stage,** the organism is called an **embryo.** The growing embryo floats within the **amnion,** a thin, clear sac filled with **amniotic fluid.** Early in this stage, the **chorion,** or outer cells of the rounded cell mass, joins with the endometrium to form the **placenta.** This vital structure provides nutrients for and removes wastes from the embryo. The chorion channels the nutrients to or receives wastes from to the embryo's **umbilical cord.**

Fetal stage

From the end of the 8th week until birth, the developing infant is called a fetus.

Childbirth

Delivery of the fetus is achieved through labor, the process in which the cervix dilates and uterine contractions act to expel the fetus from the uterus. Childbirth can be divided into three stages.

First, the fetus begins its descent and **cervical effacement** (thinning and dilation) occurs. By the end of this stage, the cervix is fully dilated. The second stage of labor begins with full cervical dilation and ends with expulsion of the fetus. The third stage begins immediately after childbirth and ends with expulsion of the placenta. After the **neonate** (newborn) is delivered, the uterus continues to contract intermittently and grows smaller.

After childbirth, the reproductive tract takes about 6 weeks to revert to its former condition in a process called **involution.** The uterus shrinks quickly during the first 2 weeks following childbirth. Postpartum vaginal discharge called **lochia** persists for several weeks, during which the discharge changes in color and consistency:

- **Lochia rubra** is a bloody discharge that appears 1 to 4 days after delivery.
- **Lochia serosa** is a pinkish brown serous discharge that appears 5 to 7 days after delivery.
- **Lochia alba** is a grayish white or colorless discharge that appears 1 to 3 weeks after delivery.

Physical examination terms

Here are terms associated with physical examination of the male and female reproductive systems:

- **Ballottement** is passive fetal movement in response to tapping of the lower portion of the uterus or cervix.
- **Braxton Hicks contraction** are episodes of light, painless, irregular tightening of the uterus during pregnancy. The condition arises during the first trimester and increases in duration and intensity by the third trimester.
- **Chadwick's sign** is a bluish coloration of the vulva and vagina after the 6th week of pregnancy resulting from local venous congestion.
- **Dysmenorrhea** is painful menstruation. This occurs at least occasionally in nearly all women. (See *Dissecting dysmenorrhea.*)
- **Dyspareunia** is a condition in women in which sexual intercourse is difficult or painful.
- **Goodell's sign,** softening of the cervix, is an indication of probable pregnancy.
- **Gravid** means pregnant.
- **Gravida** refers to a pregnant female, called gravida I during the first pregnancy, gravida II in the second pregnancy, and so on.

Beyond the dictionary

Dissecting dysmenorrhea

Dysmenorrhea is painful menstruation. The term **dysmenorrhea** is easier to remember if you dissect the word. ***Dys-*** means *difficult or painful.* ***Meno*** literally means *monthly* and refers to menstruation. The third element, ***-rrhea,*** another common Greek word element, means *flow.* So, **dysmenorrhea** is painful menstrual flow.

One root, many terms

Add a few more letters to ***meno*** and you can describe different types of menstrual flow:

- **amenorrhea**: ***a-*** means *absence*; amenorrhea is thus an *absence of menstrual flow*
- **menorrhagia**: ***-rhagia*** derives from a Greek verb meaning *to burst out* and describes an excessive flow; menorrhagia is thus *profuse menstruation*
- **menostasis**: ***-stasis*** means *stoppage,* so this word means the same thing as amenorrhea
- **oligomenorrhea**: ***oligo-*** means *scant* or *little,* so oligomenorrhea is *scant menstrual flow* or *scant menstruation.*

• **Gynecology** is the branch of medicine concerned with the health care of women, including sexual and reproductive functions and diseases of the reproductive organs.
• **Gynecomastia** is an abnormal enlargement and development of the male breast.
• **Hegar's sign,** softening of the lower portion of the uterus, occurs around the 7th week of and is considered an early sign of possible pregnancy.
• **Infertile** means having a diminished capacity to produce offspring but not necessarily sterile.
• **Leukorrhea** is a white discharge from the vagina.
• **Lightening** is a subjective sensation reported by some women as the fetus descends into the pelvic inlet and changes the shape and position of the uterus near term.
• **Linea nigra** is a line of dark pigment that appears on a pregnant woman's abdomen.
• **Mastalgia** is pain in the breast.
• **Metrorrhagia** is abnormal uterine bleeding, especially between menstrual periods.
• **Obstetrics** is the branch of surgical medicine involving pregnancy and childbirth. It includes care of the mother and fetus throughout pregnancy, childbirth, and the postpartum period.
• **Para** is a mother who has produced living offspring. Para I designates one child, para II refers to two children, and so forth.
• **Presentation** is the portion of the fetus that first enters the birth canal.
• **Priapism** is a persistent abnormal erection of the penis, without sexual desire.
• **Primigravida** refers to a woman in her first pregnancy (also called gravida I).
• **Primipara** is a woman who had one pregnancy that resulted in viable offspring, or who is giving birth for the first time (also called para I).
• **Quickening** refers to the first notable fetal movement in utero and usually occurs at 16 to 20 weeks' gestation.
• **Sterile** means the patient is unable to reproduce due to an abnormality, such as the absence of spermatogenesis in a man or fallopian tube blockage in a woman.
• **Striae gravidarum,** also called stretch marks, are red streaks that appear on a pregnant woman's abdomen.

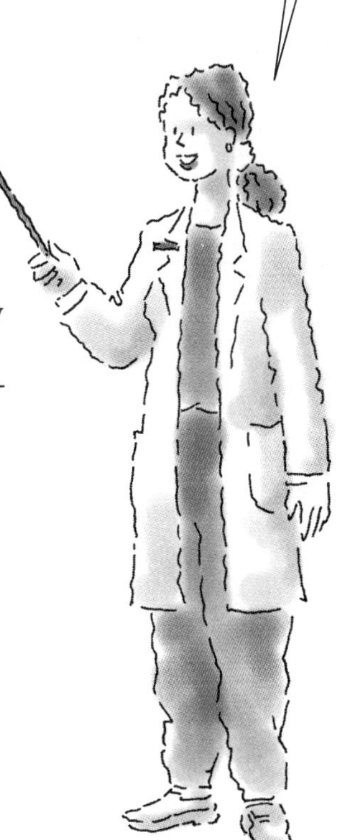
Leukorrhea is a white discharge — that makes sense. ***Leuk*** *is Greek for white and* ***-rrhea*** *means flow.*

Diagnostic tests

Diagnostic tests associated with the reproductive system include blood and fluids tests as well as radiologic and other imaging procedures.

Blood and fluid tests

Here are some common blood and fluid tests associated with the reproductive system:

- **Amniocentesis** involves the withdrawal of a sample of amniotic fluid by transabdominal puncture and needle aspiration.
- **Chorionic villus sampling** is a biopsy that samples a minute amount of the chorionic villi, fingerlike projections of the chorion that attach to the maternal endometrial tissues.
- A **darkfield examination** is a microscopic test of fluid taken from a lesion in suspected primary syphilis. A special microscope makes the syphilis organism appear bright against a dark background, therefore the term **darkfield.**
- A **Papanicolaou (Pap) smear** is widely used for early detection of cervical cancer and inflammatory tissue changes. (See *Pap smear.*)
- **Percutaneous umbilical blood sampling** is an invasive procedure that involves insertion of a spinal needle into the umbilical cord to obtain a fetal blood sample or to transfuse the fetus in utero.
- The **prostatic acid phosphatase** test measures the phosphatase enzymes, found mostly in the prostate. Above-normal levels are suspicious for prostate cancer.
- A **prostate specific antigen** blood test detects a normally occurring substance that increases with prostate diseases.
- A **semen analysis** examines seminal fluid to evaluate male fertility. The procedure includes measuring the volume of seminal fluid, counting sperm, and performing microscopic examination.
- A **serum alpha-fetoprotein (AFP)** study measures the glycoprotein AFP. An above-normal level may indicate testicular cancer. In a fetus, an above-normal level may indicate neural tube defect.

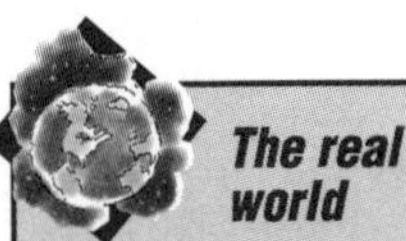
The real world

Pap smear

What everyone commonly refers to as a **Pap smear** or **Pap test** is a **Papanicolaou test.**

It's named for George Papanicolaou (1883 to 1962), the Greek doctor who immigrated to the United States and developed the test.

- **Triple screen** is a blood test performed between 15 and 20 weeks' gestation to determine whether a fetus is at increased risk for Down syndrome, a neural tube defect, or both.
- **Urine culture** uses a common culture medium to detect infectious microorganisms in the urine.
- **Venereal disease research laboratory (VDRL)** test confirms a diagnosis of syphilis.

Radiologic and other imaging procedures

Here are some common radiologic and other imaging procedures associated with the reproductive system:

- **Amniography** is an X-ray of the pregnant uterus after contrast media is injected into the amniotic sac to visualize its contents.
- During a **colposcopy,** the examiner studies the vulva, cervix, and vagina with a **colposcope,** an instrument containing a magnifying lens and a light.
- **Hysterosalpingography** allows the visualization of the uterine cavity, the fallopian tubes, and the peritubal area. (See *Making sense of hysterosalpingography.*)
- A **laparoscopy** allows visual inspection of organs in the peritoneal cavity using a fiber-optic telescope **(laparoscope)** through the abdominal wall.
- The **nonstress test** is a noninvasive test used to detect fetal heart accelerations in response to fetal movement.

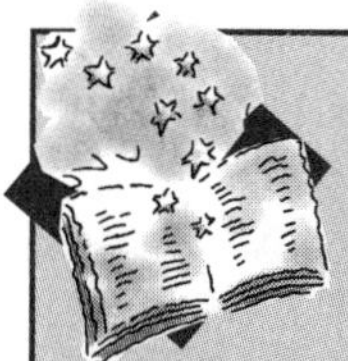

Beyond the dictionary

Making sense of hysterosalpingography

The Greek word ***hystero*** means *uterus.* ***Salpingo*** is the Greek term for *fallopian tube,* and ***-graphy*** is the term for a recording. So, **hysterosalpingography** means *examination of the uterus and fallopian tubes.*

Sometimes the Greeks got it wrong

Hysteros, the Greek word for the *uterus* or *womb,* also provided the root for another Greek word ***hysteria.*** Seems the ancient Greeks had the notion that only women became extremely emotionally upset and attributed this perceived difference from men to the presence of the uterus.

• The **oxytocin challenge test** evaluates fetal ability to withstand an oxytocin-induced contraction. The test requires I.V. administration of oxytocin in increasing doses until three high-quality uterine contractions occur within a 10-minute period.
• A **pelvic ultrasound** passes sound waves through the body. The result is electronic images of internal structures. This test can help diagnose pelvic disease or examine a developing fetus.
• The **vibroacoustic stimulation test** is a noninvasive test using 1 to 5 seconds of vibration and sound to induce fetal reactivity during a nonstress test. Vibration is produced by an artificial larynx or fetal acoustic stimulator placed above the head of the fetus.

Reproductive disorders

Common disorders associated with the reproductive system include those affecting females, those affecting males, and sexually transmitted diseases (STDs) that can affect either gender.

Female disorders

Here are some common disorders associated with the female reproductive system:
• **Endometriosis** refers to endometrial tissue appearing outside the lining of the uterine cavity.
• **Ovarian cysts** are noncancerous sacs containing fluid or semisolid material.
• **Pelvic inflammatory disease** is an infection of the oviducts and ovaries.
• **Premenstrual syndrome (PMS)** is characterized by varying symptoms appearing 7 to 10 days before menses and usually subsiding with its onset. The effects of PMS range from minimal discomfort to severe disruptive symptoms that can include nervousness, irritability, depression, and multiple somatic complaints.
• **Uterine leiomyomas,** also called **myomas, fibromyomas,** or **fibroids,** are the most common **neoplasms** (tumors) among women. They occur most often in the uterus or cervix.

• **Vaginismus** is an involuntary, spastic constriction of the lower vaginal muscles.

Male disorders

Here are some common disorders associated with the male reproductive system:

• **Cryptorchidism** is condition in which one or both testes fail to descend into the scrotum and remain in the abdomen, the inguinal canal, or at the external inguinal ring.
• **Epididymitis** is an inflammation of the epididymis.
• **Premature ejaculation** refers to a man's inability to control the ejaculatory reflex during intercourse resulting in persistently early ejaculation.
• **Prostatitis** refers to a chronic inflammation of the prostate gland, usually from infection.

Impotence

Impotence is also known as **erectile dysfunction.** A man with this problem can't attain or maintain sufficient penile erection to complete intercourse. There are two types of impotence:

• **primary impotence** — the patient has never achieved a sufficient erection to complete intercourse
• **secondary impotence** — the patient has succeeded in completing intercourse in the past.

Testicular torsion

Testicular torsion is abnormal twisting of the spermatic cord caused by rotation of the testis. Two types of testicular torsion are:

• **intravaginal torsion,** resulting from an abnormal tunica or from narrowing of the muscular support (normally, the tunica vaginalis envelops the testis and attaches to the epididymis and spermatic cord; in intravaginal torsion, testicular twisting may result from an abnormality of the tunica in which the testis is abnormally positioned or from narrowing of the muscular support)
• **extravaginal torsion,** caused by loose attachment of the tunica to the scrotal lining, which causes the spermatic cord rotation above the testis.

Sexually transmitted diseases

Here are the names of some common STDs and conditions that accompany them:

- **Chancroid,** also called **soft chancre,** is a venereal disorder marked by painful genital ulcers and inguinal lymph node inflammation.
- **Chlamydia** is the most common STD in the United States. This group of infections, which include **urethritis** (inflammation of the urethra) in men and urethritis and **cervicitis** (cervical inflammation) in women are linked to the *Chlamydia trachomatis* organism.
- **Genital herpes,** also known as **herpes simplex virus, herpes type 2,** or **venereal herpes,** is an acute, inflammatory infection that causes fluid-filled vesicles on genitalia. The vesicles rupture and develop into shallow, painful ulcers.
- **Genital warts,** also called **condylomata acuminata,** consist of painless **papillomas** (noncancerous skin tumors) with fibrous tissue overgrowth that often has a cauliflower–like appearance.
- **Gonorrhea** is a common disease caused by the *Neisseria gonorrhoeae* organism. This STD most often affects the urethra and cervix.
- **Trichomoniasis** is a protozoal infection of the lower urinary tract and reproductive system.

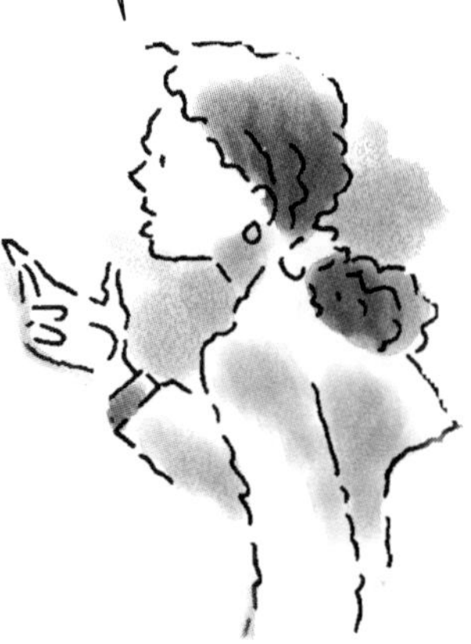

STDs were once called **venereal** after Venus, the goddess of love.

Syphilis

Syphilis is a chronic, infectious venereal disease that begins in the mucous membranes and quickly moves through the body by spreading to nearby lymph nodes and the bloodstream. The untreated disease process has four stages:

- **Primary syphilis** occurs within 3 weeks of original contact. Patients may develop **chancres** (small sores) on the body and lymph node tenderness.
- **Secondary syphilis** occurs from a few days to 8 weeks after the onset of sores. Patients develop a rash, white lesions, and flulike symptoms.
- **Latent syphilis** is characterized by an absence of symptoms.
- **Late syphilis,** also called **tertiary syphilis,** involves other organs, such as those in the cardiovascular and central nervous systems.

Other reproductive disorders

Here are some other common reproductive disorders, including disorders associated with pregnancy:

- **Abruptio placentae** is the premature separation of a normally positioned placenta in a pregnancy of at least 20 weeks' gestation. This may occur either before or during labor but always before delivery.
- **Adenomyosis of the uterus** is a condition in which endometrial tissue invades the muscular layer of the uterus.
- **Benign prostatic hyperplasia** refers to an enlargement of the prostate gland.
- **Ectopic pregnancy** is the implantation of the fertilized ovum outside the uterine cavity.
- In **hematocele,** blood collects in a body cavity, such as the scrotum, testis, or pelvis.
- **Hydatidiform mole** is an uncommon chorionic tumor of the placenta.
- **Hydrocele** is a collection of clear fluid in a testis.
- **Hydrorrhea gravidarum** is the discharge of thin, watery fluid from the pregnant uterus.
- **Hyperemesis gravidarum** is severe and unremitting nausea and vomiting that persists after the first 12 weeks of pregnancy.
- **Hyperplasia of the endometrium** is the overdevelopment of the uterine lining.
- **Mastitis** is an inflammation of the mammary glands occurring with breast-feeding.
- **Oligohydramnios** is less than a normal amount of amniotic fluid. (See *Taking apart oligohydramnios*, page 238.)
- **Oligospermia** is less than a normal amount of sperm in the semen.
- **Phimosis** is a constriction of the foreskin over the penis so that it can't be drawn back over the glans.
- **Placenta previa** is a placenta that develops in the lower segment of the uterus.
- **Precocious puberty** is the early onset of pubertal changes, such as breast development and menstruation before age 9 (in females). Males with the disorder begin to sexually mature before age 10.
- **Premature labor,** also called preterm labor, is the onset of rhythmic uterine contractions that produce cervi-

Beyond the dictionary

Taking apart oligohydramnios

Oligohydramnios is less than a normal amount of amniotic fluid. The word element ***oligo*** means *few* or *scanty*. ***Hydro*** means *water* or *fluid* and ***amnios*** refers to the amnion. Thus, **oligohydramnios** means *little fluid in the amnion.*

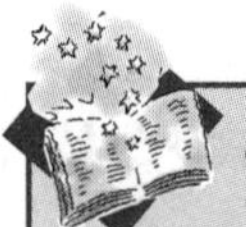

Beyond the dictionary

Salpingocele story

Salpingocele is a herniation of the fallopian tube. The Greek word ***salpinex*** for *trumpet,* a tubular instrument, gives us ***salpingo-,*** which refers to the fallopian tubes. The ***-cele*** stands for *cavity,* and thus refers to a hernia.

cal change after fetal viability but before fetal maturity, usually between the 20th and 37th week of gestation.

- **Premature rupture of membranes** is a spontaneous break or tear in the amniotic sac before the onset of regular contractions.
- **Prolapse of uterus** is the protrusion of the uterus thought the vaginal opening.
- **Pruritus vulvae** is intense itching of the vulva.
- **Salpingocele** is a hernial protrusion of the fallopian tube. (See *Salpingocele story.*)
- **Spermatocele** is a cyst containing sperm cells near the epididymis.
- **Spontaneous abortion** is a premature loss of an embryo or nonviable fetus from the uterus.

Treatments

Here are terms relating to surgeries and other treatments of the male and female reproductive systems:

- **Abortion** is the termination of a pregnancy.
- **Artificial insemination** is the placement of seminal fluid into the patient's vaginal canal or cervix. The procedure is coordinated with ovulation.
- **Cervical suturing,** also called **cerclage,** is when a purse-string suture is used to reinforce the cervix.
- A **cervicectomy** is removal of the cervix.
- **Cesarean section** is an incision made through the abdominal and uterine walls to deliver a neonate.
- **Circumcision** is the removal of all or part of the **prepuce** (foreskin) of the glans penis.

- In **dilatation of the uterine cervix and curettage** (scraping) **of the endometrium (D&C)** the doctor dilatates (expands) the cervix to access the endocervix and uterus. A **curette** (an instrument with sharp edges) is used to scrape away endometrial tissue. (See *Just say "D&C."*)
- In **dilatation and evacuation,** suction is used to remove the uterine contents.
- **Episiotomy** is an incision made to the vulva to prevent tearing during delivery of a neonate.
- With **in vitro fertilization,** an ovum is removed from the body and fertilized with sperm in a laboratory culture medium. The resulting embryo is then transferred into the woman's body.
- In a **laparoscopy,** surgical instruments are inserted through a laparoscope to remove small lesions.
- A **laparotomy** is a surgical incision through the abdomen made to provide access to the peritoneal cavity.
- **Oophorectomy** is excision of one or both ovaries.
- An **orchiectomy** is removal of one of the testes.
- **Vasectomy** is excision of the vas deferens. When done bilaterally, this results in sterility.

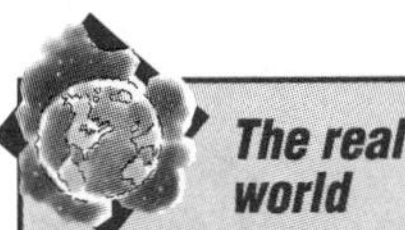

Just say "D&C"

In the "real world," **dilatation** of the uterine cervix and **curettage** of the endometrium is known as a "D and C." A **dilatation and evacuation,** in which suction is used to remove the uterine contents, is referred to as a "D and E."

Hysterectomy

A hysterectomy is removal of the uterus. There are four types:

- **Total hysterectomy,** also called a **panhysterectomy,** is removal of the entire uterus and cervix.
- **Subtotal hysterectomy** is removal of only part of the uterus, leaving the cervix intact.
- **Radical hysterectomy** is removal of all of the reproductive organs and supporting structures.
- **Vaginal hysterectomy** is excision of the uterus through the vagina.

Remember, the word **hystero** means uterus and **-ectomy** means surgical removal. Therefore a **hysterectomy** is removal of the uterus.

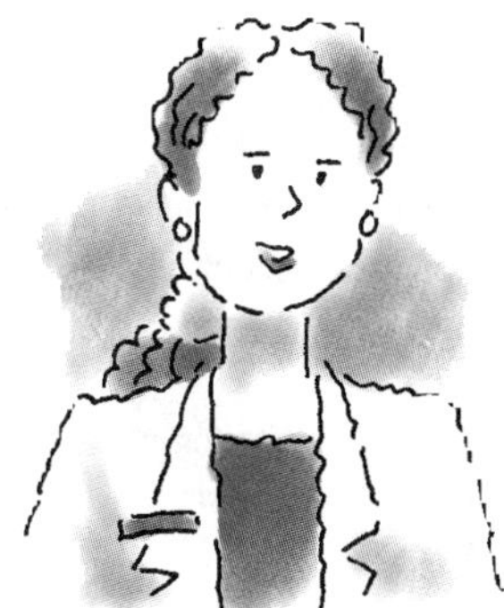

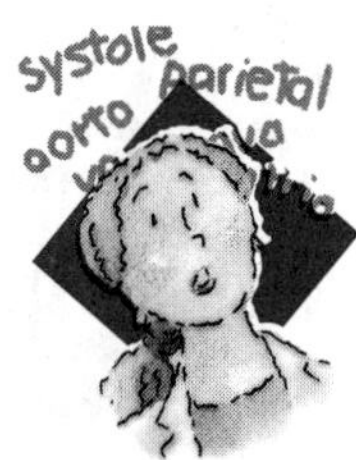

Vocabulary builders

At a crossroads

Completing this crossword puzzle will help you produce the correct terms for the reproductive system. Good luck!

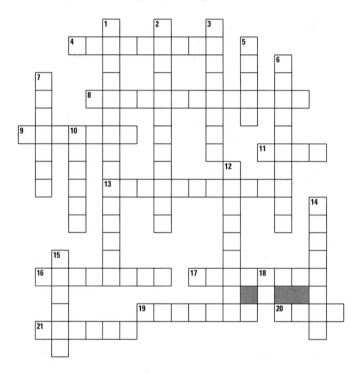

Across

4. Erectile dysfunction
8. Aspiration of amniotic fluid
9. Mammary glands
11. Abbreviation for a venereal disease test
13. Lining of the uterus
16. Skin that covers tip of the penis
17. Female sex hormone
19. Hormone produced after menopause
20. Female sex cell
21. Upper uterus

Down

1. Sperm formation
2. Male sex hormone
3. Area between anus and vulva
5. Tissue covering the vaginal opening
6. A duct system in the testes
7. Two almond-shaped female organs
10. An embryo floats within it
12. Lactogenic hormone
14. Visible female genitals
15. Main body of the uterus
18. Mouth of the cervix

Answers are on page 244.

Match game

Match each description of a reproductive disorder to its name.

Clues	Choices
1. Testicular torsion ____	A. Constriction of foreskin
2. Endometriosis ____	B. Enlargement of male breast
3. Fibroid tumor ____	C. Leiomyoma
4. Trichomoniasis ____	D. Ectopic uterine tissue
5. Genital warts ____	E. Termination of a pregnancy
6. Gynecomastia ____	F. Papillomas
7. Phimosis ____	G. Twisting of the spermatic cord
8. Abortion ____	H. Protozoal infection

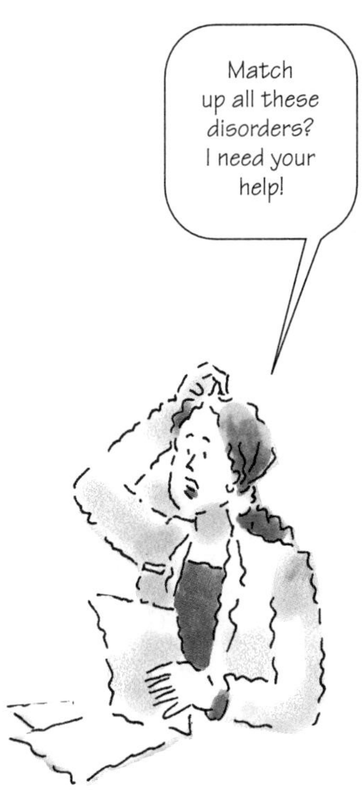

Match up all these disorders? I need your help!

Answers are on page 244.

Finish line

Fill in the blanks below with the appropriate word(s).

1. Each ______ _____ is enclosed by a spermatic cord.
2. ________ stimulates milk production.
3. Surgical removal of the uterus is called a ________.
4. ________ sign is softening of the cervix and is a probable sign of pregnancy.
5. A procedure to visualize pelvic organs is called a _______.
6. The process of uniting a sperm and an egg in a culture dish is known as _________ fertilization.
7. The process of instilling seminal fluid into a patient's vaginal canal is called ________ insemination.
8. Patients with erectile dysfunction due to spinal cord injury may have a ________ inserted into the penis.
9. A suturing procedure to reinforce the cervix is called _______.
10. An ________ procedure surgically secures the testis in the scrotum and is used to treat an undescended testis.

Are there any hormones that stimulate answer production?

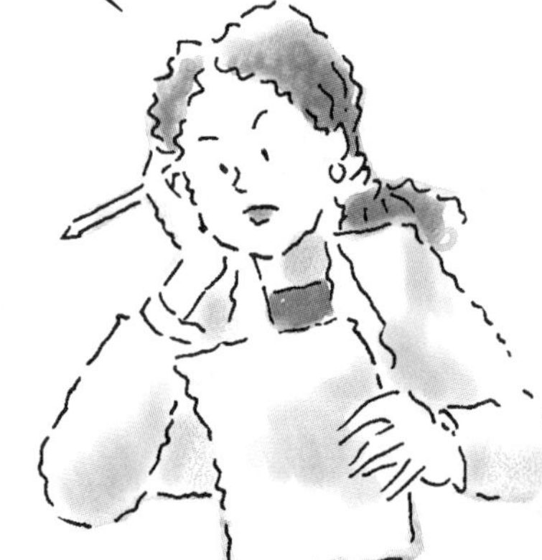

Answers are on page 244.

Scrambled or overeasy

Fill in the answers for the following questions, then unscramble the circled letters to find the answer to the puzzle.

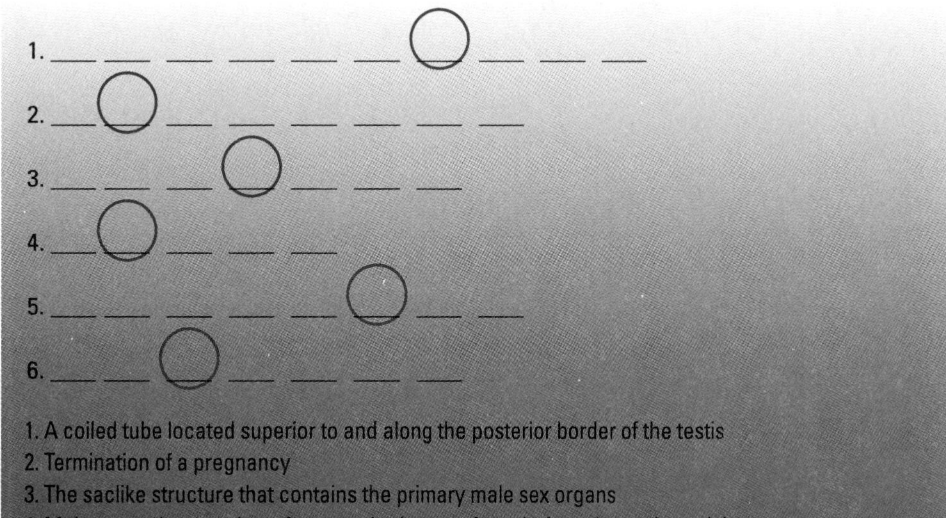

1. A coiled tube located superior to and along the posterior border of the testis
2. Termination of a pregnancy
3. The saclike structure that contains the primary male sex organs
4. Male organ that consists of an attached root, a free shaft, and an enlarged tip
5. Female organ that contains erectile tissue and sensory corpuscles that are stimulated during sexual activity
6. Specialized accessory glands that secrete milk

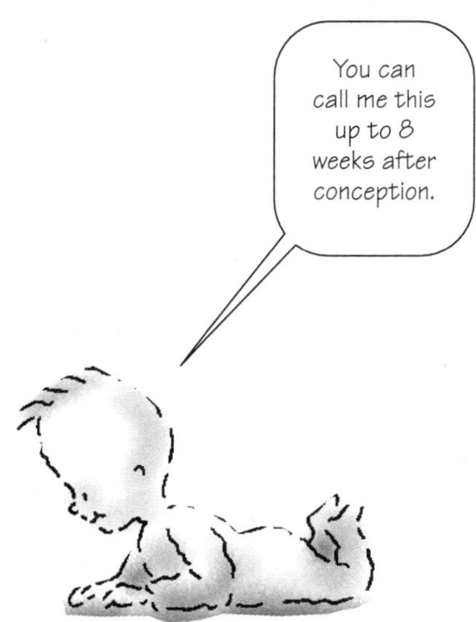

You can call me this up to 8 weeks after conception.

Answers are on page 244.

Answers

At a crossroads

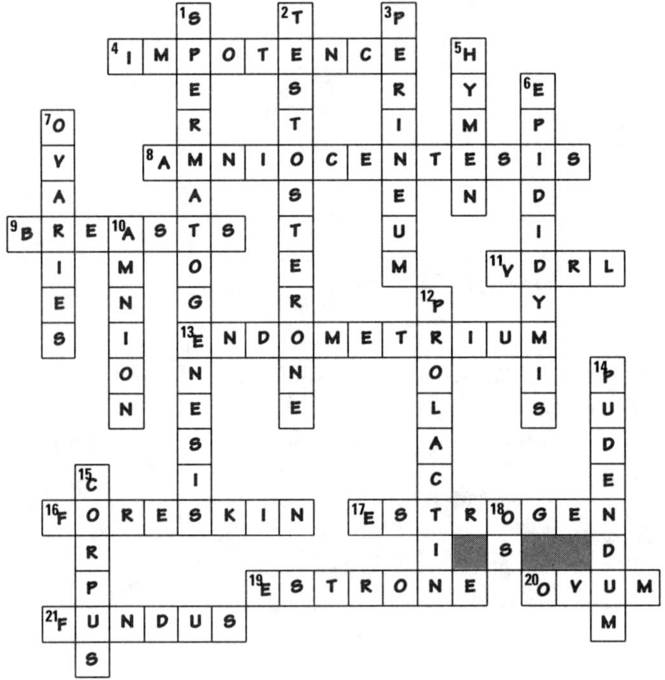

Match game

1. G; 2. D; 3. C; 4. H; 5. F; 6. B; 7. A; 8. E.

Finish line

1. Vas deferens; 2. Prolactin; 3. Hysterectomy; 4. Goodell's; 5. Laparoscopy; 6. In vitro; 7. Artificial; 8. Prosthesis; 9. Cerclage; 10. Orchiopexy.

Scrambled or overeasy

1. Epididymis; 2. Abortion; 3. Scrotum; 4. Penis; 5. Clitoris; 6. Mammary.
Answer to puzzle — Embryo

Neurologic system

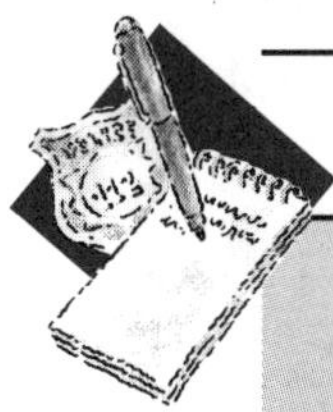

Just the facts

In this chapter, you'll review:

- terminology related to the structure and function of the neurologic system
- terminology needed for physical examination
- tests that help diagnose common neurologic disorders
- neurologic system disorders and their treatments.

Neurologic structure and function

The nervous system coordinates all body functions, enabling a person to adapt to changes in internal and external environments. It has two main types of cells — neurons and neuroglia — and two main divisions — the **central nervous system (CNS)** and the **peripheral nervous system.** (See *Pronouncing key neurologic system terms,* page 246.)

Cells of the nervous system

The nervous system is packed with intertwined cells.

Neurons — the naked truth

Neurons, the conducting cells of the nervous system, respond to stimuli and transmit responses by means of electromechanical messages.

These highly specialized cells don't reproduce. The main parts of a neuron are the **cell body** and its **cytoplasmic processes** (parts that project from the cyto-

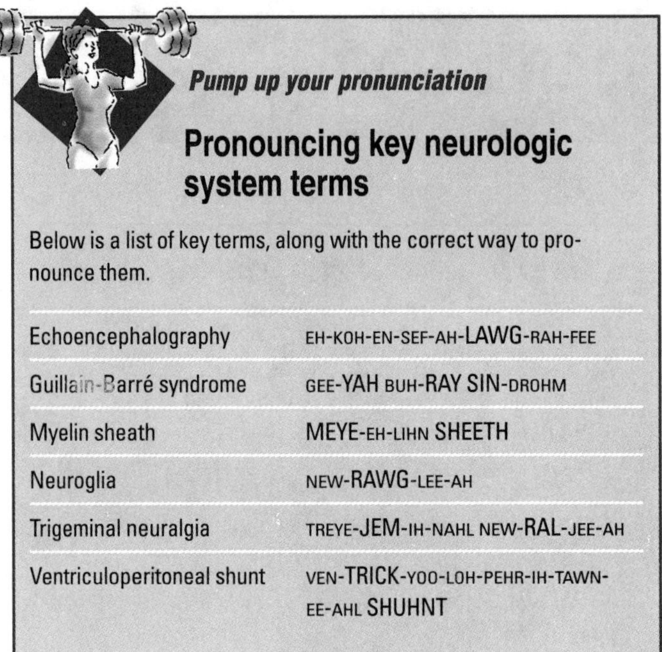

Pump up your pronunciation

Pronouncing key neurologic system terms

Below is a list of key terms, along with the correct way to pronounce them.

Echoencephalography	EH-KOH-EN-SEF-AH-LAWG-RAH-FEE
Guillain-Barré syndrome	GEE-YAH BUH-RAY SIN-DROHM
Myelin sheath	MEYE-EH-LIHN SHEETH
Neuroglia	NEW-RAWG-LEE-AH
Trigeminal neuralgia	TREYE-JEM-IH-NAHL NEW-RAL-JEE-AH
Ventriculoperitoneal shunt	VEN-TRICK-YOO-LOH-PEHR-IH-TAWN-EE-AHL SHUHNT

plasm) called axons and dendrites. In a typical neuron, one axon and many dendrites extend from the cell body. (See *Parts of a neuron.*)

Shipping and receiving

Axons conduct nerve impulses away from the cell body. **Dendrites** conduct impulses toward the cell body.

The axon may vary from quite short to very long — up to $3\frac{1}{4}'$ (1 m). A typical axon has **terminal branches** and is wrapped in a white, fatty segmented covering called a **myelin sheath.** The myelin sheath is produced by **Schwann cells,** made up of phagocytic cells (cells capable of engulfing and digesting microorganisms and cellular debris) separated by gaps called **nodes of Ranvier.** (See *Schwann and Ranvier,* page 248.)

Dendrites are short, thick, diffusely branched extensions that receive impulses arriving at the neuron from other cells.

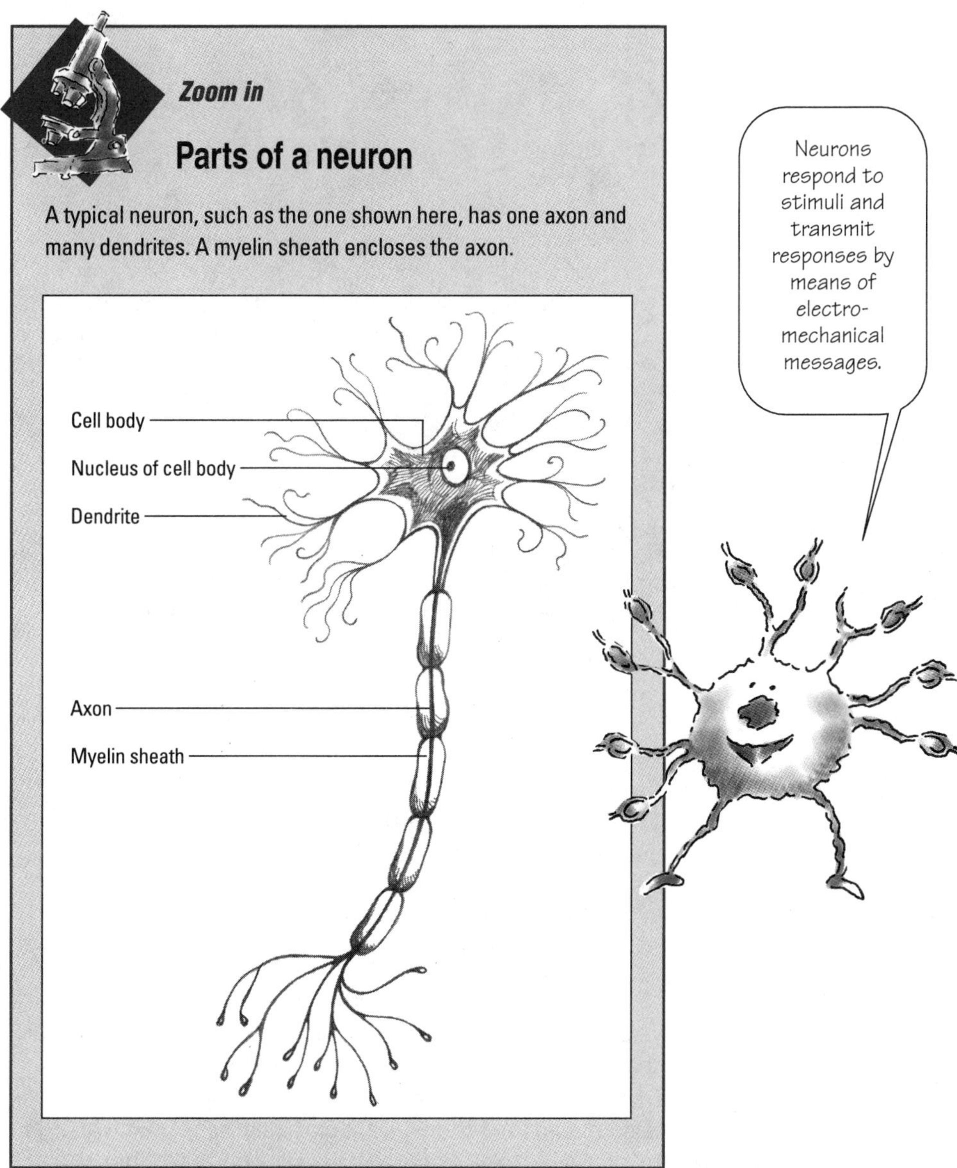

Zoom in
Parts of a neuron
A typical neuron, such as the one shown here, has one axon and many dendrites. A myelin sheath encloses the axon.
Cell body
Nucleus of cell body
Dendrite
Axon
Myelin sheath
Neurons respond to stimuli and transmit responses by means of electro-mechanical messages.

Being impulsive

The action of neurons is responsible for **neurotransmission** — the conduction of electrochemical impulses throughout the nervous system. Neuron activity may be provoked by mechanical stimuli, such as touch and pressure; by thermal stimuli, such as heat and cold; or by chemical stimuli, such as external chemicals and chemicals released by the body such as histamine.

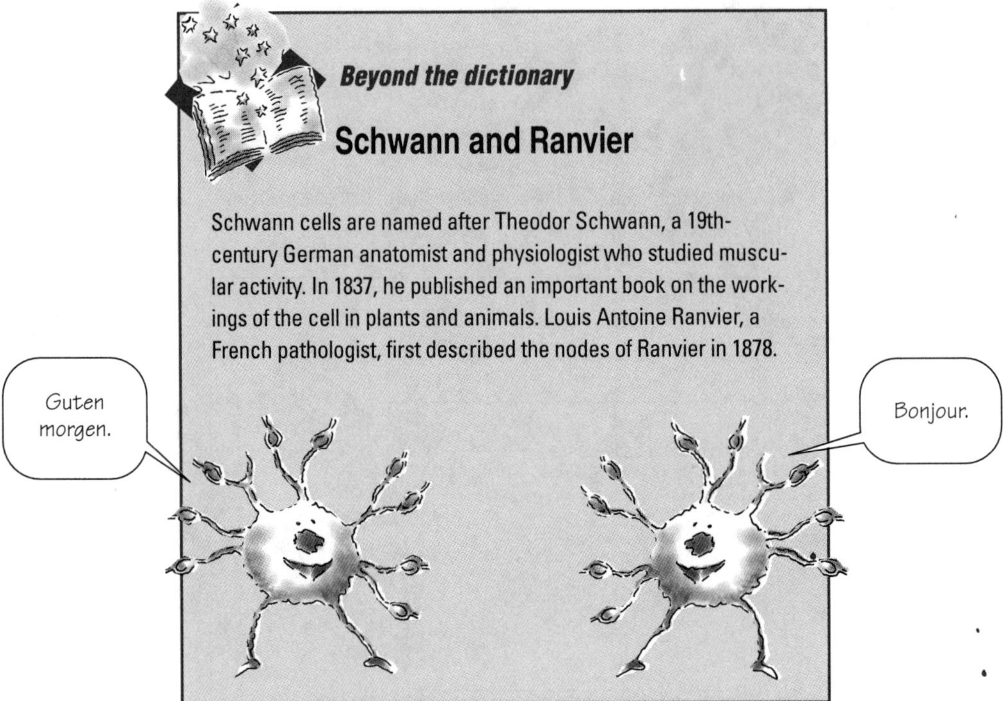

Beyond the dictionary
Schwann and Ranvier
Schwann cells are named after Theodor Schwann, a 19th-century German anatomist and physiologist who studied muscular activity. In 1837, he published an important book on the workings of the cell in plants and animals. Louis Antoine Ranvier, a French pathologist, first described the nodes of Ranvier in 1878.
Guten morgen.
Bonjour.

Neuro-glue

The supportive cells of the nervous system, **neuroglia,** are also called **glial cells. Glial** is derived from the Greek word for *glue* — these cells hold the neurons together and form roughly 40% of the brain's bulk. Four types of neuroglia exist.

- **Astroglia,** or **astrocytes,** exist throughout the nervous system. They supply nutrients to neurons and help them maintain their electrical potential. Astrocytes also form part of the **blood-brain barrier** that separates CNS tissue from the bloodstream and guards against invasion by disease-causing organisms and other harmful substances.

- A second type of neuroglia, **ependymal cells,** line the **ventricles,** four small cavities in the brain, as well as the **choroid plexuses,** vascular structures that form a network in the pia mater of the brain and project into the third, lateral, and fourth ventricles. These cells help produce **cerebrospinal fluid (CSF).**

Microglia are phagocytic cells that ingest and digest microorganisms and waste products from injured neurons.

Oligodendroglia support and electrically insulate CNS axons by forming protective myelin sheaths.

Brain

The CNS includes the spinal cord and the brain. The brain consists of the cerebrum, cerebellum, brain stem, and primitive structures that lie below the cerebrum — the diencephalon, limbic system, and reticular activating system. (See *Major structures in the brain*, page 250.)

You're so cerebral

The cerebrum has right and left hemispheres. The **corpus callosum —** a mass of nerve fibers — bridges the hemispheres, allowing communication between corresponding centers in each. The rolling surface of the cerebrum is made up of **gyri** (convolutions) and **sulci** (creases or fissures). The thin surface layer, the **cerebral cortex,** consists of **gray matter** (unmyelinated nerve fibers). Within the cerebrum lie **white matter** (myelinated nerve fibers) and islands of internal gray matter.

Lots of lobes

Each cerebral hemisphere is divided into four lobes, based on anatomic landmarks and functional differences. The lobes are named for the cranial bones that lie over them — frontal, temporal, parietal, and occipital:

- The **frontal lobe** influences personality, judgment, abstract reasoning, social behavior, language expression, and movement.
- The **temporal lobe** controls hearing, language comprehension, and storage and recall of memories (although memories are stored throughout the entire brain).
- The **parietal lobe** interprets and integrates sensations, including pain, temperature, and touch. It also interprets size, shape, distance, and texture. The parietal

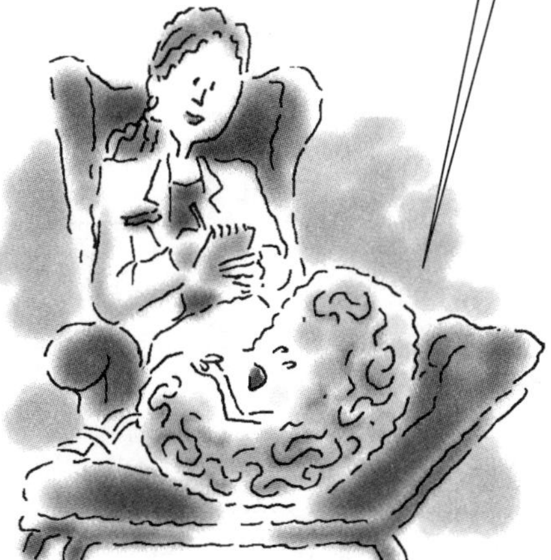
Let's talk about communication.
Okay. The **corpus callosum** bridges my right and left hemispheres, allowing communication between them.

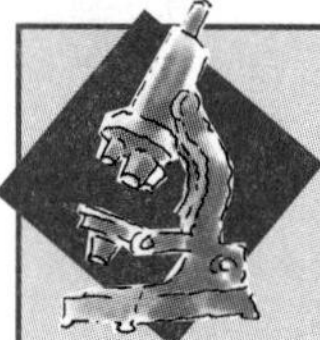

Zoom in

Major structures in the brain

This illustration shows the two largest structures of the brain — the cerebrum and cerebellum. Note the locations of the four cerebral lobes and of the sensory cortex and motor cortex.

The illustration below shows a cross section of the brain, from its outermost portion (cerebrum) to its innermost (diencephalon).

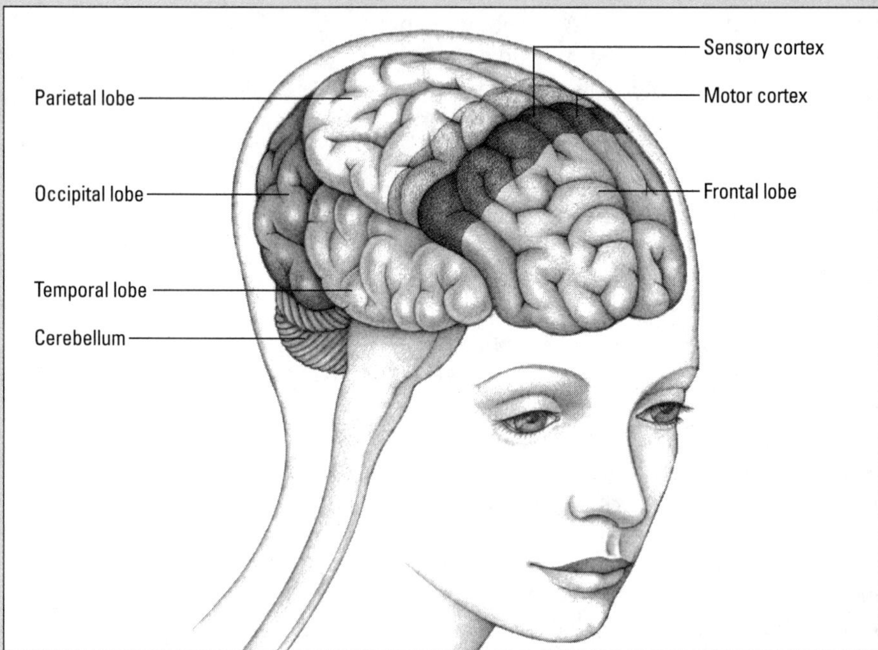

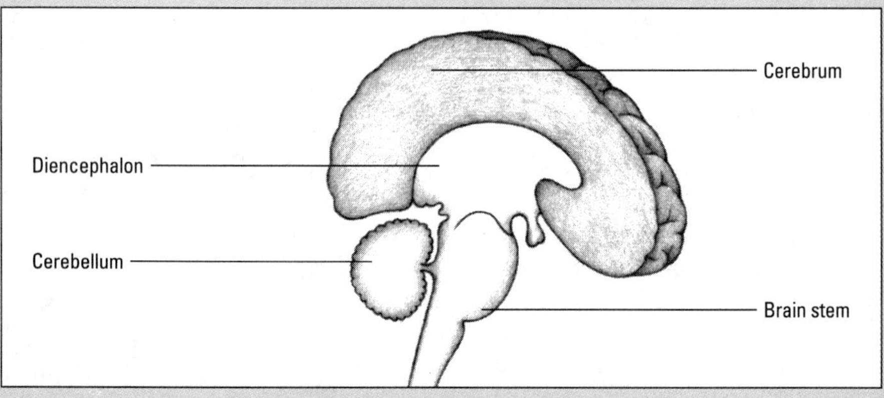

lobe of the nondominant hemisphere is especially important for awareness of one's own body shape.

- The **occipital lobe** functions mainly to interpret visual stimuli.

Celebrating the cerebellum

The **cerebellum,** the second largest brain region, lies posterior and inferior to the cerebrum. Like the cerebrum, it has two hemispheres, an outer cortex of gray matter and an inner core of white matter. The cerebellum functions to maintain muscle tone, coordinate muscle movement, and control balance.

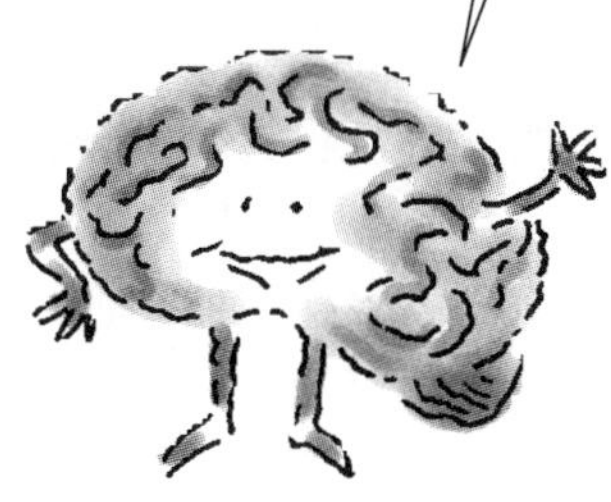

My lobes are named for the cranial bones that lie over them — frontal, temporal, parietal, and occipital.

Brain stem

The **brain stem** lies immediately inferior to the cerebrum, just anterior to the cerebellum. It's continuous with the cerebrum superiorly and with the spinal cord inferiorly.

Composed of the midbrain, pons, and medulla oblongata, the brain stem relays messages between the parts of the nervous system. It has three main functions:

- It produces the rigid autonomic behaviors necessary for survival, such as increasing the heart rate and stimulating the adrenal medulla to produce epinephrine.
- It provides pathways for nerve fibers between higher and lower neural centers.
- It serves as the origin for 10 of the 12 pairs of cranial nerves.

The **reticular activating system (RAS),** a diffuse network of hyperexcitable neurons, fans out from the brain stem through the cerebral cortex. After screening all incoming sensory information, the RAS channels it to appropriate areas of the brain for interpretation. RAS activity also stimulates wakefulness.

Where nerves volunteer

The **midbrain** connects dorsally with the cerebellum. It contains large voluntary motor nerve tracts running between the brain and spinal cord.

The pons pathway

The **pons** connects the cerebellum with the cerebrum and links the midbrain to the medulla oblongata.

In addition to housing one of the brain's respiratory centers, the pons acts as a pathway between brain centers and the spinal cord and serves as the exit point for cranial nerves V, VI, and VII.

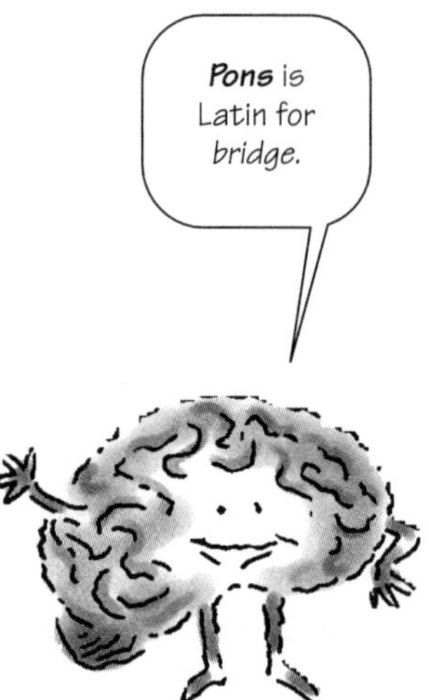
Pons is Latin for *bridge.*

Inferior, not unimportant

The **medulla oblongata,** the most inferior portion of the brain stem, is a small, cone-shaped structure. It joins the spinal cord at the level of the **foramen magnum,** an opening in the occipital portion of the skull. The medulla oblongata serves as an autonomic reflex center to maintain homeostasis, regulating respiratory, vasomotor, and cardiac functions.

Primitive structures

The **diencephalon** consists of the thalamus and hypothalamus, which lie beneath the surface of the cerebral hemispheres. The **thalamus** relays all sensory stimuli (except olfactory) as they ascend to the cerebral cortex. Its functions include primitive awareness of pain, screening of incoming stimuli, and focusing of attention. The **hypothalamus** controls or affects body temperature, appetite, water balance, pituitary secretions, emotions, and autonomic functions (including sleep and wakeful cycles).

Limbo with the limbic system

The **limbic system** is a primitive brain area deep within the temporal lobe. In addition to initiating basic drives, such as hunger, aggression, and emotional and sexual arousal, the limbic system screens all sensory messages traveling to the cerebral cortex. (See *Limbic system and brain stem.*)

Spinal cord

A cylindrical structure in the vertebral canal, the **spinal cord** extends from the foramen magnum at the base of the skull to the upper lumbar region of the vertebral column. The spinal nerves arise from the cord. At the cord's inferior end, nerve roots cluster in the **cauda equina.**

Zoom in

Limbic system and brain stem

The major structures of the limbic system and brain stem, shown here, are associated with such emotions as anger, fear, and sexual arousal.

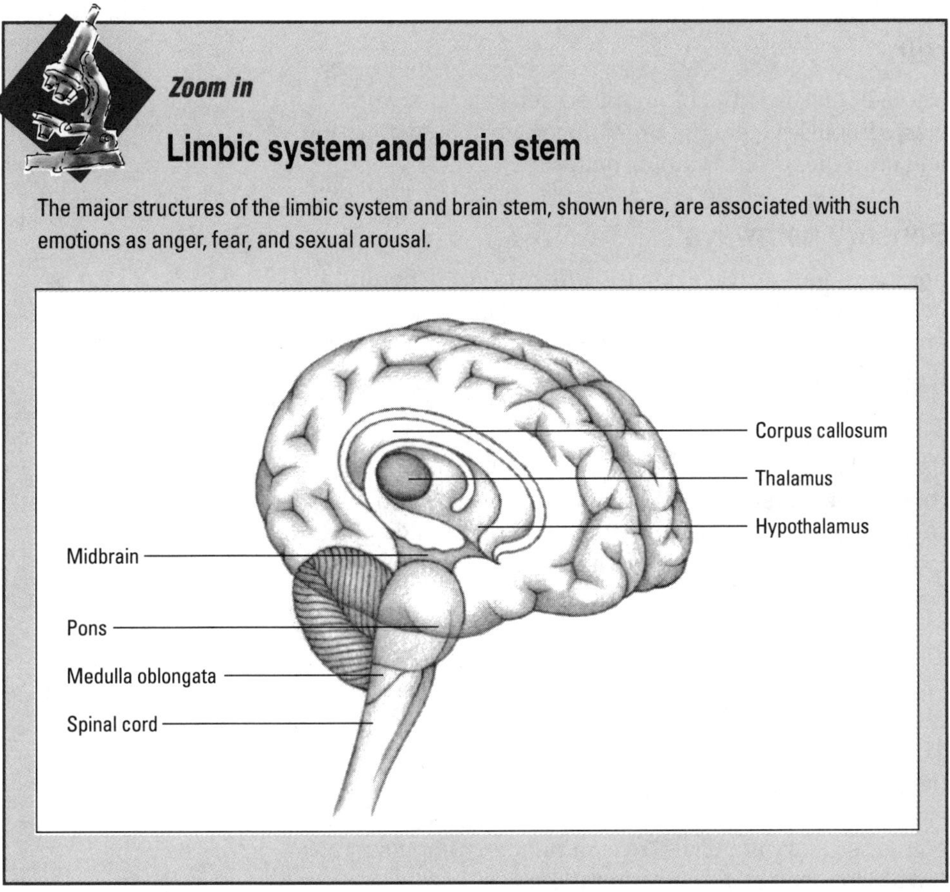

Horn of sensation, horn of activity

Within the spinal cord, the H-shaped mass of gray matter is divided into horns, which consist mainly of neuron cell bodies. Cell bodies in the **posterior horn** primarily relay sensations; those in the **anterior horn** play a part in voluntary and reflex motor activity. White matter surrounding the outer part of these horns consists of myelinated nerve fibers grouped functionally in vertical columns, or **tracts.**

Impulse conductor

The spinal cord conducts sensory nerve impulses to the brain and conducts motor impulses from the brain. It also controls such reflexes as the knee-jerk (patellar) reaction to a reflex hammer.

Pathways in the brain

Nerve impulses to the brain follow sensory pathways. Nerve impulses from the brain that control body function and movement follow motor pathways.

Sensory pathways

Sensory impulses travel via the **afferent,** or **ascending,** neural pathways to the brain's sensory cortex in the parietal lobe where they're interpreted. These impulses use two major pathways.

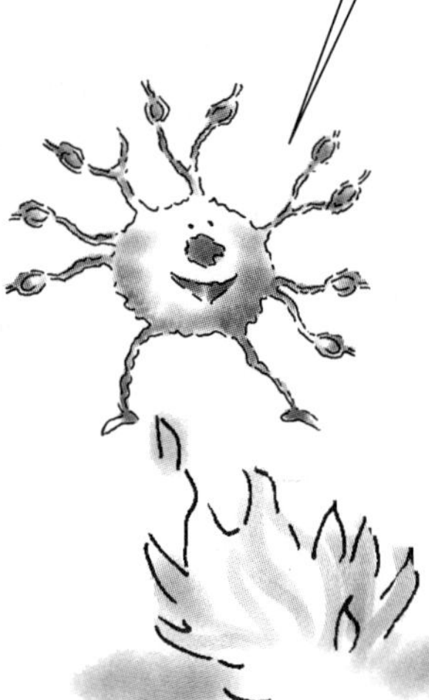
That's hot! Better alert the spinothalamic tract.

Ouch!

Pain and temperature sensations enter the spinal cord through the dorsal horn. After immediately crossing over to the opposite side of the cord, these stimuli then travel to the thalamus via the **spinothalamic tract.**

Touch-feely with the ganglia

Tactile, pressure, and vibration sensations enter the cord via relay stations called **ganglia,** knotlike masses of nerve cell bodies on the dorsal roots of spinal nerves. These stimuli then travel up the cord in the dorsal column to the medulla, where they cross to the opposite side and enter the thalamus. The thalamus relays all incoming sensory impulses (except olfactory impulses) to the sensory cortex for interpretation.

Flex...

Motor impulses travel from the brain to the muscles via **efferent,** or **descending,** pathways. Originating in the motor cortex of the frontal lobe, these impulses reach the lower motor neurons of the peripheral nervous system via **upper motor neurons.** Upper motor neurons originate in the brain and form two major systems:

- The **pyramidal system,** also called the **corticospinal tract,** is responsible for fine motor movements of skeletal muscle. Impulses in this system travel from the motor cortex through the internal capsule to the medulla, where they cross to the opposite side and continue down the spinal cord.
- The **extrapyramidal system,** or **extracorticospinal tract,** controls gross motor movements. Impulses originate in the premotor area of the frontal lobe and travel to

(Text continues on page 259.)

Incredibly Easy miniguide: The brain

The cerebrum has right and left hemispheres. Each cerebral hemisphere is divided into four lobes.

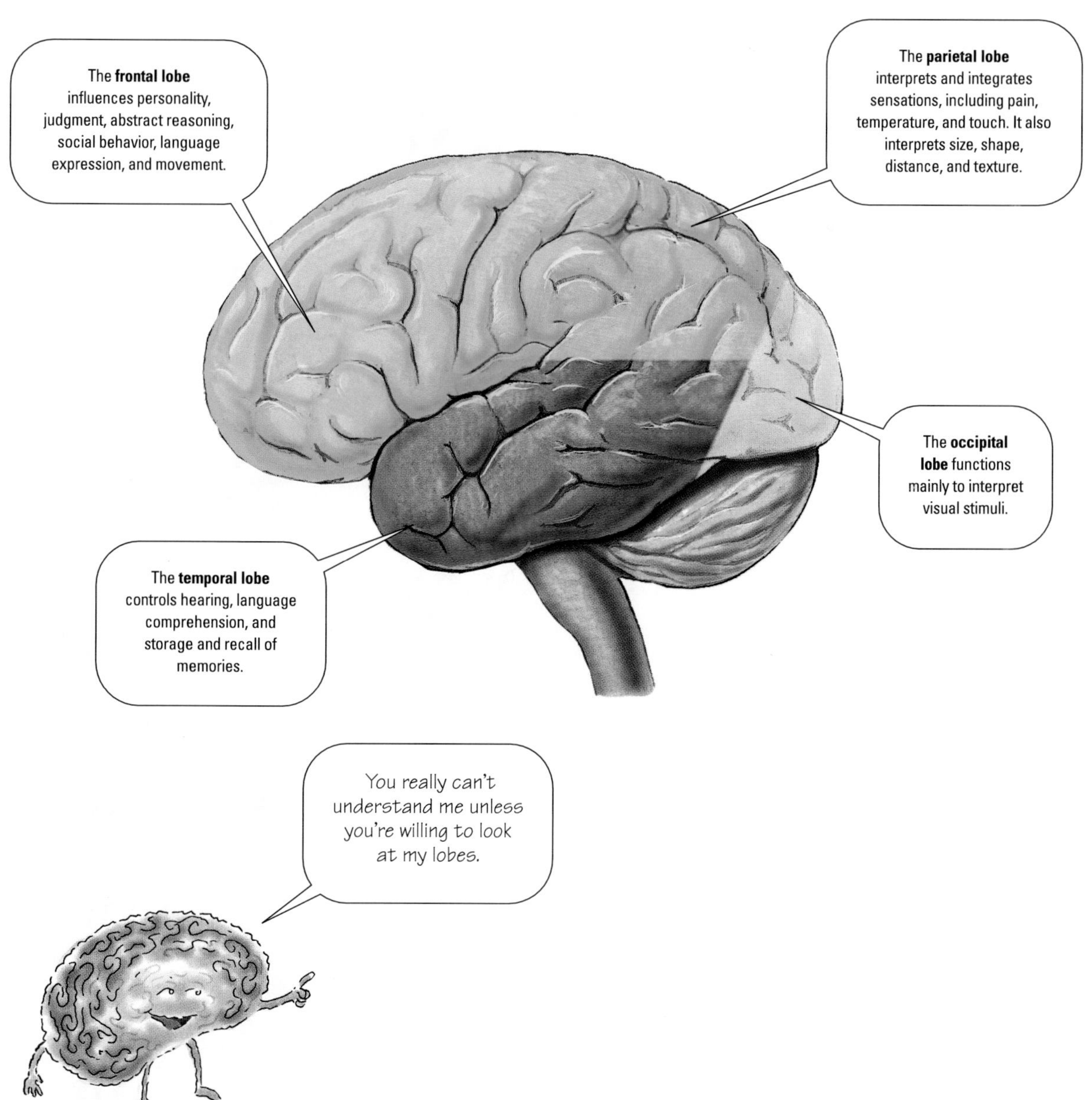
The **frontal lobe** influences personality, judgment, abstract reasoning, social behavior, language expression, and movement.
The **parietal lobe** interprets and integrates sensations, including pain, temperature, and touch. It also interprets size, shape, distance, and texture.
The **occipital lobe** functions mainly to interpret visual stimuli.
The **temporal lobe** controls hearing, language comprehension, and storage and recall of memories.
You really can't understand me unless you're willing to look at my lobes.

Incredibly Easy miniguide: The brain

This illustration of the inferior surface of the brain shows the anterior and posterior arteries, which join with smaller arteries to form the circle of Willis.

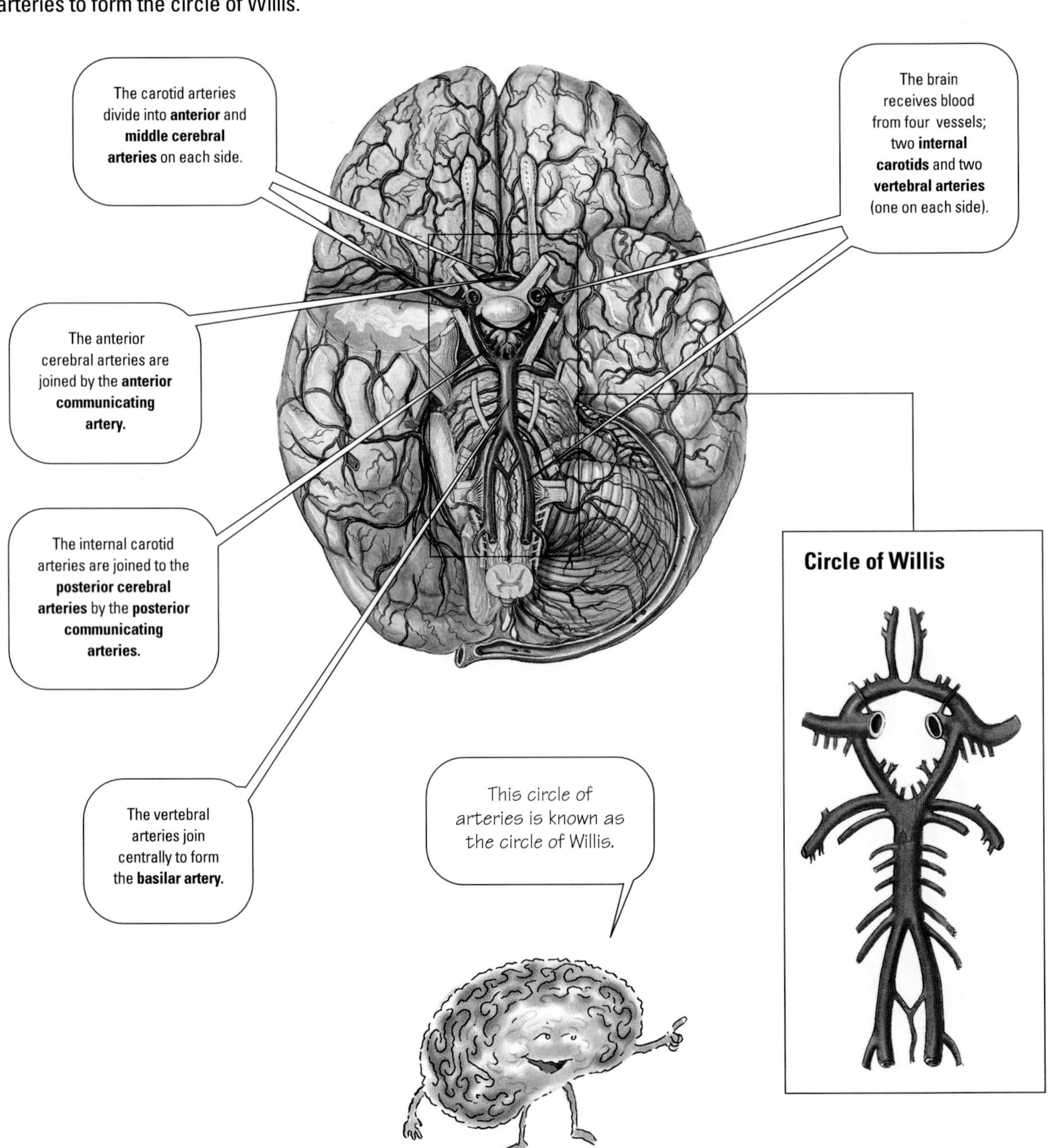

The carotid arteries divide into **anterior** and **middle cerebral arteries** on each side.
The brain receives blood from four vessels; two **internal carotids** and two **vertebral arteries** (one on each side).
The anterior cerebral arteries are joined by the **anterior communicating artery.**
The internal carotid arteries are joined to the **posterior cerebral arteries** by the **posterior communicating arteries.**
The vertebral arteries join centrally to form the **basilar artery.**
This circle of arteries is known as the circle of Willis.
Circle of Willis

Incredibly Easy miniguide: The brain

The meninges cover and protect the brain. They consist of three layers of connective tissue—the dura mater, arachnoid, and pia mater.

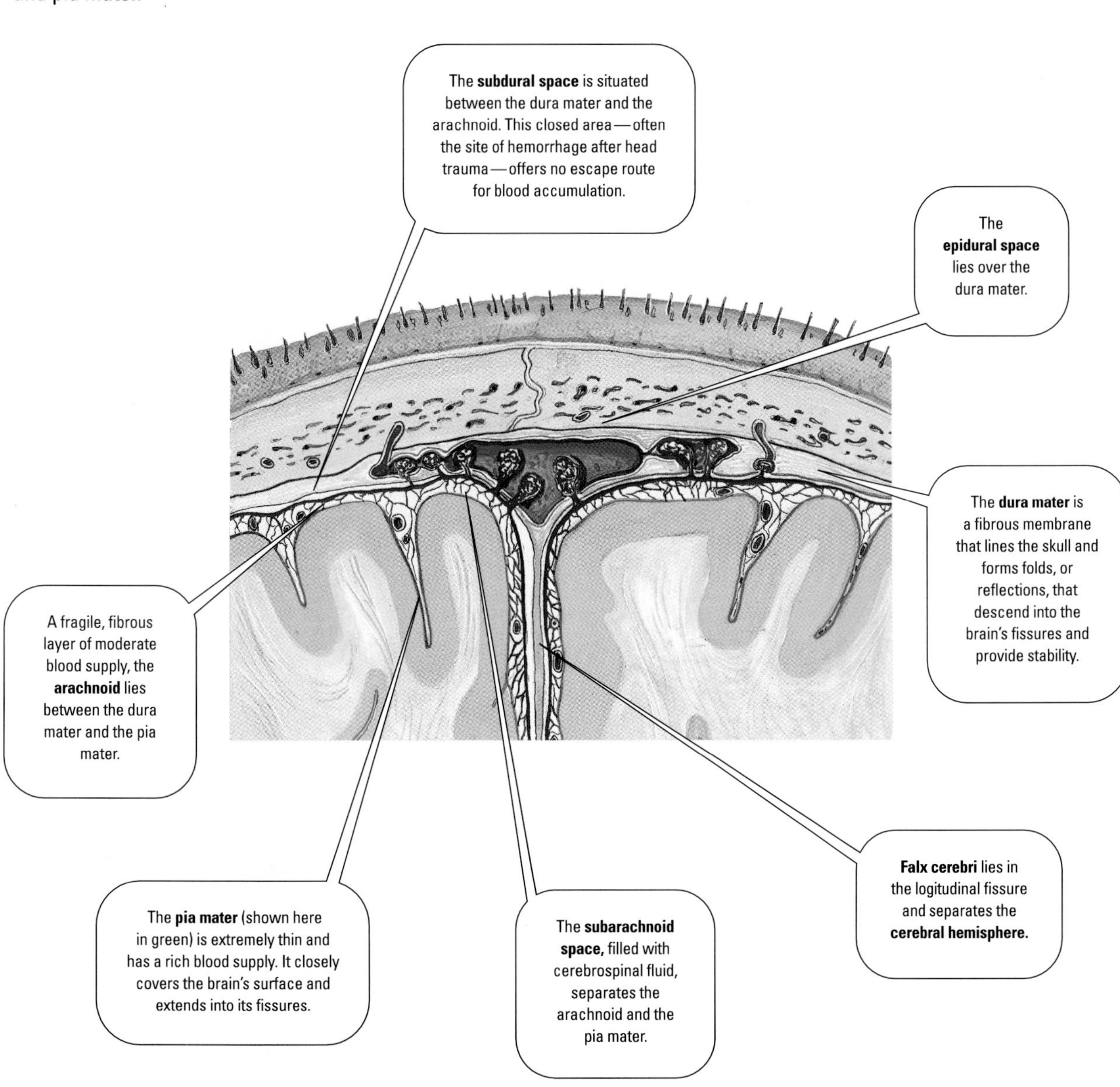

The **subdural space** is situated between the dura mater and the arachnoid. This closed area—often the site of hemorrhage after head trauma—offers no escape route for blood accumulation.
The **epidural space** lies over the dura mater.
The **dura mater** is a fibrous membrane that lines the skull and forms folds, or reflections, that descend into the brain's fissures and provide stability.
A fragile, fibrous layer of moderate blood supply, the **arachnoid** lies between the dura mater and the pia mater.
The **pia mater** (shown here in green) is extremely thin and has a rich blood supply. It closely covers the brain's surface and extends into its fissures.
The **subarachnoid space,** filled with cerebrospinal fluid, separates the arachnoid and the pia mater.
Falx cerebri lies in the logitudinal fissure and separates the **cerebral hemisphere.**

Incredibly Easy miniguide: The brain

The 12 pairs of cranial nerves transmit motor messages, sensory messages, or both, primarily between the brain or brainstem and the head and neck.

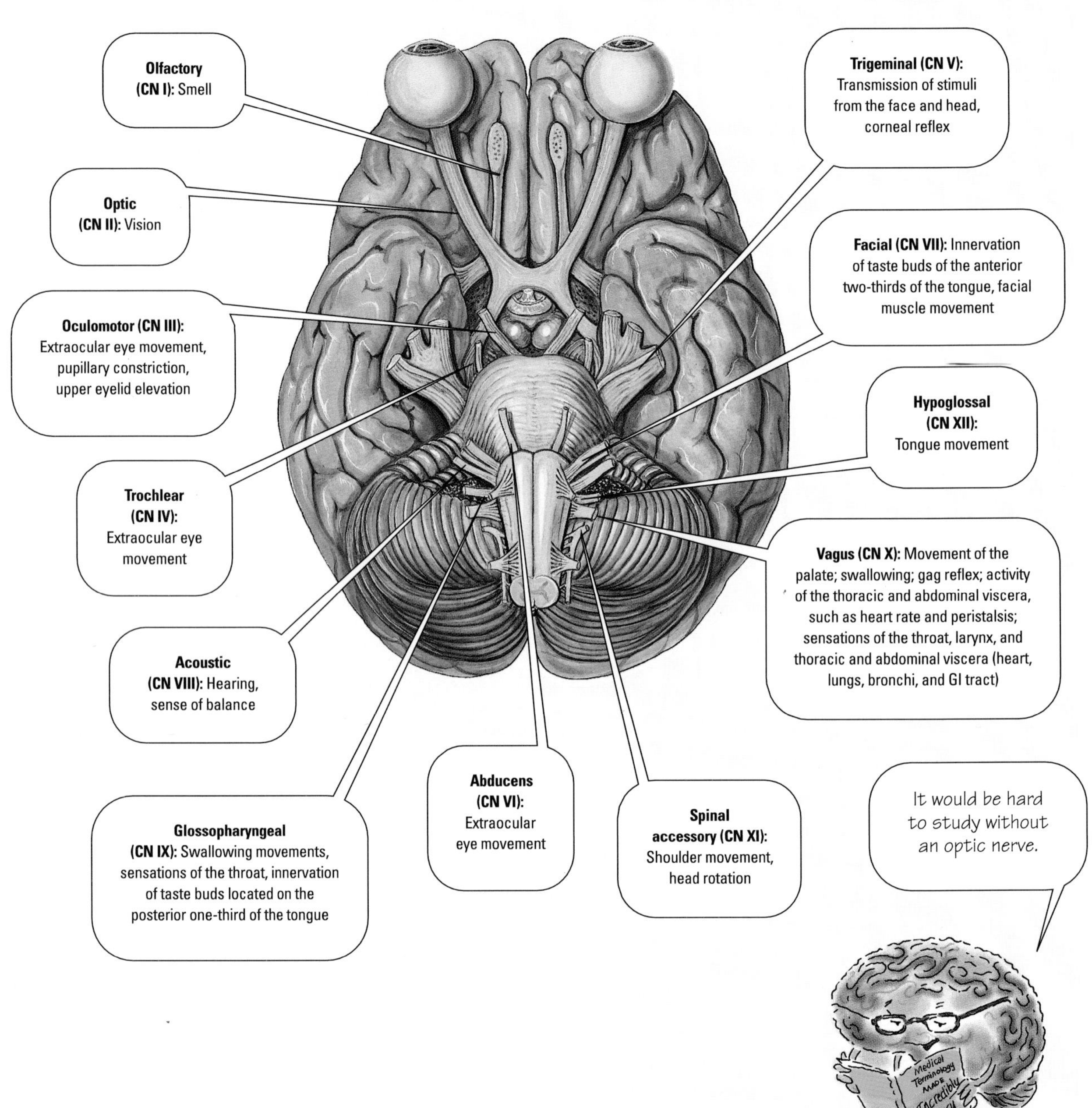

Olfactory (CN I): Smell
Optic (CN II): Vision
Oculomotor (CN III): Extraocular eye movement, pupillary constriction, upper eyelid elevation
Trochlear (CN IV): Extraocular eye movement
Acoustic (CN VIII): Hearing, sense of balance
Glossopharyngeal (CN IX): Swallowing movements, sensations of the throat, innervation of taste buds located on the posterior one-third of the tongue
Abducens (CN VI): Extraocular eye movement
Spinal accessory (CN XI): Shoulder movement, head rotation
Trigeminal (CN V): Transmission of stimuli from the face and head, corneal reflex
Facial (CN VII): Innervation of taste buds of the anterior two-thirds of the tongue, facial muscle movement
Hypoglossal (CN XII): Tongue movement
Vagus (CN X): Movement of the palate; swallowing; gag reflex; activity of the thoracic and abdominal viscera, such as heart rate and peristalsis; sensations of the throat, larynx, and thoracic and abdominal viscera (heart, lungs, bronchi, and GI tract)
It would be hard to study without an optic nerve.
Medical Terminology MADE Incredibly Easy

the pons, where they cross to the opposite side. Then the impulses travel down the spinal cord to the anterior horn, where they're relayed to the lower motor neurons. These neurons, in turn, carry the impulses to the muscles.

...and reflex

Reflex responses occur automatically, without any brain involvement, to protect the body. Spinal nerves, which have both sensory and motor portions, mediate **deep tendon reflexes** — involuntary contractions of a muscle after brief stretching caused by tendon percussion — and **superficial reflexes** — withdrawal reflexes elicited by noxious or tactile stimulation of the skin, cornea, or mucous membranes.

A simple reflex, such as the **knee-jerk reflex,** requires an **afferent** (sensory) neuron and an **efferent** (motor) neuron.

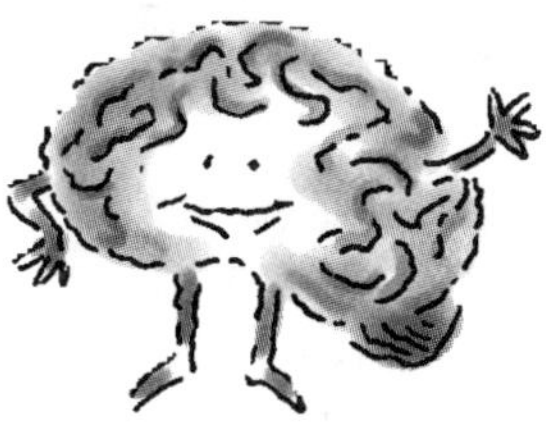
The extrapyramidal system controls gross motor movements.

Protective structures of the CNS

The brain and spinal cord are protected from shock and infection by bones, the meninges, several additional cushioning layers, and CSF.

Bones

The **skull,** formed of cranial bones, completely surrounds the brain. It opens at the foramen magnum, where the spinal cord exits.

The **vertebral column** protects the spinal cord. Its 30 vertebrae are separated from each other by an intervertebral disk that allows flexibility.

Meninges

The **meninges** cover and protect the cerebral cortex and spinal column. They consist of three layers of connective tissue: the dura mater, arachnoid membrane, and pia mater. (See *Protective membranes of the CNS,* page 260.)

Skull lining

The **dura mater** is a fibrous membrane that lines the skull and forms reflections, or folds, that descend into the brain's fissures and provide stability. The dural folds include:

- the **falx cerebri,** which lies in the longitudinal fissure and separates the cerebral hemispheres

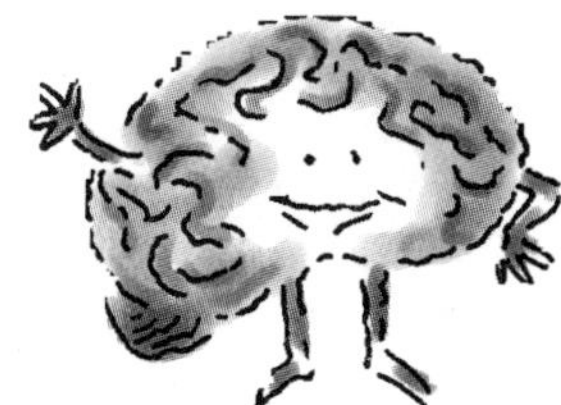
The spinal cord and I are protected by bones, the meninges, several additional cushioning layers, and CSF.

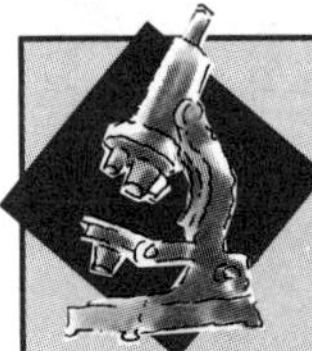

Zoom in

Protective membranes of the CNS

Three membranes — dura mater, arachnoid membrane, and pia mater — help protect the central nervous system (CNS). The arachnoid villi project from the arachnoid membrane into the superior sagittal and transverse sinuses. The subarachnoid space, filled with cerebrospinal fluid, separates the arachnoid membrane and the pia mater.

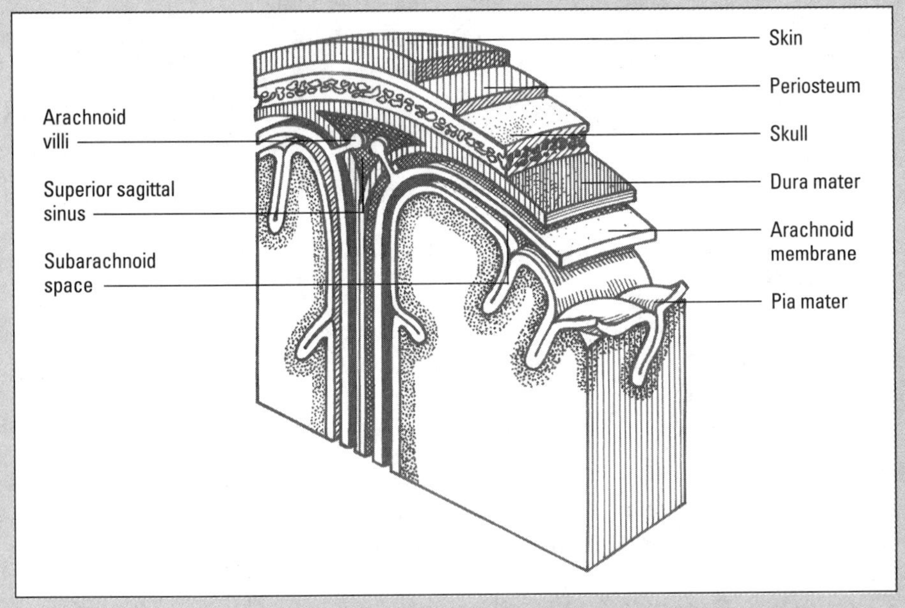

- the **tentorium cerebelli,** which separates the cerebrum from the cerebellum
- the **falx cerebelli,** which separates the two lobes of the cerebellum.

The **arachnoid villi,** projections of the dura mater into the superior sagittal and transverse sinuses, serve as the exit points for CSF drainage into the venous circulation.

Fragile layer

A fragile, fibrous layer of moderate vascularity, the **arachnoid membrane** lies between the dura mater and the pia mater.

Vascular layer

Extremely thin, the **pia mater** has a rich blood supply. It adheres to the brain's surface and extends into its fissures.

Cushioning layers

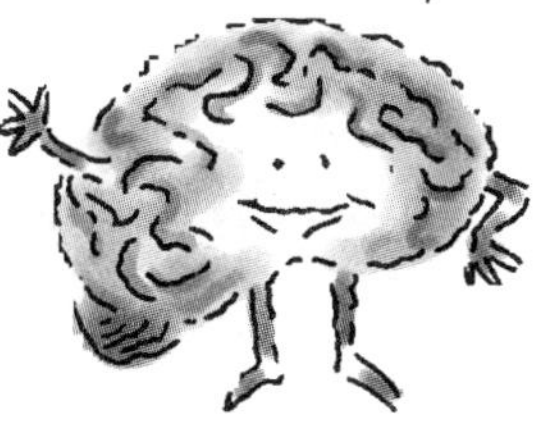

The epidural space, subdural space, and subarachnoid space protect me against injury.

Three layers of space further cushion the brain and spinal cord against injury. The **epidural space** (actually, a potential space) lies over the dura mater. The **subdural space** is situated between the dura mater and arachnoid membrane. This closed area — often the site of hemorrhage after head trauma — offers no escape route for blood accumulation. The **subarachnoid space,** filled with CSF, separates the arachnoid membrane and pia mater.

Cerebrospinal fluid

CSF is a colorless fluid that arises from blood plasma and has a similar composition. It cushions the brain and spinal cord, nourishes cells, and transports metabolic waste.

Fluid factory

CSF forms continuously in clusters of capillaries called the **choroid plexuses,** located in the roof of each ventricle. The choroid plexuses produce approximately 500 ml of CSF each day.

Open to flow

From the lateral ventricles, CSF flows through the **interventricular foramen,** commonly known as the **foramen of Monro,** to the third ventricle of the brain. A foramen is a term used to describe a natural opening or passage. The foramen of Monro is named after the man who first described it: Alexander Monro II, a professor of anatomy at the University of Edinburgh. (See *Three men of Monro,* page 262.)

From there, it reaches the subarachnoid space and then passes under the base of the brain, upward over the brain's upper surfaces, and down around the spinal cord. Eventually, it reaches the arachnoid villi, where it's reabsorbed into venous blood at the venous sinuses on top of the brain.

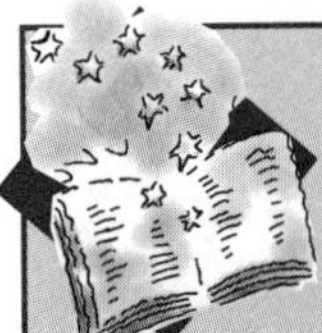

Beyond the dictionary

Three men of Monro

The foramen of Monro is named after Alexander Monro II (1733 to 1817), the man who first described it. Monro II was the second professor of anatomy at the University of Edinburgh (and the second named Alexander Monro). He succeeded his father in this position and was succeeded by his own son, Alex III.

Peripheral nervous system

The peripheral nervous system consists of the cranial nerves, spinal nerves, and **autonomic nervous system (ANS).**

Message lines: neck and above

The 12 pairs of **cranial nerves** transmit motor or sensory messages or both, primarily between the brain or brain stem and the head and neck. All cranial nerves except the olfactory and optic nerves exit from the midbrain, pons, or medulla oblongata of the brain stem. (See *A look at the 12 cranial nerves.*)

Message lines: spine to body

The 31 pairs of **spinal nerves** are named for the vertebra immediately below each nerve's exit point from the spinal cord; thus, they're designated from top to bottom as C1 through S5 and the coccygeal nerve. Each spinal nerve consists of afferent and efferent neurons, which carry messages to and from particular body regions, called **dermatomes.**

Autonomic nervous system

The vast ANS innervates all internal organs. Sometimes known as **visceral efferent nerves,** the nerves of the ANS carry messages to the viscera from the brain stem and neuroendocrine regulatory centers. The ANS has two major subdivisions: the **sympathetic (thoracolumbar)** nervous system and **parasympathetic (craniosacral)** nervous system. (See *On autonomic pilot,* page 264.)

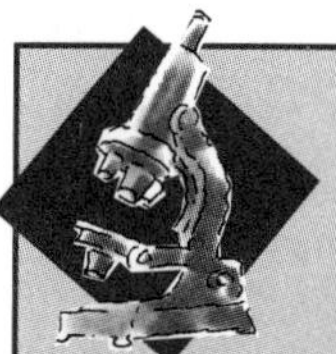

Zoom in

A look at the 12 cranial nerves

As this illustration reveals, 10 of the 12 pairs or cranial nerves (CNs) exit from the brain stem. The remaining two pairs — the olfactory and optic nerves — exit from the forebrain.

Olfactory (CN I) *Sensory:* smell

Optic (CN II) *Sensory:* vision

Trochlear (CN IV) *Motor:* extraocular eye movement (inferior medial)

Vagus (CN X) *Motor:* movement of the palate, swallowing, gag reflex, activity of the thoracic and abdominal viscera, such as heart rate and peristalsis; *Sensory:* sensations of the throat, larynx, and thoracic and abdominal visceral (heart, lungs, bronchi, and GI tract)

Trigeminal (CN V) *Sensory:* transmitting stimuli from face and head, corneal reflex; *Motor:* chewing, biting, and lateral jaw movements

Facial (CN VII) *Sensory:* taste receptors (anterior two-thirds of the tongue); *Motor:* facial muscle movement, including muscles of expression (those in the forehead and around the eyes and mouth)

Acoustic (CN VIII) *Sensory:* Hearing, sense of balance

Glossopharyngeal (CN IX) *Motor:* swallowing movements; *Sensory:* sensations of the throat, taste receptors (posterior one-third of the tongue)

Hypoglossal (CN XII) *Motor:* tongue movement

Spinal accessory (CN XI) *Motor:* shoulder movement, head rotation

Abducens (CN VI) *Motor:* extraocular eye movement

Oculomotor (CN III) *Motor:* extraocular eye movement (superior, medial, and inferior lateral), pupillary constriction, upper eyelid elevation

Most of the cranial nerves transmit either **motor** or **sensory** information. A few, such as the **vagus nerve,** do both.

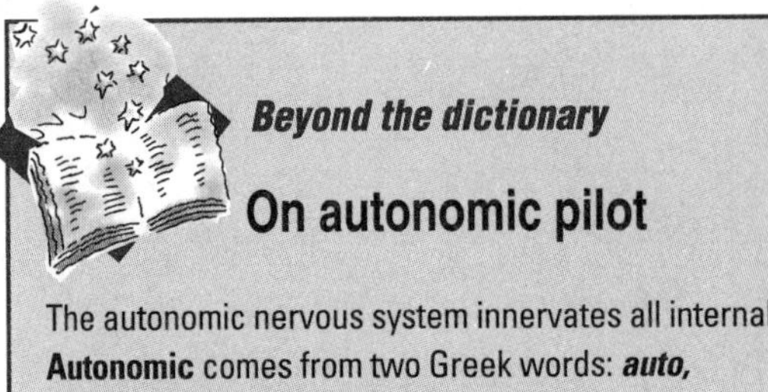

Beyond the dictionary

On autonomic pilot

The autonomic nervous system innervates all internal organs. **Autonomic** comes from two Greek words: ***auto,*** meaning *self,* and ***nomos,*** meaning *law.* So, this nervous system operates according to its own law, or without conscious control.

Think of the autonomic nervous system as being on autopilot.

System response: General

Sympathetic nerves called **preganglionic neurons** exit the spinal cord between the levels of the first thoracic and second lumbar vertebrae. After they leave the spinal cord, these nerves enter small ganglia near the cord. The ganglia form a chain that spreads the impulse to **postganglionic neurons,** which reach many organs and glands and can produce widespread, generalized physiologic responses.

System response: Specific

Fibers of the parasympathetic nervous system leave the CNS by way of the cranial nerves from the midbrain and medulla and the spinal nerves between the second and fourth sacral vertebrae (S2 to S4).

After leaving the CNS, the long preganglionic fiber of each parasympathetic nerve travels to a ganglion near a particular organ or gland; the short postganglionic fiber enters the organ or gland. This creates a more specific response involving only one organ or gland.

Physical examination terms

Here are terms associated with procedures and observations one might encounter in a physical examination relating to the neurologic system:

- **Absence seizure** is marked by a sudden, momentary loss of consciousness, typically accompanied by loss of muscle control or spasms and a vacant facial expression.

• **Aphasia** is a loss or impairment of the ability to communicate through speech, written language, or signs, resulting from brain disease or trauma.
• **Aphonia** is a loss of the ability to speak.
• **Apraxia** is a complete or partial inability to perform purposeful movements in the absence of sensory or motor impairment.
• **Ataxia** is impairment of the ability to coordinate voluntary muscle movement.
• **Ataxic speech** is characterized by faulty formation of sounds, resulting from neuromuscular disease.
• **Athetosis** is a condition characterized by constant, slow, writhing, involuntary movements of the extremities, especially the hands.
• **Aura** are sensations that occur before a paroxysmal attack, such as a seizure or migraine headache.
• **Battle's sign** is discoloration of the skin behind the ear following the fracture of a bone in the lower skull.
• **Biot's respiration** is an abnormal, unpredictable breathing pattern characterized by irregular periods of apnea alternating with periods of four or five breaths having the same depth. Biot's respiration indicates meningitis, a lesion in the medulla, or increased intracranial pressure.
• **Bradylalia** refers to abnormally slow speech, caused by a brain lesion.
• **Brudzinski's sign** is flexion of the hips and knees in response to passive flexion of the neck. A positive Brudzinski's sign signals meningeal irritation.
• A **coma** is a state of unconsciousness from which the patient can't be aroused.
• **Decerebrate posturing** is associated with a lesion of the upper brain stem or severe bilateral lesions in the cerebrum. The patient typically lies with legs extended, head retracted, arms adducted and extended, wrists pronated, and the fingers, ankles, and toes flexed.
• **Decorticate posturing** is associated with a lesion of the frontal lobes, cerebral peduncles, or internal capsule. The patient lies with arms adducted and flexed, wrists and fingers flexed on the chest, legs stiffly extended and internally rotated, and feet plantar flexed.
• **Delirium** is a disorientation to time and place; the patient may also experience illusions and hallucinations.
• **Dementia** is an organic mental syndrome marked by general loss of intellectual abilities, with chronic person-

Biot's (BEE-OHZ) **respiration** is named after Camille Biot, a 19th-century French doctor.

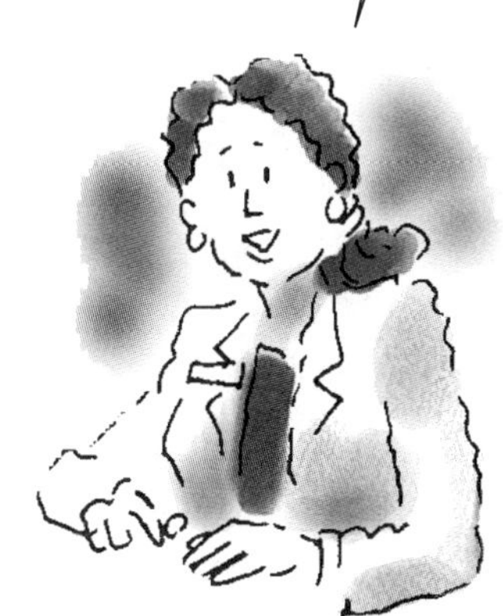

ality disintegration, confusion, disorientation, and stupor. It doesn't include states of impaired intellectual functioning resulting from delirium or depression.

- **Dysphagia** is difficulty swallowing.
- **Dysphasia** is impairment of speech involving failure to arrange words in their proper order, usually resulting from injury to the speech area in the cerebral cortex.
- **Dyspraxia** is a partial loss of the ability to perform coordinated movements, with no associated defect in motor or sensory functions.
- **Generalized tonic-clonic (grand mal) seizure** is an **epileptic seizure** frequently preceded by an aura and characterized by loss of consciousness and muscle spasms (tonic phase), followed by convulsive movement of the limbs (clonic phase).
- The **Glasgow Coma Scale** is commonly used to assess a patient's level of consciousness. It was designed to help determine a patient's chances for survival and recovery after a head injury. The scale scores three observations — eye opening response, best motor response, and best verbal response. Each response receives a point value. If a patient is alert, can follow simple commands, and is well-oriented, his score will total 15 points. If the patient is comatose, his score will be 7 or less. The lowest possible score, 3, indicates deep coma and a poor prognosis.
- **Headache** is diffuse pain in different portions of the head and not confined to any nerve distribution area.
- **Hemiparesis** refers to paralysis or muscular weakness affecting only one side of the body.
- **Hemiplegia** is paralysis of one side of the body.
- **Hyperpathia** is an exaggerated response to stimuli.
- **Intracranial pressure (ICP)** is the pressure created by the CSF in the subarachnoid space between the skull and brain. ICP increases as a result of head trauma, brain tumor, stroke, or infection in the brain. (See *ICP*.)
- **Kernig's sign** elicits both resistance and hamstring muscle pain when the examiner attempts to extend the knee while the hip and knee are both flexed 90 degrees. This sign is usually present in meningitis or subarachnoid hemorrhage.
- **Neuralgia** is severe pain that occurs in a nerve or nerves.

Dysphasia
failure words
is proper order
in arrange to.

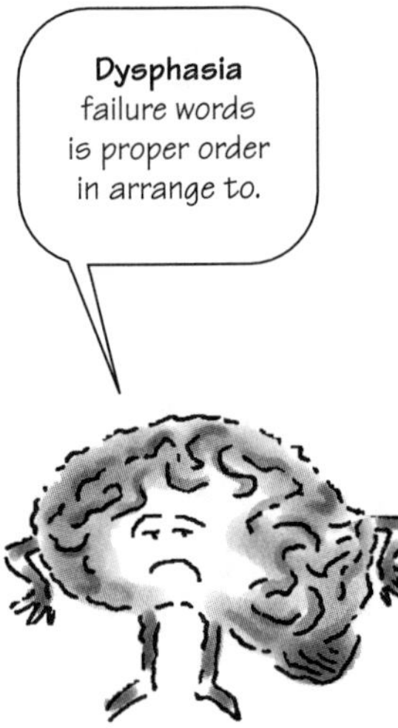

Reflexes

Reflexes, involuntary responses to stimuli, are discussed here:

- **Achilles tendon reflex** produces plantar flexion when the Achilles tendon is tapped.
- **Babinski's reflex** is dorsiflexion of the big toe in response to scraping the sole of the foot.
- **Biceps reflex** causes contraction of the biceps muscles when the tendon is tapped.
- **Corneal reflex** is closure of the eyelids when the cornea is touched.
- Absent **doll's eye sign** or a negative oculocephalic reflex is an indicator of brain stem dysfunction. The absence of the doll's eye sign is detected by rapid, but gentle turning of the patient's head from side to side. The eyes remain fixed in a straight-ahead position instead of moving in the opposite direction that the head is turned.
- **Gag reflex** is elicited by touching the soft palate or the back of the pharynx; response is elevation of the palate, retraction of the tongue, and contraction of the constrictor muscle of the pharynx.
- **Knee-jerk reflex** is a kick reflex produced by sharply tapping the patellar ligament.
- **Pupillary reflex** is the contracting of the pupil in response to light.

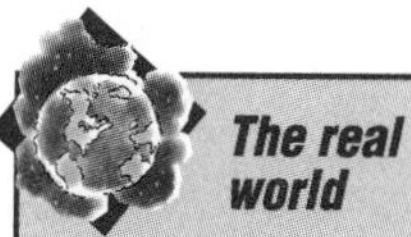

The real world

ICP

A rise in a patient's **intracranial pressure** is typically referred to as "increased ICP."

Diagnostic tests

Diagnostic tests associated with the neurologic system include radiographic and imaging studies, electrophysiologic studies, and CSF and blood tests.

Radiographic and imaging studies

Here are some common radiographic and imaging studies:

- **Cerebral angiography** is a radiographic procedure that employs injected radiopaque contrast material to allow visualization of the vascular system of the brain.
- **Computed tomography** combines radiology and computer analysis of tissue density to study structures inside the skull and spinal cord.

- **Digital subtraction angiography** traces the cerebral vessels by using a type of computerized fluoroscopy. The technician takes an image of the area being studied and stores it in the computer's memory. Additional images are taken after the patient receives a contrast medium. By subtracting the original picture from the later images, the computer produces high-resolution images for interpretation.
- **Echoencephalography** is a diagnostic technique that uses ultrasound waves to study structures within the brain.
- **Magnetic resonance angiography** is a noninvasive method of scanning that allows visualization of blood flowing through the cerebral vessels.
- **Magnetic resonance imaging,** also called **nuclear magnetic resonance,** is a noninvasive method of scanning using an electromagnetic field and radio waves, which provides visual images on a computer screen.
- In **myelography,** dye or air is injected into the patient's subarachnoid space after lumbar puncture and X-rays are taken.
- A **positron emission tomography** scan determines the brain's metabolic activity after the infusion of radioactive materials.
- **Pneumoencephalography (PEG)** visualizes the fluid-filled structures of the brain after CSF is intermittently withdrawn through lumbar puncture and replaced by air, oxygen, or helium. (See *Getting around PEG.*)
- **Skull X-rays** use high-energy radiography to detect fractures, bony tumors, or vascular abnormalities and are typically taken from two angles: **anteroposterior** and **lateral. Waters' projection** examines the frontal and maxillary sinuses, facial bone, and eye orbits. **Towne's projection** examines the occipital bone.
- **Spinal X-rays** detect spinal fractures, displacement of the spine, destructive lesions, structural abnormalities, and other conditions.
- **Stereotaxic neuroradiography** is an X-ray procedure used during neurosurgery to guide a needle or electrodes into a specific area of the brain. (See *Understanding stereotaxic neuroradiography.*)

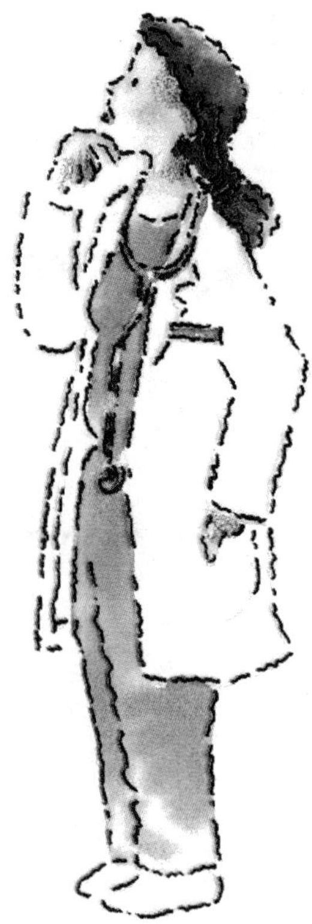

The root ***echo*** in ***echoencephalography*** tells you that this test uses sound waves.

Beyond the dictionary

Understanding stereotaxic neuroradiography

This phrase is easy when you break it down into its components. ***Stereo*** is a familiar term from Greek that refers to something that is *solid,* meaning it has three dimensions. ***Taxic*** refers to *movement in response to a stimulus.* ***Neuro*** refers to the nervous system. **Radiography** is an X-ray study. Thus, **stereotaxic neuroradiography** involves movement in three dimensions (of a needle or electrode) accompanied by X-ray photography of the brain.

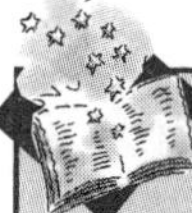

Beyond the dictionary

Getting around PEG

Pneumoencephalography is a long word but can easily be broken down.

Pneumo- means *air.* The prefix ***en-*** means *within,* and ***cephal*** is a Greek term for *head.* So **encephal** literally means *within the head* and thus refers to the brain. The suffix **-graphy** refers to a method of recording, in this case X-ray photography. So, the term means *an X-ray photography of air (or gas) in the brain.*

Electrophysiologic studies

Here are some common electrophysiologic studies associated with the neurologic system:

- **Electroencephalography,** also called **EEG,** records the brain's continuous electrical activity.
- **Evoked potential testing** evaluates the integrity of visual, somatosensory, and auditory nerve pathways by measuring evoked potentials — the brain's electrical response to stimulation of the sensory organs or peripheral nerves. This testing is used to detect neurologic lesions and to evaluate multiple sclerosis as well as various vision and hearing disorders.
- **Magnetoencephalography** is a noninvasive test that directly measures the magnetic fields produced by electrical currents in the brain.

CSF and blood tests

Three common tests of CSF and of the blood are described here:

- The **amyloid beta-protein precursor test** checks CSF for levels of a substance that produces the protein plaques seen in the brain of patients with Alzheimer's disease.
- **Coccidioidomycosis antibodies** is a blood test to identify a fungal infection that affects CNS and other body parts.
- **CSF analysis** shows the presence of blood, infection, and other abnormalities.

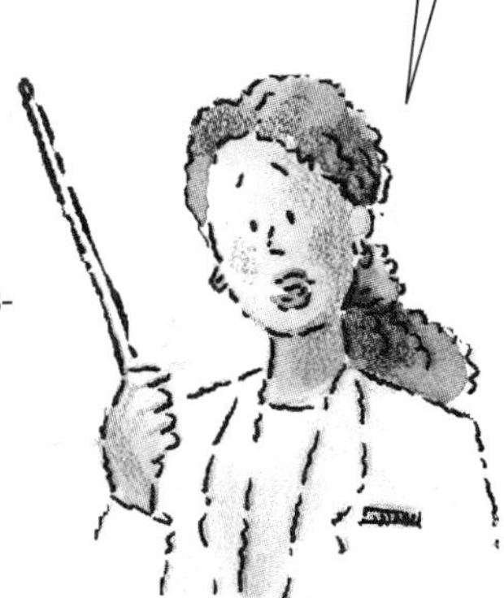
Evoked potential? That's the brain's electrical response to stimulation from sensory organs or peripheral nerves.

Neurologic disorders

This section discusses brain and spinal cord disorders, cranial nerve disorders, degenerative disorders, head trauma, vascular disorders, and miscellaneous neurologic disorders.

Brain and spinal cord disorders

Here are some common brain and spinal cord disorders, including CNS infections and neural tube defects:

- **Cerebral palsy** is a permanent disorder of motor function resulting from nonprogressive brain damage or a brain lesion.
- **Epilepsy** refers to a group of neurologic disorders marked by uncontrolled electrical discharge from the cerebral cortex and typically manifested by seizures with clouding of consciousness. **Status epilepticus** describes a continuous seizure state, which is life-threatening and can occur with any type of seizure.
- **Hydrocephalus** is a condition marked by excess CSF within the brain's ventricles. Two types exist; they are named according to the cause. **Noncommunicating hydrocephalus** results from obstruction of CSF flow. **Communicating hydrocephalus** is caused by faulty reabsorption of CSF. (See *Too much water.*)
- **Migraine headache** is a throbbing, vascular headache that is associated with constriction and dilation of arteries within the brain.
- A **subarachnoid hemorrhage** is an intracranial hemorrhage into the subarachnoid space.
- **Subdural hematoma** is accumulation of blood in the subdural space of the brain.

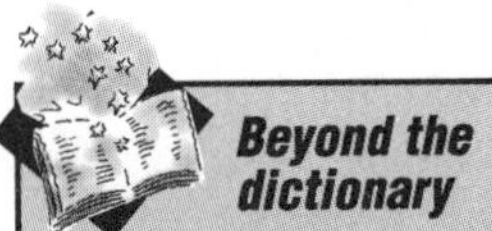

Too much water

Hydrocephalus is a condition marked by excess cerebrospinal fluid within the brain's ventricles. The term **hydrocephalus** originated from the Greek words ***hydro,*** meaning *water* or *fluid* and ***kephale,*** meaning *head.*

CNS infections

CNS infections include encephalitis, meningitis, rabies, and other infections:

- **Brain abscess,** also known as an intracranial abscess, is a free or encapsulated collection of pus usually found in the temporal lobe, cerebellum, or frontal lobe.
- **Encephalitis** is an inflammatory disorder of the brain commonly caused by the bite of an infected mosquito.

• **Meningitis** refers to the inflammation of the meninges of the brain and spinal cord caused by bacterial, viral, or fungal infection.
• **Myelitis** is an inflammation of the spinal cord.
• **Poliomyelitis** is an acute viral infection and inflammation of the gray matter of the spine, usually caused by poliovirus.
• **Rabies,** is an acute, usually fatal CNS disease spread by animals to people through contaminated saliva, blood, or tissue. (See *Afraid of the water.*)

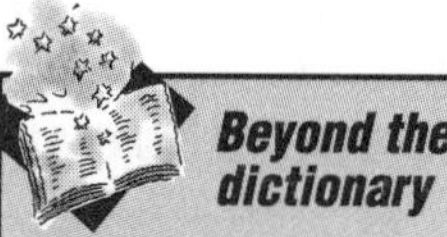

Afraid of the water

Rabies is also called **hydrophobia** — meaning *fear of water* — because this condition produces muscle spasms in the throat when the patient drinks water.

Neural tube defects

Neural tube defects are serious birth defects involving the spine or brain that result from failure of the neural tube to close approximately 28 days after conception.

The most common forms of neural tube defects are spina bifida, anencephaly, and encephalocele:
• In **anencephaly,** part of the top of the skull is missing, severely damaging the brain.
• In **encephalocele,** a saclike portion of the meninges and brain protrudes through a defective opening in the skull.
• **Spina bifida occulta** is incomplete closure of one or more vertebrae, causing spinal contents to protrude in an external sac.
• **Spina bifida with meningocele** is a form of spina bifida in which the sac contains meninges and CSF.
• **Spina bifida with myelomeningocele (meningomyelocele)** is a form of spina bifida in which the sac contains meninges, CSF, and a portion of the spinal cord or nerve roots.

Remember, **-itis** refers to inflammation. So **meningitis** is an inflammation of the meninges.

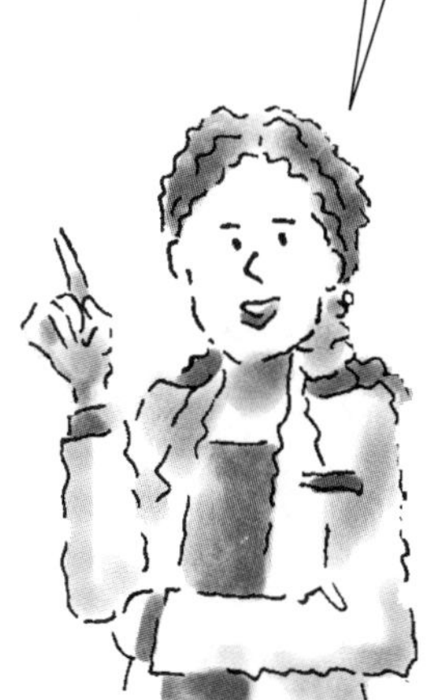

Cranial nerve disorders

Cranial nerve disorders include Bell's palsy and trigeminal neuralgia:
• **Bell's palsy** is a unilateral facial paralysis of sudden onset attributable to a lesion of the facial nerve.
• **Trigeminal neuralgia,** also called **tic douloureux,** is a painful disorder affecting one or more branches of the fifth cranial (trigeminal) nerve. On stimulation of a trigger zone, the patient experiences paroxysmal attacks of excruciating facial pain.

Degenerative disorders

Degenerative disorders of the brain include Alzheimer's disease, multiple sclerosis, Parkinson's disease, and others:

- **Alzheimer's disease** produces three hallmark features in the brain: neurofibrillary tangles, neuritic plaques, and granulovascular degeneration. Early signs progress to severe deterioration in memory, language, and motor function.
- **Amyotrophic lateral sclerosis,** also called **Lou Gehrig disease** or **Charcot syndrome,** is an incurable disease affecting the spinal cord and the medulla and cortex of the brain, characterized by progressive degeneration of motor neurons. Such degeneration leads to weakness and wasting of the muscles, increased reflexes, and severe muscle spasms. Death typically occurs within 2 to 5 years.
- **Huntington's disease,** also called **Huntington's chorea,** is a hereditary disorder causing degeneration in the cerebral cortex and basal ganglia. Degeneration leads to chronic, progressive **chorea** (rapid, jerky movements) and mental deterioration and ends with dementia and death.
- **Multiple sclerosis** is a progressive demyelination of white matter of the brain and spinal cord that results in weakness, incoordination, paresthesia, speech disturbances, and visual complaints.
- **Myasthenia gravis** is abnormal muscle weakness and fatigability, especially in the muscles of the face and throat, resulting from a defect in the conduction of nerve impulses at the myoneural junction.
- **Parkinson's disease** is a slowly progressive, degenerative neurologic disorder that produces progressive muscle rigidity, akinesia, and involuntary tremor.

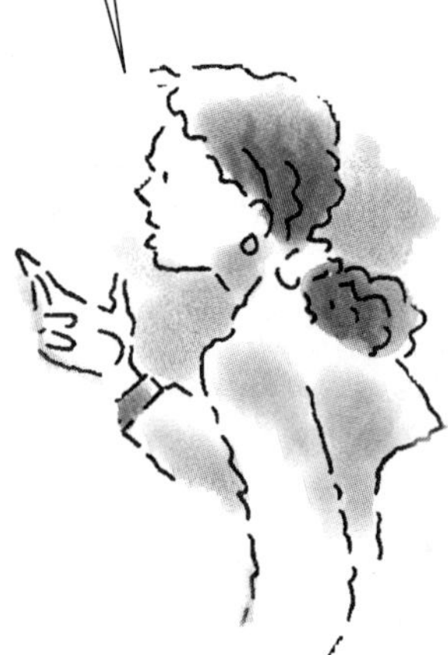
Asthenia is Greek for *weakness.* **Myasthenia gravis** is abnormal muscle weakness, particularly in the face and throat.

Head trauma

Head traumas can range from concussion to tentorial herniation:

- **Cerebral contusion** is a bruising of the brain tissue as a result of a severe blow to the head. More severe than a concussion, a contusion disrupts normal nerve function in the bruised area and may cause loss of consciousness, hemorrhage, edema, and even death.

• **Concussion,** the most common head injury, results from a blow to the head hard enough to jostle the brain and cause it to strike the skull. This causes temporary neural dysfunction.
• An **epidural hematoma** is the rapid accumulation of blood between the skull and the dura mater.
• **Tentorial herniation** occurs when injured brain tissue swells and squeezes through the tentorial notch (an area that contains the midbrain), constricting the brainstem.

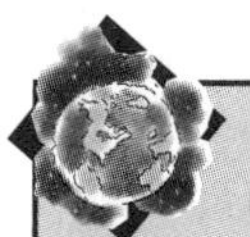

The real world

CVA

A **cerebrovascular accident** is rarely referred to by its proper name in the real world. Rather, it's referred to as a "CVA" or "stroke."

Vascular disorders

Vascular disorders include cerebral aneurysm, cerebrovascular accident, and others:
• **Arteriovenous malformation (AVM)** is a congenital malformation characterized by a tangled mass of dilated cerebral vessels that form an abnormal communication between the arterial and venous systems.
• A **cerebral aneurysm** is a localized dilation (ballooning) of a cerebral artery caused by weakness in the arterial wall.
• **Cerebrovascular accident,** also called a **stroke** or **brain attack,** is a condition of sudden onset in which a cerebral blood vessel is occluded by an embolus or cerebrovascular hemorrhage. The resulting ischemia of brain tissue normally perfused by the affected vessel may lead to permanent neurologic damage. (See *CVA.*)
• **Transient ischemic attack** is a recurrent neurologic episode lasting less than 1 hour. It doesn't cause neurologic deficit but is usually considered a warning sign of an impending CVA.

Miscellaneous neurologic disorders

Other neurologic disorders include Reye's syndrome, tetanus, and Tourette's disease:
• **Guillain-Barré syndrome** is an acute febrile polyneuritis that occurs after a viral infection. It's marked by rapidly ascending paralysis that begins as paresthesia of the feet.
• **Neurofibromatosis** is a genetic trait characterized by several neurofibromas (fibrous tumor of peripheral nerves resulting from abnormal proliferation of Schwann

cells) of the nerves and skin, café-au-lait spots on the skin and, sometimes, developmental anomalies of the muscles, bones, and visceral tissue.

• **Reye's syndrome** is an acute childhood illness that causes fatty infiltration of the liver with concurrent elevated blood ammonia levels, encephalopathy, and increased ICP.

• **Tetanus** refers to an acute, often fatal, infection caused by the anaerobic bacillus *Clostridium tetani*, which usually enters the body through a contaminated puncture wound.

• **Tetany** refers to the hyperexcitability of nerves and muscles caused by low calcium levels.

• **Tourette disease** or **syndrome** is a condition characterized by facial and vocal tics, generalized lack of coordination, and **coprolalia** (uncontrollable urge to say obscenities).

Treatments

The terminology discussed here describes treatments (including surgeries) that may be employed when caring for a patient with a neurologic disorder.

Treatments of the brain

Treatments can include craniotomy, lobotomy, placement of a ventriculoperitoneal shunt, and different methods of intracranial pressure monitoring:

• **Cerebellar stimulator implantation** uses electrical impulses from surgically implanted electrodes in the patient's brain to regulate uncoordinated neuromuscular activity. It has also been used to prevent seizures.

• **Craniectomy** removes a part of the skull.

• A **craniotomy** is the creation of a surgical incision into the skull to expose the brain for treatment.

• **Hemicraniectomy** exposes half of the brain for surgery.

• **Intracranial hematoma aspiration** requires a craniotomy to reduce high ICP caused by a collection of blood around the surface of the brain.

• **Lobectomy** removes a lobe of the brain.
• **Lobotomy** is incision into the frontal lobe of the brain through holes drilled in the skull.
• A **ventriculoperitoneal shunt** is a surgical treatment for hydrocephalus in which a catheter drains CSF from the ventricular system for absorption. The shunt extends from the cerebral ventricle to the scalp, where it's tunneled under the skin to the peritoneal cavity. Shunting lowers ICP and prevents brain damage by draining excess CSF or relieving blockage.
• **Volumetric interstitial brachytherapy** utilizes radioactive materials, which are implanted into the skull and left in place for several days to deliver radiation to a brain tumor.

Lobectomy or lobotomy? I'm confused.

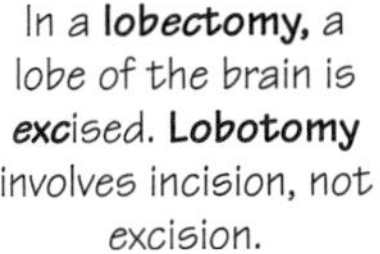

In a **lobectomy,** a lobe of the brain is **exc**ised. **Lobotomy** involves incision, not excision.

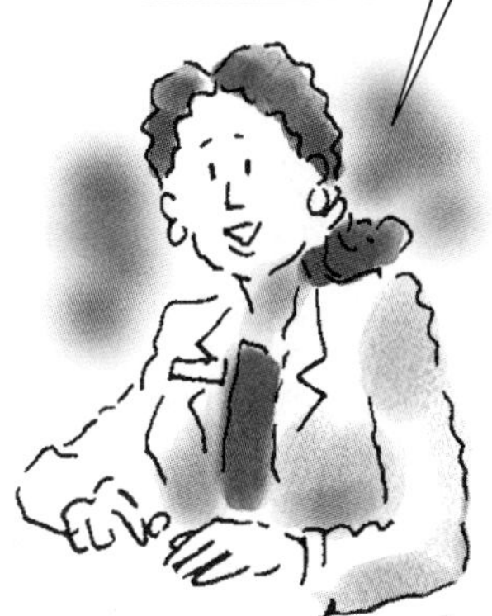

Intracranial pressure monitoring

ICP monitoring is an important part of neurologic treatment because increased ICP can lead to fatal brain herniation. Invasive ICP monitoring is accomplished in one of several ways:
• An **epidural probe** is a tiny fiber-optic sensor inserted in the brain's epidural space through a burr hole in the skull.
• A **subarachnoid screw** is a small hollow steel screw with a sensor tip, inserted through a burr hole, that monitors pressure in the subarachnoid space.
• A **ventricular catheter,** consisting of a small polyethylene cannula and external drainage and collection system, is inserted through a burr hole into a lateral ventricle.

Spinal and nerve surgery

Here are some common surgeries on the spine or spinal nerves:
• **Chordotomy** is any operation on the spinal cord.
• **Myelomeningocele repair** fixes a congenital spinal defect to prevent infection. The surgeon isolates neural

tissue from the rest of the myelomeningocele sac and fashions a flap from surrounding tissue.
- **Neurectomy** removes part of a nerve.
- **Neuroplasty** repairs a nerve.
- **Sympathectomy** resects a sympathetic nerve or ganglion.
- **Vagotomy** transects the vagus nerve.

Other neurologic treatments

Here are some other common neurologic treatments:
- **AVM embolization** is a noninvasive technique to treat AVMs when surgery isn't an option. To lower the risk of rupture and hemorrhage, a flexible catheter is threaded into the AVM site and small, heat-resistant silicon beads or a rapid-setting plastic polymer is inserted. The beads or polymer lodge in the feeder artery and occlude blood flow to the AVM.
- An induced **barbiturate coma** is a treatment of last resort for patients experiencing sustained or acute episodes of high ICP. The patient receives large doses of a short-acting barbiturate such as pentobarbitol to induce a coma. The drug reduces the metabolic rate and cerebral blood volume, possibly reducing ICP and protecting cerebral tissue.
- **Drug therapy** includes anticonvulsants to control seizures, corticosteroids to decrease inflammation and edema, osmotic diuretics to promote diureses and reduce cerebral edema, and antibiotics to treat infection.
- **Plasmapheresis** removes plasma from withdrawn blood and reinfuses formed blood elements mixed with a plasma replacement solution. In some methods, the plasma is filtered to remove a specific disease mediator and then returned to the patient. Plasmapheresis cleans the blood of harmful substances and is used for Guillain-Barré syndrome, multiple sclerosis, and myasthenia gravis.

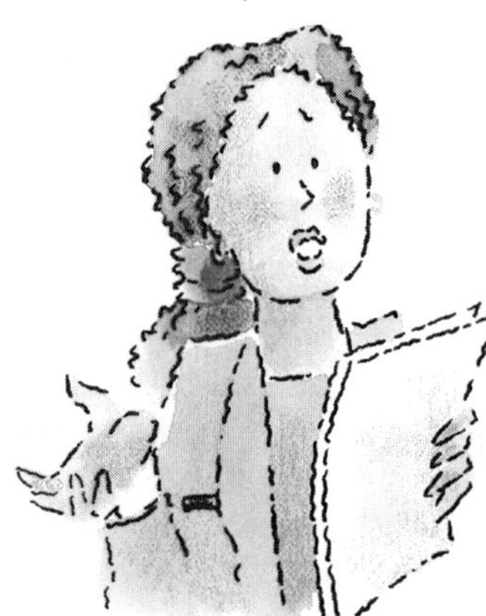

Think you've got a handle on neurologic terms? Try some games on the next page.

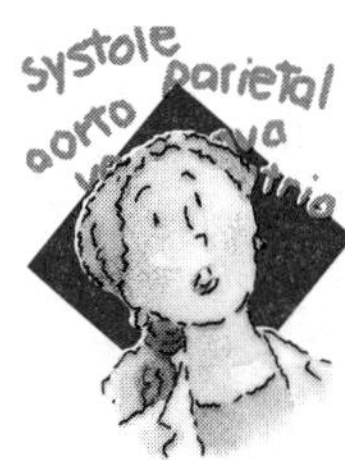

Vocabulary builders

At a crossroads

Completing this crossword puzzle will help test your nerve with the nervous system. Good luck!

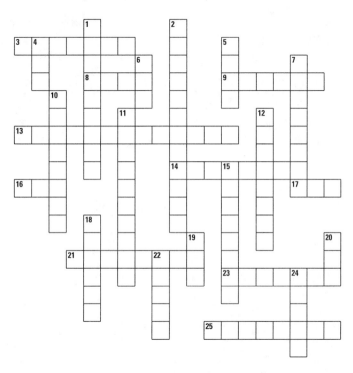

Across

3. Neurons outside the brain
8. Carries impulses away from the cell
9. Neurons within the brain
13. "Water on the brain"
14. Another name for sensory neurons
16. Cerebrovascular accident abbreviation
17. Records the brain's electrical activity
21. Membranes enclosing the CNS
23. Basic cells of the nervous system
25. Headaches preceded by an aura

Down

1. First cranial nerve
2. Controls body temperature
4. Arteriovenous malformation abbreviation
5. Serves as a bridge
6. Central nervous system abbreviation
7. Carries impulses to the cell
10. Another name for mesencephalon
11. Infection of the meninges
12. Largest part of the brain
15. Another name for motor neurons
18. Sheath covering nerve cells
19. Cerebrospinal fluid abbreviation
20. The brain's switchboard
22. Gluelike cells
24. Second cranial nerve

Answers are on page 280.

Match game

Match each sensory description with the nerve responsible for its function.

Clues	Choices
1. Sense of smell ____	A. Oculomotor nerve
2. Vision ____	B. Trigeminal nerve
3. Eye movement ____	C. Glossopharyngeal nerve
4. Hearing ____	D. Olfactory nerve
5. Taste and swallowing ____	E. Vestibular nerve
6. Balance and equilibrium ____	F. Optic nerve
7. Muscles of the tongue ____	G. Acoustic nerve
8. Largest cranial nerve ____	H. Hypoglossal nerve

Finish line

Fill in the blanks below with the appropriate word(s).

1. The most common head injury is a _____.
2. A patient who loses the ability to speak or write has _____.
3. Patients often experience an _____ just before a migraine headache.
4. Creation of a surgical incision into the skull is a _____.
5. Holes drilled into the skull are known as _____ holes.
6. A subarachnoid screw is used to monitor a patient's __________ __________.
7. __________ __________ is the surgical treatment of hydrocephalus.
8. Plasmapheresis is the therapeutic removal of _____ from the patient's body.

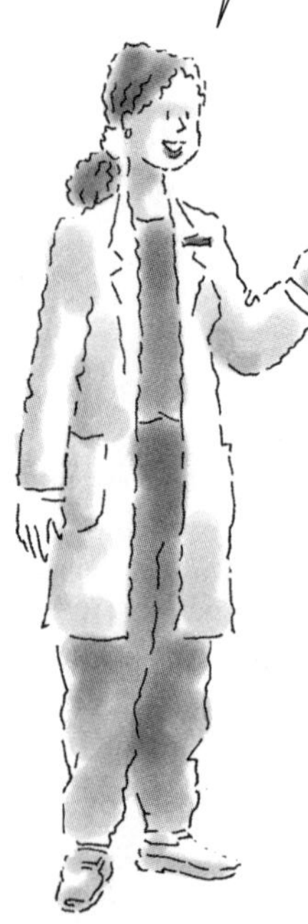
Here's a hint: -otomy indicates an incision.

Answers are on page 280.

Scrambled or overeasy

Fill in the answers for the following questions, then unscramble the circled letters to find the answer to the puzzle.

1. __ __ __ __ __ (__)
2. __ __ __ __ (__) __ __
   __ __ __ __ __ (__) __ __ __
3. __ __ __ (__) __ __ __ __
4. __ __ __ (__) __ __ __ __ __ __ (__) __
5. (__) __ __ __ __ __
6. (__) __ __ __ __ __ (__) __ __ __ __ __

1. Highly specialized cells that detect and transmit stimuli electromechanically
2. Autonomic reflex center that maintains homeostasis, regulating respiratory, vasomotor, and cardiac functions
3. Covers and protects the cerebral cortex and spinal column
4. Controls or affects body temperature, appetite, water balance, pituitary secretions, and emotions
5. Acute, usually fatal central nervous system disease spread by animals to people through contaminated saliva, blood, or tissue
6. An inflammatory disorder of the brain commonly caused by the bite of an infected mosquito

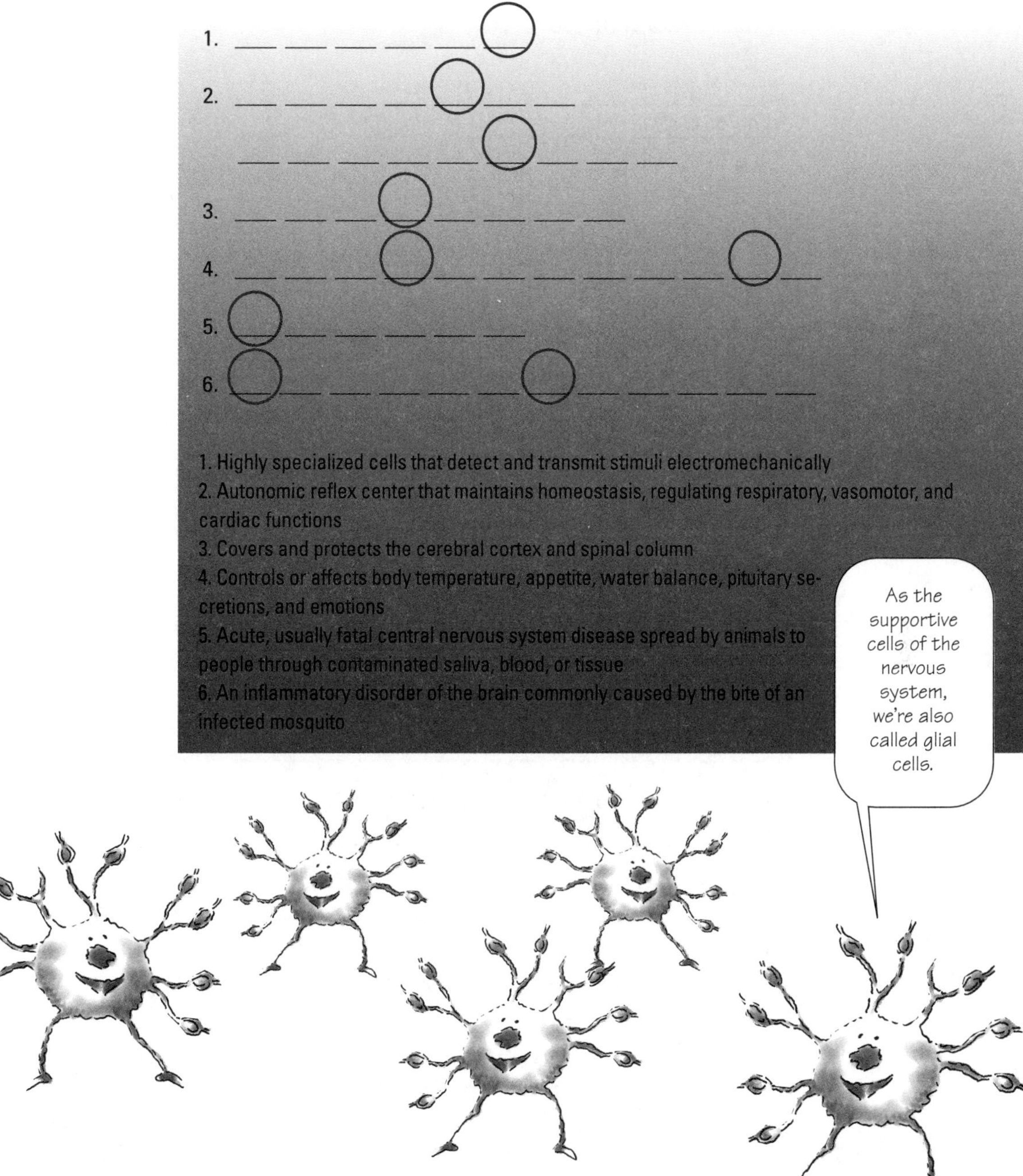

As the supportive cells of the nervous system, we're also called glial cells.

Answers are on page 280.

Answers

At a crossroads

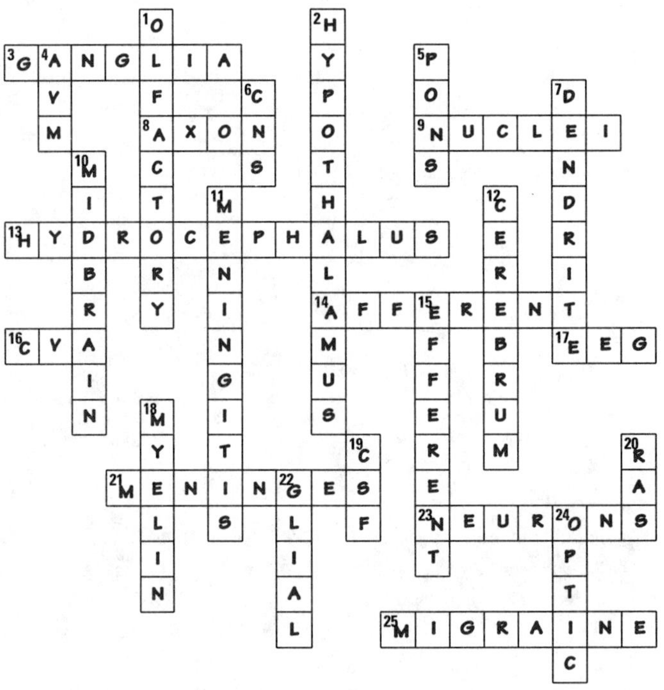

Match game

1. D; 2. F; 3. A; 4. G; 5. C; 6. E; 7. H; 8. B.

Finish line

1. Concussion; 2. Aphasia; 3. Aura; 4. Craniotomy; 5. Burr; 6. Intracranial pressure; 7. Ventricular shunting; 8. Plasma.

Scrambled or overeasy

1. Neuron; 2. Medulla oblongata; 3. Meninges; 4. Hypothalamus; 5. Rabies; 6. Encephalitis.
Answer to puzzle — Neuroglia

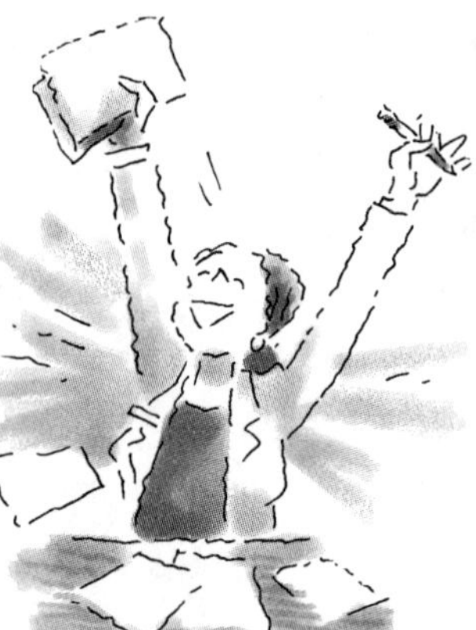

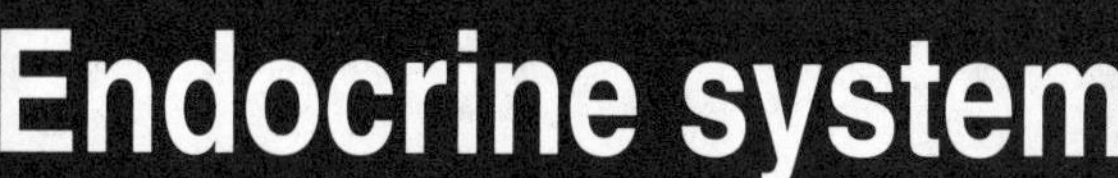

Endocrine system

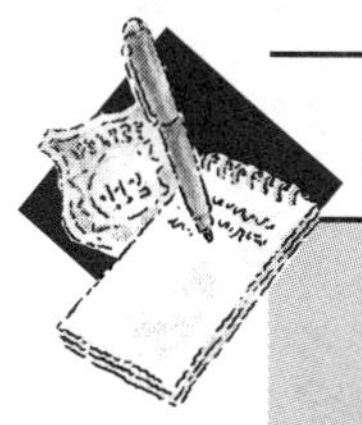

Just the facts

In this chapter, you'll review:

- terminology related to the structure and function of the endocrine system
- terminology needed for physical examination
- tests that help diagnose common endocrine disorders
- endocrine system disorders and their treatments.

Endocrine structure and function

The endocrine system controls complicated body activities by discharging secretions into the circulatory system. Its major components are glands and hormones:

- **Glands** are specialized cell clusters or organs.
- **Hormones** are chemical substances secreted by the glands in response to stimulation.

Glands in a major key

The major glands of the endocrine system include the pituitary gland, thyroid gland, parathyroid glands, adrenal glands, pancreas, thymus, pineal body, and the gonads (ovaries and testes). (See *Pronouncing key endocrine system terms*, page 282, and *Endocrine system structures*, page 283.)

Pituitary gland

The **pituitary gland,** also known as the **hypophysis,** is no larger than a pea and lies at the base of the brain in a depression of the sphenoid bone called the **sella turcica.**

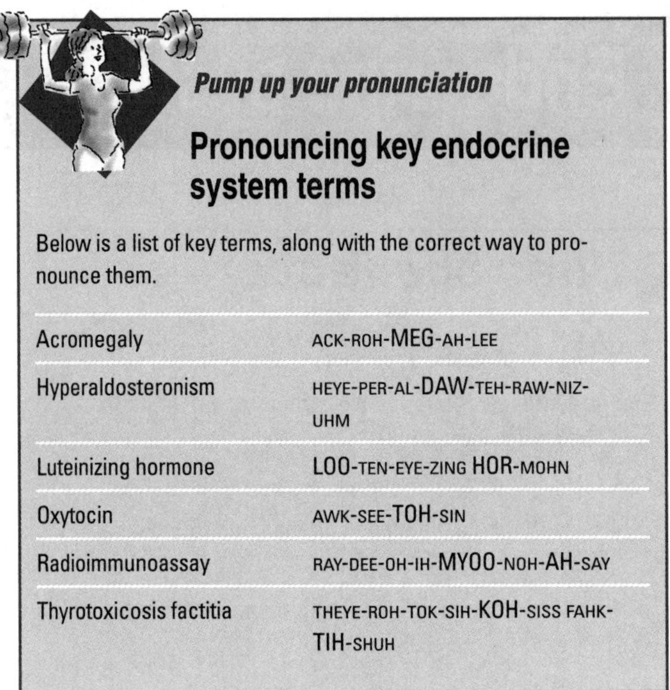

Pump up your pronunciation

Pronouncing key endocrine system terms

Below is a list of key terms, along with the correct way to pronounce them.

Acromegaly	ACK-ROH-MEG-AH-LEE
Hyperaldosteronism	HEYE-PER-AL-DAW-TEH-RAW-NIZ-UHM
Luteinizing hormone	LOO-TEN-EYE-ZING HOR-MOHN
Oxytocin	AWK-SEE-TOH-SIN
Radioimmunoassay	RAY-DEE-OH-IH-MYOO-NOH-AH-SAY
Thyrotoxicosis factitia	THEYE-ROH-TOK-SIH-KOH-SISS FAHK-TIH-SHUH

Cover and connection

The **pituitary diaphragm,** an extension of the dura mater (the membrane covering the brain), extends over the pituitary gland and protects it. The **pituitary stalk,** a stemlike structure, provides a connection to the hypothalamus part of the brain.

Master gland

The pituitary is also called the "master gland" because it controls all the other glands. It's divided into two regions: the anterior pituitary lobe and the posterior pituitary lobe.

Courtesy of the anterior pituitary

The largest region of the pituitary, the **anterior pituitary lobe (adenohypophysis)** produces at least seven hormones. (See *The history of pituitary*, page 284.) These are:

- **Growth hormone (GH),** or **somatotropin,** promotes the growth of bony and soft tissues.

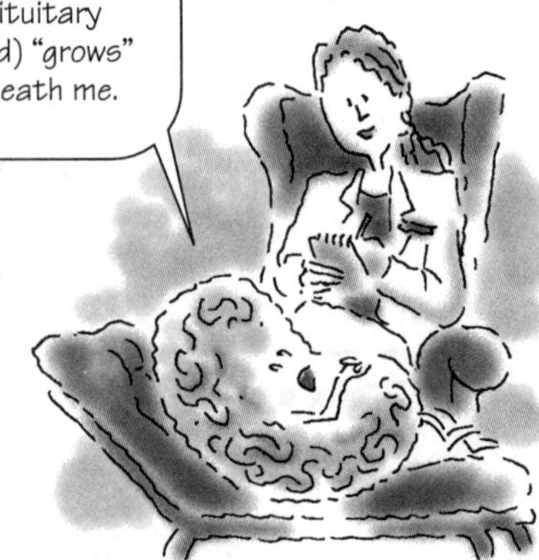

Hypo means beneath; physis means to grow.
The hypophysis (pituitary gland) "grows" beneath me.

Body shop

Endocrine system structures

Endocrine glands secrete hormones directly into the bloodstream to regulate body function. This illustration shows the location of the major endocrine glands (except the gonads).

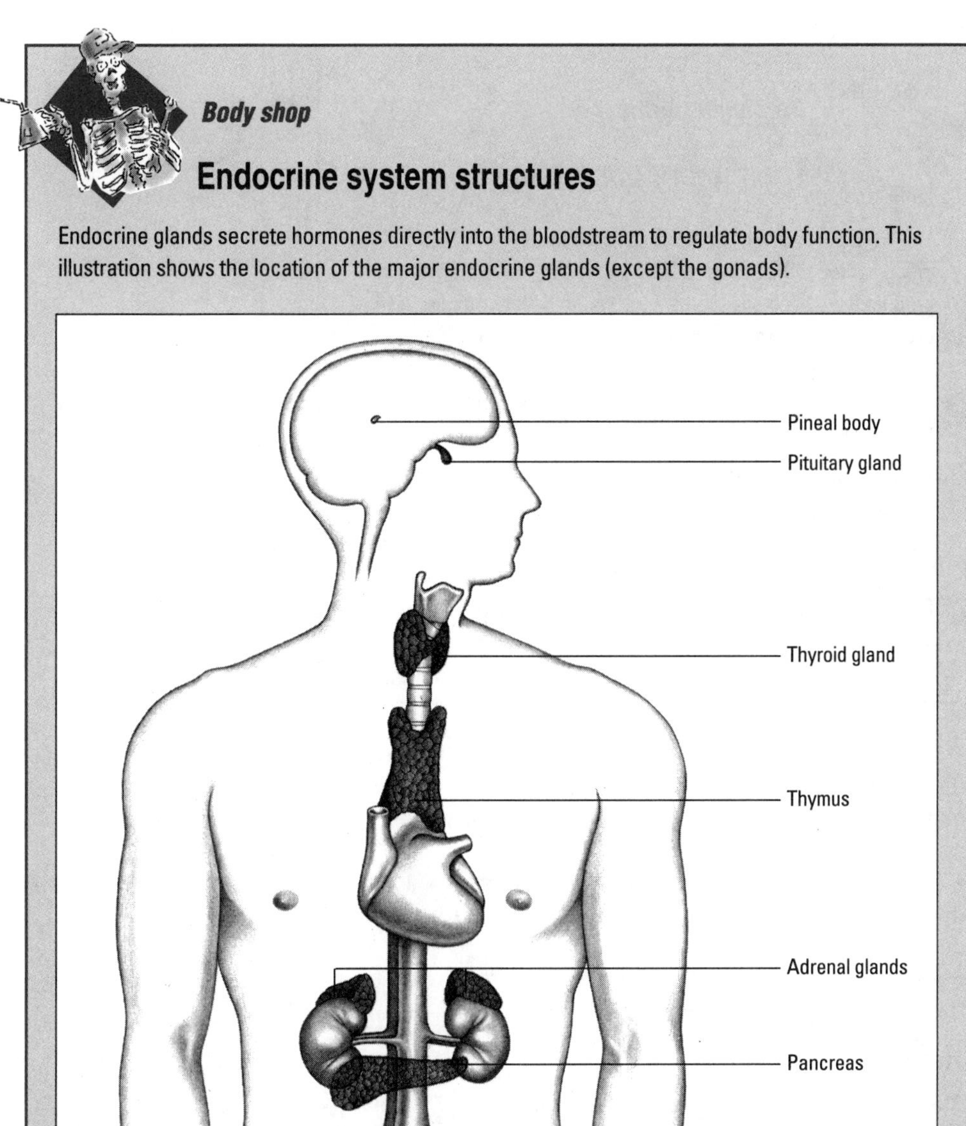

- **Thyrotropin,** or **thyroid-stimulating hormone (TSH),** influences secretion of the thyroid hormone.
- **Corticotropin,** or **adrenocorticotropic hormone (ACTH),** stimulates the adrenal cortex to produce cortisol.
- **Follicle-stimulating hormone (FSH)** stimulates the growth of graafian follicles as well as estrogen secretion in females and the development of sperm cells in males.

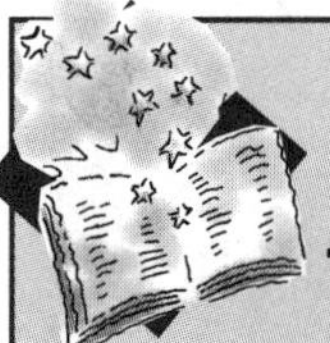

Beyond the dictionary

The history of pituitary

The word **pituitary** derives from Latin ***pituita,*** which means *phlegm (mucous)* and was based on the belief that phlegm was produced by this gland. In the doctrine of the four humors, a theory of physiology and psychology commonly held through the 17th century, too much of the humor phlegm in one's body resulted in a listless, cold, apathetic personality — in other words, a **phlegmatic** individual.

Turning on to tropins

The word **tropin,** sometimes **trophin,** appears in the name of a number of hormones produced by the pituitary gland (for example, *somatotropin* and *mammotropin*). The word derives from a Greek word meaning *to turn.* In reference to a hormone, the sense is that a tropin turns or changes something.

- **Luteinizing hormone (LH)** stimulates maturation of the ovarian follicle and the ovum, and ovulation in females. It stimulates production and secretion of testosterone in males.
- **Prolactin,** or **mammotropin,** stimulates breast development during pregnancy and is responsible for the production of milk.
- **Melanocyte-stimulating hormone** is responsible for formation of melanin pigment in the skin.

The posterior plays its part

The **posterior pituitary lobe** (neurohypophysis) makes up about 25% of the gland. It stores and releases oxytocin and antidiuretic hormone after they're produced by the hypothalamus. **Antidiuretic hormone (ADH),** also called **vasopressin,** stimulates water reabsorption by the kidneys to limit production of large volumes of urine. **Oxytocin** stimulates the ejection of breast milk into the mammary ducts and contraction of the uterus after pregnancy.

Thyroid gland

The **thyroid gland** lies directly below the larynx and partially in front of the trachea. Its two lobes are joined by a narrow tissue bridge called the **isthmus,** which gives the thyroid its butterfly shape.

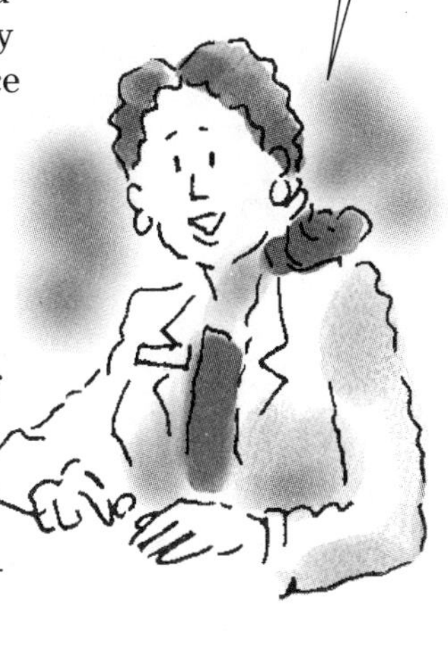
Thyroid, from Greek, literally means *shield-shaped* and refers to the shields that ancient Greek soldiers carried.

Two lobes work together

The lobes function as one unit to produce the thyroid hormones **thyroxine (T_4), triiodothyronine (T_3),** and **thyrocalcitonin (calcitonin).** T_3 and T_4 are collectively known as thyroid hormones. Thyroid hormones influence many metabolic processes, including cellular heat production, protein synthesis, and carbohydrate metabolism.

I dine on iodine

Iodine is an essential element of thyroid hormones; many thyroid disorders are caused by overproduction of thyroid hormones and the iodine-containing substances they contain. The iodine within thyroid hormones combines with a protein in the blood to form **protein-bound iodine.** The components separate, however, when the hormone enters the tissues.

Parathyroid glands

Four parathyroid glands lie on the posterior surface of the thyroid, one on each corner. (***Para*** means *alongside.*)

Checking calcium

Like the thyroid lobes, the parathyroid glands work together as a single unit, producing **parathyroid hormone (PTH).** This hormone regulates the calcium and phosphorus content of the blood and bones. PTH promotes calcium absorption in the blood and antagonizes (works opposite) the hormone calcitonin produced by the thyroid gland. Together, these two hormones maintain calcium balance.

Adrenal glands

The two **adrenal glands** sit on top of the two kidneys. Each gland contains two distinct structures that function as separate endocrine glands.

Mandatory medulla

The inner portion, or **medulla,** produces the catecholamines **epinephrine** and **norepinephrine.** Because these hormones are vital to the autonomic nervous system, the adrenal medulla is also considered a neuroendocrine structure. The adrenal medulla is essential to life but the cortex isn't.

Zoning in

The much larger outer layer — the **cortex** — has three zones and produces hormones called **corticoids:**

- The outermost zone is the **zona glomerulosa,** which produces mineralocorticoid hormones, primarily aldosterone.
- The **zona fasciculata,** the middle and largest zone, produces glucocorticoids and small amounts of the sex hormones estrogen and androgen.
- The inner zone, the **zona reticularis,** produces mainly glucocorticoids and some sex hormones.

Classifying corticoids

The corticoid hormones are classified into three groups:

- **Glucocorticoids** are secreted mainly by the middle zone and include **cortisol (hydrocortisone)** and **corticosterone.** These hormones affect all cells in the body, but specialize in controlling the metabolism of carbohydrates, fats, and proteins; stress resistance; antibody formation; lymphatic functions; and recovery from injury and inflammation.
- **Mineralocorticoids** are secreted by the outer zone and control the regulation and secretion of sodium and potassium. **Aldosterone** is the principle mineralocorticoid and is responsible for electrolyte and water balance.
- **Sex hormones** are secreted by the inner and middle zone of the cortex. They include small amounts of the male hormone **androgen,** which promotes such secondary sex characteristics as facial hair and a low-pitched voice.

Get me some **glucocorticoids.** They specialize in helping me recovery from injury.

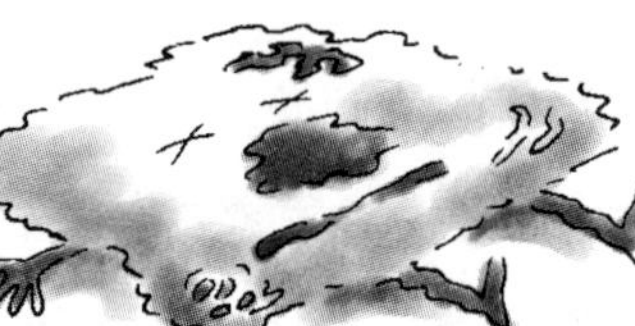

Can't do it without ACTH

The adrenal cortex can't secrete androgens and cortisol without the pituitary hormone ACTH.

Pancreas

The **pancreas** lies along the back of the abdominal wall in the upper left quadrant behind the stomach. The **islets of Langerhans,** which perform the endocrine functions of this gland, contain specialized cells that secrete hormones.

The **islets of Langerhans** are named for Paul Langerhans, the German pathologist who first described these structures in 1869.

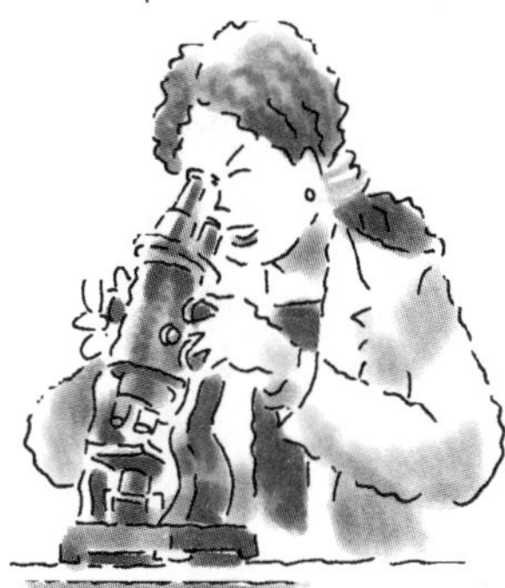

Products of the pancreas

Pancreatic hormones include:

- **insulin,** the hormone responsible for the storage and use of carbohydrates and for decreasing the body's blood glucose levels that is produced by **beta cells** in the pancreas
- **glucagon,** which increases blood glucose levels and is produced by **alpha cells** in the pancreas
- **somatostatin**, a neurotransmitter released by **delta cells** in the pancreas, which inhibits the release of glucagon and insulin.

Pineal body

The tiny **pineal body** lies at the back of third ventricle of the brain and is a neuroendocrine gland. (See *Pining away for the pineal body.*)

Makin' melatonin

This gland produces the hormone **melatonin,** which is involved in the reproductive system and the body's **circadian** (24-hour) rhythms.

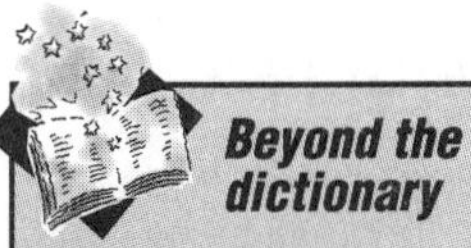

Pining away for the pineal body

The name **pineal** is derived from the structure's resemblance to a pine cone.

Thymus

Located below the sternum, the **thymus** contains lymphatic tissue.

Extra! Extra! Get your T cells here

Although the thymus produces the hormones **thymosin** and **thymopoietin,** its major role involves the immune system. T cells, important in cell-mediated immunity, are created within the thymus.

Physical examination terms

Here are terms relating to examination of patients with endocrine disorders.

Physical findings

These physical findings are significant in the diagnosis of endocrine disorders:

- **Buffalo hump** is an accumulation of **cervicodorsal fat** (fat in the neck and back). The condition may indicate hypercortisolism or Cushing's syndrome.
- **Exophthalmos** is the abnormal protrusion of one or both eyeballs. The condition may be the result of thyrotoxicosis.
- **Goiter** is an enlarged thyroid gland, usually evident as a swelling in the front of the neck.
- **Hirsutism** is an excessive growth of dark hair. Its occurrence on a woman's body results from excessive androgen production.
- **Moon face,** usually caused by hypercortisolism, results in marked roundness of the face, double chin, and a fullness in the upper lip.
- **Polydipsia** is excessive thirst, a symptom of diabetes mellitus.
- **Polyphagia** is excessive hunger, also a symptom of diabetes mellitus.
- **Polyuria** is the increased excretion of urine by the kidneys; it's a sign of diabetes mellitus and diabetes insipidus.

Polydipsia refers to excessive thirst.

Serum studies

Specific tests are used to measure the blood level of hormones or other substances and monitor the functioning of endocrine glands. Among these tests are:

- A **fasting plasma glucose** test is used to measure plasma glucose levels after a 12- to 14-hour fast. This test is commonly used to screen for diabetes mellitus.
- **Glycosylated hemoglobin** monitoring provides information about the average blood glucose level during the preceding 2 to 3 months. This test requires one venipunc-

ture every 6 to 8 weeks and can, therefore, be used to evaluate long-term effectiveness of diabetes therapy.
- The **oral glucose tolerance test** measures plasma and urine glucose levels 3 hours after ingestion of glucose to assess insulin secretion and the body's ability to metabolize glucose.
- Quantitative analysis of **plasma cortisol** levels is used to test for pheochromocytoma or adrenal medullary tumors.
- Quantitative analysis of **plasma catecholamines** is used to test for adrenal dysfunction.
- The **plasma LH** test, typically ordered for anovulation and infertility studies in women, is a quantitative analysis of plasma LH.
- **Provocative testing** stimulates an underactive gland or suppresses an overactive gland, depending on the patient's suspected disorder. A hormone level that doesn't increase despite stimulation confirms primary hypofunction. Hormone secretion that continues after suppression confirms hyperfunction.
- **Radioimmunoassay (RIA)** is the technique used to determine most hormone levels. This test incubates blood or urine (or a urine extract) with the hormone's antibody and a radiolabeled hormone tracer (antigen). Antibody-tracer complexes can then be measured. (See *Dissecting radioimmunoassay.*)
- **Serum calcium** analysis measures blood levels of calcium to detect bone and parathyroid disorders.
- **Serum FSH** analysis measures gonadal function, especially in women.
- The **serum human growth hormone (hGH)** test is a quantitative analysis of plasma hGH levels that detects hyposecretion or hypersecretion of this hormone.

Indirect tests measure the substance a particular hormone controls, not the hormone itself.

Beyond the dictionary

Dissecting radioimmunoassay

The word **radioimmunoassay** can be broken down into three readily understandable units: **radio** refers to the radioactive tracer; **immuno** refers to the hormone's antibody (which creates an immunologic response); and **assay** means *test.*

• **Serum phosphates** analysis measures serum levels of phosphates, the primary anion in intracellular fluid.
• **Serum PTH** measurement evaluates parathyroid function.
• **Serum TSH** levels are measured by RIA, which can detect primary hypothyroidism and determine whether the hypothyroidism results from thyroid gland failure or from pituitary or hypothalamic dysfunction.
• **T_4** measurement determines the total circulating T_4 level.
• **T_3** measurement determines total serum content of T_3 to investigate thyroid dysfunction.

Urine studies

These tests are used to analyze urine samples for evidence of endocrine dysfunction:
• **Catecholamines** analysis utilizes a 24-hour urine specimen to measure levels of the major catecholamines — epinephrine, norepinephrine, and dopamine — to assess adrenal medulla function.
• **17-ketosteroids (17-KS)** assay determines urine levels of 17-KS. This test is used to diagnose adrenal dysfunction.
• **17-hydroxycorticosteroids (17-OHCS)** test measures urine levels of 17-OHCS — metabolites of the hormones that regulate glyconeogenesis.

Radiologic and imaging studies

These tests are used to create images of body structure and assess function:
• **Computerized tomography scans** provide high-resolution, three-dimensional images of a gland's structure by registering radiation levels absorbed by tissues.
• **Magnetic resonance imaging** uses magnetic waves and radiofrequency waves. The deflection of the waves is interpreted by computer to provide detailed, three-dimensional images of soft tissues.
• **Radioactive iodine uptake** test evaluates thyroid function by measuring the amount of orally ingested iodine isotope that accumulates in the thyroid.

• In **radionuclide thyroid imaging,** the thyroid is studied by a gamma camera after the patient receives a radioisotope.
• **Thyroid ultrasonography** is a noninvasive procedure to detect cysts and tumors of the thyroid by directing ultrasonic pulses at the gland.
• Routine **X-rays** evaluate how an endocrine dysfunction affects body tissues, although they don't reveal the endocrine glands.

Endocrine disorders

Endocrine problems are caused by **hyperfunction,** resulting in excess hormone effects, or **hypofunction,** resulting in hormone deficiency. **Primary dysfunction** is caused by disease within an endocrine gland. **Secondary dysfunction** occurs when endocrine tissue is affected by dysfunction of a nonendocrine organ. **Functional hyperfunction** or **functional hypofunction** results from disease in a nonendocrine tissue or organ.

Pituitary disorders

Terms used to describe pituitary dysfunction are discussed here:
• **Adiposogenital dystrophy** is marked by increased body fat and underdevelopment of secondary sex characteristics in males. This disorder is caused by damage to the hypothalamus, with a decrease in secretion of gonadotropic hormones from the anterior pituitary gland.
• **Diabetes insipidus** is caused by deficiency of circulating ADH, or vasopressin. Lack of ADH leads to extreme polyuria. Patients can urinate up to 30 L of dilute urine per day because the kidneys can't concentrate urine.
• **Hypopituitarism** (called **dwarfism** when it begins in childhood), is a complex syndrome that leads to metabolic problems, sexual immaturity, and growth retardation. These complications are caused by a deficiency of hormones secreted by the anterior pituitary gland.
• **Panhypopituitarism** refers to a generalized condition caused by partial or total failure of all six of the pituitary gland's vital hormones: ACTH, TSH, LH, FSH, GH, and prolactin.

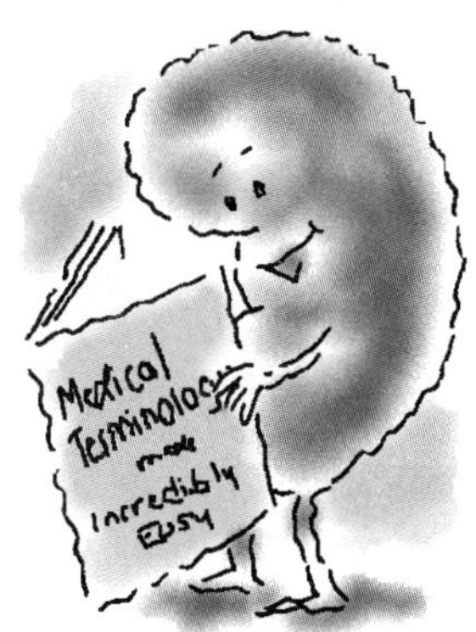
I had better get back to work. If I fail to concentrate urine, it leads to **polyuria.**
Medical Terminology made Incredibly Easy

Gonadotrophic hormone excess

Gonadotrophic hormone excess is a chronic, progressive disease marked by excess GH, tissue overgrowth, and hyperpituitarism. It appears in two forms: gigantism and acromegaly. These forms are described here:
- **Gigantism** begins while the bones are still growing and causes proportional overgrowth of all body tissues.
- **Acromegaly** occurs after bone growth is complete, causing bones and organs to thicken. Bones of the face, jaw, and extremities gradually enlarge with acromegaly.

Thyroid disorders

Two types of thyroid dysfunction, hyperthyroidism and hypothyroidism, are detailed here.

Hyperthyroidism

Hyperthyroidism results from excess thyroid hormone. The most common form of this disorder is **Graves' disease,** which increases T_4 production, enlarges the thyroid gland **(goiter),** and causes metabolic changes.

Seven subtypes

Forms of hyperthyroidism include:

1. **thyroid storm,** an acute exacerbation of hyperthyroidism that is a medical emergency and may lead to cardiac failure
2. **toxic adenoma,** a small, benign nodule in the thyroid gland that secretes thyroid hormone
3. **thyrotoxicosis factitia,** which results from chronic ingestion of thyroid hormone, sometimes by persons who are trying to lose weight
4. **functioning metastatic thyroid carcinoma,** a rare disease that causes excess production of thyroid hormone
5. **TSH-secreting pituitary tumor,** which causes overproduction of thyroid hormone

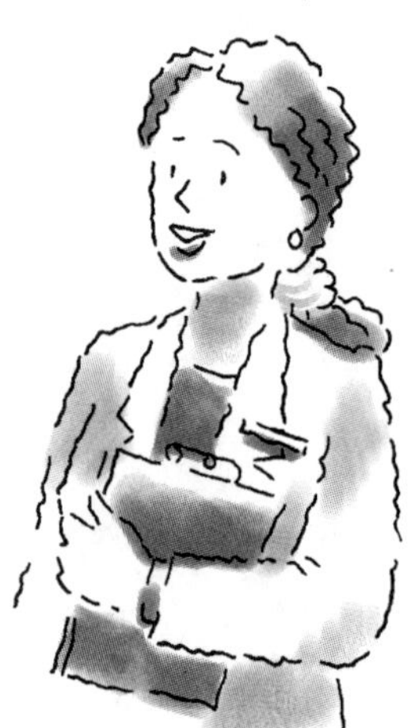

Why is **silent thyroiditis** called "silent"? Because it has no inflammatory symptoms.

subacute thyroiditis, a viral inflammation of the thyroid gland, which produces short-term hyperthyroidism associated with flulike symptoms

silent thyroiditis, a self-limiting form of hyperthyroidism with no inflammatory symptoms.

Hypothyroidism

Hypothyroidism results from low serum thyroid hormone or cellular resistance to the thyroid hormone. It's caused by insufficiency of the hypothalamus or pituitary or thyroid gland. Here are two related terms:

- **Hashimoto's thyroiditis** is an inflammation of the thyroid gland caused by antibodies to thyroid antigens in the blood. It causes inflammation and lymphocytic infiltration of the thyroid, leading to thyroid tissue destruction and hypothyroidism.
- **Myxedema coma** is a life-threatening complication of hypothyroidism marked by depressed respirations, decreased cardiac output, and hypotension.

Parathyroid disorders

Parathyroid disorders include:

- **Hypoparathyroidism** stems from a deficiency of PTH. Because PTH regulates calcium balance, a PTH deficiency causes **hypocalcemia** (low blood levels of calcium), which leads to neuromuscular symptoms, such as **paresthesia** (tingling of the extremities) and **tetany** (muscle rigidity).
- **Hyperparathyroidism,** overactivity of one or more of the parathyroid glands and production of excess PTH, promotes bone resorption and leads to **hypophosphatemia** and **hypercalcemia** (low blood phosphate and elevated blood calcium levels). With **primary hyperparathyroidism,** the glands enlarge. In **secondary hyperparathyroidism,** the glands produce excessive PTH to compensate for low calcium levels in the blood caused by some other abnormality.

Pancreatic disorders

These diseases are associated with the pancreas:

• **Diabetes mellitus** is a chronic insulin deficiency or resistance to insulin by the cells. This form of diabetes causes problems with carbohydrate, protein, and fat metabolism. Diabetes mellitus is classified as type 1 — insulin-dependent, or type 2 — non-insulin-dependent — the more prevalent form. (See *Distinguishing mellitus from insipidus.*)
• **Gestational diabetes** is a form of diabetes mellitus that occurs during pregnancy. Usually, the patient's condition returns to normal after delivery

When diabetes gets complicated

These complications can occur with diabetes:
• **Diabetic ketoacidosis** is a life-threatening form of metabolic acidosis that may arise as a complication of uncontrolled diabetes mellitus. Accumulation of ketone bodies leads to urinary loss of water, potassium, ammonium, and sodium, resulting in hypovolemia, electrolyte imbalances, an extremely high blood glucose level and, commonly, coma.
• **Hyperosmolar hyperglycemic nonketotic syndrome** is a complication of diabetes mellitus in which the level of blood glucose is increased but ketosis doesn't occur; coma results when the high concentration of blood glucose causes dehydration of brain tissues.
• **Hypoglycemia** is characterized by an abnormally low blood glucose level. This condition occurs when glucose is used too rapidly, when the rate of glucose release falls

Beyond the dictionary

Distinguishing mellitus from insipidus

Diabetes mellitus and **diabetes insipidus** are two distinct diseases with similar symptoms, especially profuse urine excretion. The word **mellitus** derives from the Latin word for *honey* — diabetes mellitus refers to the sweet smell of a patient's urine due to excess amounts of glucose. Diabetes insipidus produces no such sweetness and is therefore called **insipidus,** meaning *bland.*

behind demand, or when excess insulin enters the bloodstream.

Adrenal disorders

Here are names of important adrenal gland disorders:

- **Addisonian crisis,** an acute adrenal crisis, occurs when the body's stores of glucocorticoids are exhausted, leading to hypotension, hypoglycemia, electrolyte imbalances, cardiac arrhythmias, and death. (See *Addison and Cushing.*)
- **Adrenal hyperfunction,** also called **Cushing's syndrome,** results from excessive levels of adrenocortical hormones, especially cortisol. This condition can be caused by hypersecretion of ACTH by the pituitary gland, an ACTH-secreting tumor of another organ, or the use of glucocorticoid medications.
- **Adrenal hypofunction,** also called **Addison's disease,** is the most common sign of adrenal insufficiency, seen when 90% of the gland is destroyed. In this autoimmune process, circulating antibodies react against adrenal tissue, leading to decreased secretion of androgens, glucocorticoids, and mineralocorticoids.
- **Hyperaldosteronism** results when the adrenal cortex secretes excess amounts of aldosterone. It can be a primary disease of the adrenal cortex or a response to other disorders. Excessive aldosterone in the bloodstream instructs the kidneys to reabsorb too much sodium and water and excrete too much potassium. The fluid retention and hypokalemia caused by this disorder lead to hypertension, decreased hematocrit, muscle weakness, tetany, excess thirst, and many other symptoms.
- **Pheochromocytoma** refers to a vascular tumor of the chromaffin tissue found in the adrenal medulla. This condition is characterized by secretion of epinephrine and norepinephrine, causing hypertension associated with attacks of palpitations, nausea, headache, dyspnea, anxiety, pallor, and profuse sweating. (See *Focus on pheochromocytoma*, page 296.)

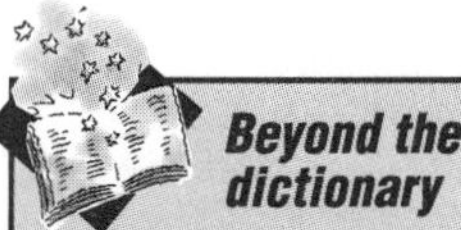

Beyond the dictionary

Addison and Cushing

Addison's disease is named after the British doctor Thomas Addison (1793 to 1860), who described this form of adrenal insufficiency in 1849. Harvey Cushing (1869 to 1939), an American physiologist, was the first to note the changes in body appearance — development of fat deposits on the face, neck, and trunk and purple **striae** (streaks) on the skin — associated with pituitary tumors **(Cushing's syndrome).**

Beyond the dictionary

Focus on pheochromocytoma

Pheochromocytoma refers to a vascular tumor of the chromaffin tissue found in the adrenal medulla. To better understand pheochromocytoma, break down the word:

- **pheo** means *dusky*
- **chromo** means *color*
- **cyt** refers to *cell*
- ***-oma*** is a suffix that means *tumor.*

Thus, **pheochromocytoma** is *a tumor of the dusky colored cells of the adrenal glands.*

Treatments

Treatments for endocrine disorders include surgery, radiation therapy, and drug therapy.

Surgery

Surgeries to correct diseases affecting the endocrine systems are described here:

- **Adrenalectomy** is a resection or removal of one or both adrenal glands.
- **Hypophysectomy** is the surgical removal of pituitary tumors. In a procedure called **transsphenoidal hypophysectomy,** the tumor is removed by entering the inner aspect of the upper lip through the sphenoid sinus.
- **Pancreatectomy** is removal of the pancreas after more conservative measures have failed.
- **Parathyroidectomy** is the surgical removal of one or more of the four parathyroid glands and is used to treat hyperparathyroidism. The number of glands removed depends on the underlying cause of excessive hormone secretion.
- A **subtotal thyroidectomy** surgically removes a portion of the thyroid gland.
- **Total bilateral adrenalectomy** excises both adrenal glands and eliminates the body's reserve

Out I go. **Pancreatectomy** is removal of the pancreas, which occurs after more conservative measures have failed.

of corticosteroids, which are synthesized in the adrenal cortex. Adrenalectomy is performed only when treatment of the pituitary gland is impossible.

- **Total parathyroidectomy** removes all of the parathyroid glands. In such cases, the patient requires lifelong treatment for hypoparathyroidism.
- A **total thyroidectomy** removes the entire thyroid gland.

Radiation therapy

There are two radiation treatments for endocrine disorders:

- **Pituitary radiation** controls the growth of a pituitary tumor or relieves its signs and symptoms.
- **^{131}I administration** uses an isotope of iodine to treat hyperthyroidism or thyroid cancer. It shrinks functioning thyroid tissue, decreases levels of thyroid hormone in the body, and destroys malignant cells.

Drug therapy

Here are some common drug therapies for endocrine disorders:

- **Corticosteroids** and **hormone replacement** are administered to combat hormone deficiencies.
- **Insulin** or **oral antidiabetic agents** may be administered to control glucose levels.

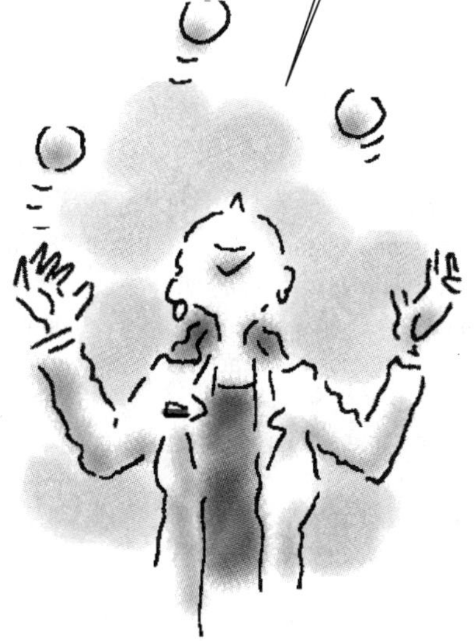
Get ready
for some fun
and games!

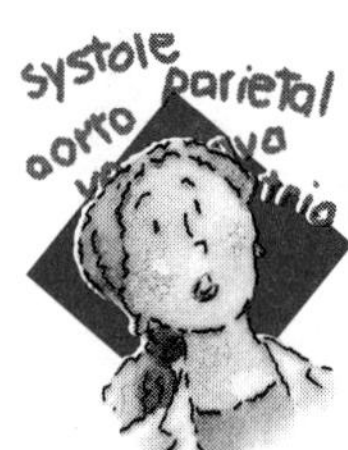

Vocabulary builders

At a crossroads

Completing this crossword puzzle will help stimulate your excretion of correct endocrine system terms. Good luck!

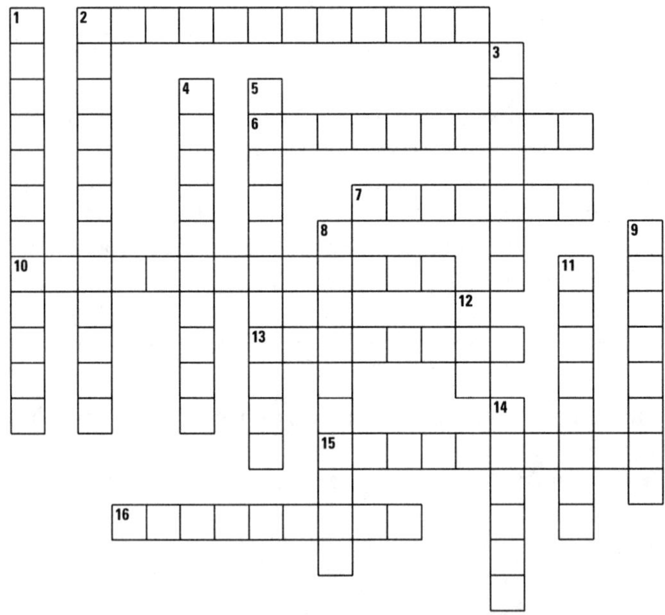

Across

2. Enlarged spleen
6. Also known as the pituitary gland
7. Inner portion of the adrenal gland
10. Stimulates the adrenal cortex
13. Stimulates the ejection of breast milk into mammary ducts
15. Excessive hunger
16. Proportional overgrowth of body tissues

Down

1. Condition characterized by abnormally low blood glucose level
2. Promotes the growth of bony and soft tissues
3. Hormone that decreases blood glucose levels
4. Hormones produced by the cortex
5. Influences secretion of the thyroid hormone
8. Excessive thirst (a sign of diabetes mellitus)
9. Organ that lies along the back of the abdominal wall behind the stomach
11. Hormone that increases blood glucose levels
12. Abbreviation for radioimmunoassay
14. Gland located below the sternum

Answers are on page 300.

Match game

Match each hormone or organ with its other name.

Clues	Choices
1. Pituitary gland ____	A. Somatotropin
2. Growth hormone ____	B. Prolactin
3. Antidiuretic hormone ____	C. Hypophysis
4. Mammotropin ____	D. Vasopressin

Finish line

Fill in the blanks with the appropriate treatment or surgical intervention.

1. Removal of the entire thyroid gland is known as ______ ______.
2. ______ removes the pancreas after more conservative measures have failed.
3. The resection or removal of one or both adrenal glands is known as ______.
4. ______ ______ controls the growth of a pituitary tumor or relieves its signs and symptoms.
5. When only a portion of the thyroid gland is surgically removed it's called a ______ ______.
6. The surgical removal of pituitary tumors is known as ______.

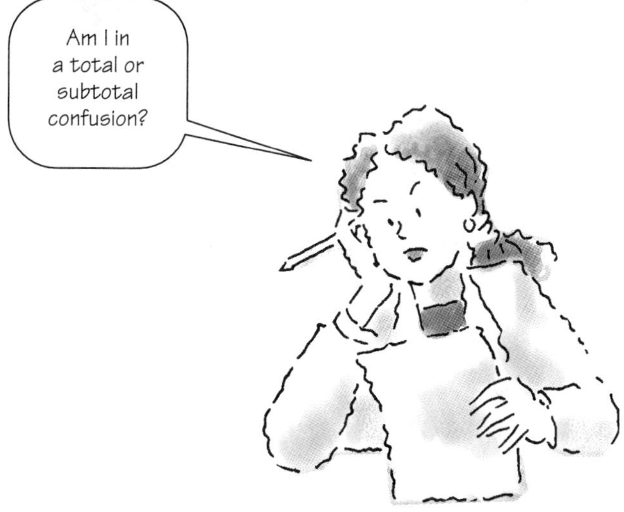
Am I in a total or subtotal confusion?

Answers are on page 300.

Answers

At a crossroads

[1] H		[2] S	P	L	E	N	O	M	E	G	A	L	Y					
Y		O												[3] I				
P		M			[4] C		[5] T							N				
O		A			O		[6] H	Y	P	O	P	H	Y	S	I	S		
G		T			R		Y							U				
L		O			T		R			[7] M	E	D	U	L	L	A		
Y		T			I		O		[8] P					I				[9] P
[10] C	O	R	T	I	C	O	T	R	O	P	I	N		N		[11] G		A
E		O			O		R		L				[12] R			L		N
M		P			I		[13] O	X	Y	T	O	C	I	N		U		C
I		I			D		P		D				A			C		R
A		N			S		I		I					[14] T		A		E
							N		[15] P	O	L	Y	P	H	A	G	I	A
									S					Y		O		S
			[16] G	I	G	A	N	T	I	S	M			M		N		
									A					U				
														S				

Match game

1. C; 2. A; 3. D; 4. B.

Finish line

1. Total thyroidectomy; 2. Pancreatectomy; 3. Adrenalectomy; 4. Pituitary radiation; 5. Subtotal thyroidectomy; 6. Hypophysectomy.

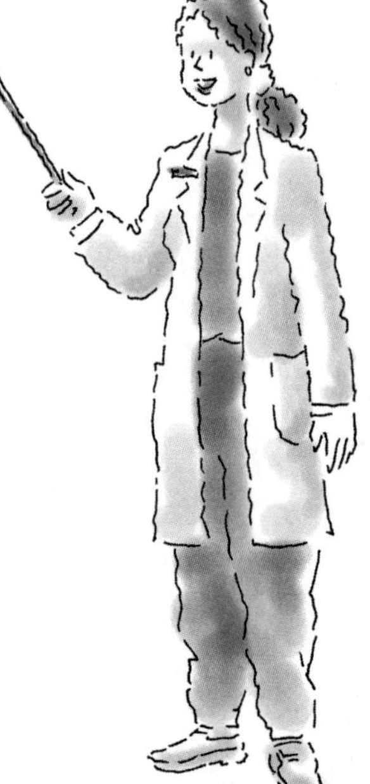

Lymphatic and immune system

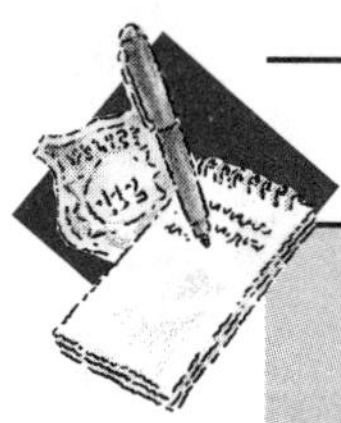

Just the facts

In this chapter, you'll review:

- terminology related to the structure and function of the lymphatic and immune system
- terminology needed for physical examination
- tests that help diagnose lymphatic and immune system disorders
- lymphatic and immune system disorders and their treatments.

Lymphatic and immune structure and function

I'm a **pluripotential** stem cell. That means I have the **potential** to take many **(pluri-)** forms.

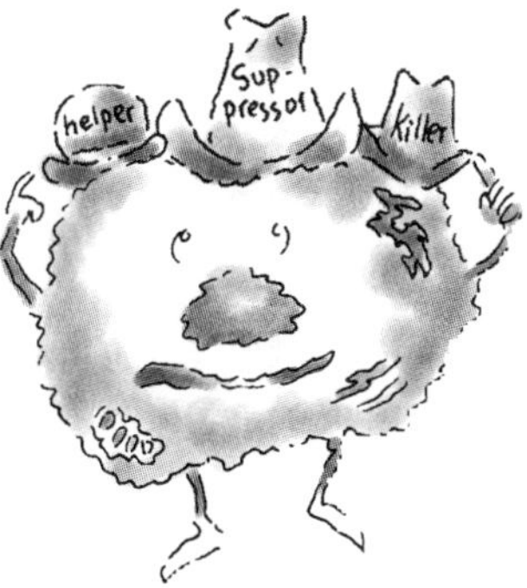

The **immune system** is diverse and complicated, with specialized cells and structures that defend the body against invasion of harmful organisms or chemical toxins. The blood is an important part of this protective system. Although the immune system and blood are distinct entities, they're closely related. For example, their cells share a common origin in the bone marrow, and the immune system uses the bloodstream to transport its components. (See *Pronouncing key immune system terms*, page 302.)

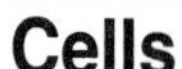

Cells

Special cells located in the bone marrow, called **pluripotential stem cells,** develop into immune system and

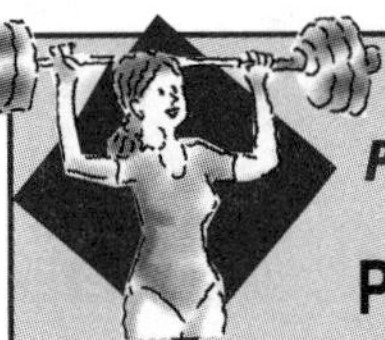

Pump up your pronunciation

Pronouncing key immune system terms

Here is a list of key terms, along with the correct way to pronounce them.

Hypogammaglobulinemia	HIGH-POH-GAM-AH-GLOB-YOO-LIH-NEE-MEE-AH
Immunoelectrophoresis	IHM-YOO-NOH-EH-LECK-TROH-FOR-EE-SISS
Lymphadenopathy	LIHM-FAD-EH-NAWP-AH-THEE
Phagocytosis	FAG-OH-SIGH-TOE-SISS
Splenomegaly	SPLEE-NOH-MEG-AH-LEE
Thymus	THEYE-MUSS
Trabeculae	TRAH-BECK-YOU-LEE

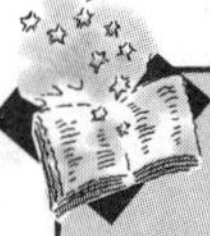

Beyond the dictionary

Blood formation

Hematopoiesis may seem like a difficult word at first glance, but break it down and the difficulty disappears.

In Greek, ***hematos*** is the word for *blood* and ***poiesis*** means *formation.* Together they form the word for *blood formation* — **hematopoiesis.**

blood cells through a process called **hematopoiesis.** (See *Blood formation.*)

Some stem cells destined to produce immune system cells serve as sources of **lymphocytes** (a type of white blood cell), whereas others develop into **phagocytes** (cells that engulf and digest microorganisms and cellular debris). Those that become lymphocytes are differentiated to become either B cells (which mature in the bone marrow) or T cells (which travel to the thymus and mature there).

B cells and T cells are distributed throughout the lymphoid organs, especially the lymph nodes and spleen.

In the **thymus** (a lymph structure located in the mediastinum), T cells undergo a process called **T-cell education,** in which the cells are "trained" to recognize other cells from the same body (**self cells**) and distinguish them from all other cells (**nonself cells**).

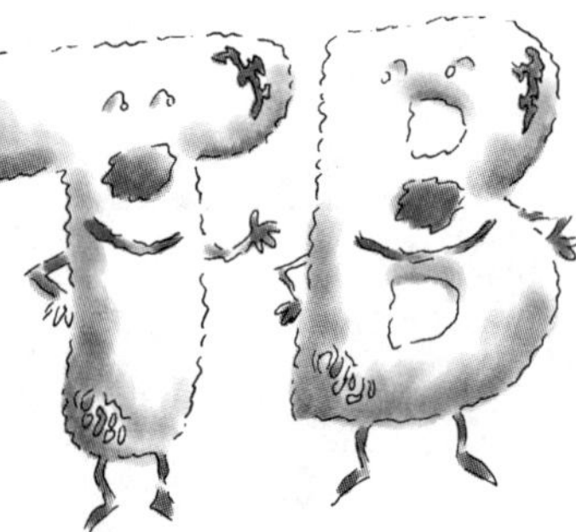

I'm a T cell and this is my friend, a B cell. We're both lymphocytes, but I grew up in the thymus...
...and I grew up in the bone marrow — that is how we got our names.

Organs and tissues of the immune system

The term **lymphoid** is used to refer to immune system organs and tissues because they're all involved in some way in the growth, development, and dissemination of lymphocytes (or white blood cells [WBCs]). (See *How nymph became lymph.*)

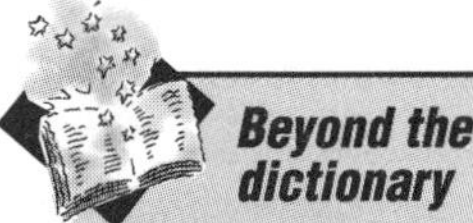

Beyond the dictionary

How nymph became lymph

Lymph fluid is a clear, transparent liquid found in the **lymphatic vessels,** which take their name from this substance. In Greek, ***nymph*** was the name for a goddess of lower rank usually associated with a river or lake. In turn, the Greeks applied the term to young women, "pure as a virgin river," of marriageable age. Latin borrowed the term, but the ***n*** mutated to an ***l*** and it became applied to a fluid thought to be as pure and clear as the nymphs of long ago.

Lymph nodes

The small, oval-shaped **lymph nodes** contain **lymphatic tissue** and are located along a network of lymphatic channels. They release lymphocytes, the primary cells of the immune system, and help remove and destroy antigens circulating in the blood and lymphatic vessels. Each lymph node is surrounded by a fibrous capsule that extends **trabeculae** (bands of connective tissue) into the node.

Function is an emphatic issue for lymphatic tissue

When lymph fluid enters the node, it's filtered through sinuses before draining into the single exit vessel. The filtration process removes bacteria and other foreign bodies or particles, including malignant cells.

Another function of lymph nodes is **phagocytosis,** the destruction of invading cells or particles. Lymphatic tissue is also the site of final maturation for lymphocytes that migrate from the bone marrow.

Location, location, location

Locations of lymph nodes include:

- **axillary**— underarm and upper chest
- **cervical**—neck
- **inguinal**— groin area
- **popliteal**—behind the knee
- **submandibular**— floor of the mouth and lower jaw.

Lymphatic fluid

Lymphatic fluid (also **lymph fluid** or **lymph**) is a transparent, usually slightly yellow liquid found within the lymphatic vessels. It's collected from all parts of the body and returned to the blood after filtration in the lymph nodes.

Lymphatic vessels

Lymphatic vessels intertwine with blood vessels and distribute lymphatic fluid throughout the body.

Lymphatic vessels located in the small intestine are called **lacteals.** They absorb fats and other nutrients, producing a milky lymph fluid called **chyle,** from the Greek word ***chylos,*** or *juice.*

Lymphatic vessels remove proteins and water from the interstitial spaces and return them to the bloodstream.

The word **lacteal** probably will remind you of the word **lactate,** which means to *produce milk.* Lacteals produce a "milky" lymph fluid.

Spleen

The **spleen** is a lymphoid organ located in the left upper quadrant of the abdomen beneath the diaphragm. The largest structure of the lymphatic system, the spleen initiates an immune response, filters and removes bacteria and other foreign substances from the bloodstream, destroys worn-out blood cells, and serves as a blood reservoir. (See *History of* spleen.)

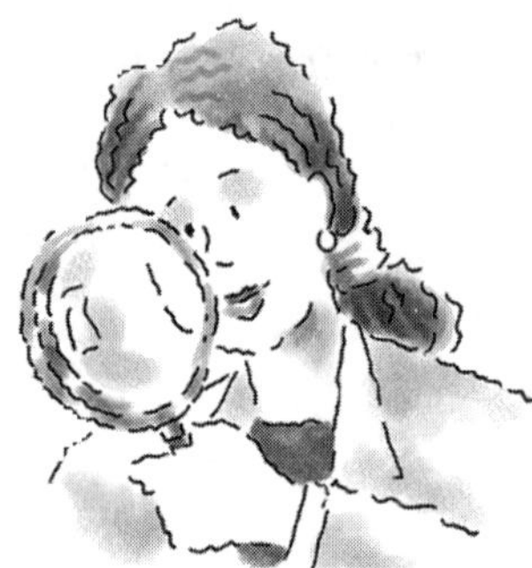

Accessory lymphoid organs and tissues

The tonsils, adenoids, appendix, thymus, and Peyer's patches remove foreign debris in much the same way lymph nodes do. They're located in food and air passages—areas where microbial access is more likely to occur.

Fighting disease

Immunity is the body's capacity to resist invading organisms and toxins, thereby preventing tissue and organ damage. The immune system's cells and organs are designed to recognize, respond to, and eliminate foreign substances, including bacteria, viruses, and parasites. The immune system also preserves the body's internal environment by scavenging dead or damaged cells and by patrolling antigens.

Specific immune responses

All foreign substances elicit the same response in general host defenses. In contrast, particular microorganisms or molecules activate specific immune responses and initially can involve specialized sets of immune cells. Such specific responses, classified as either humoral immunity or cell-mediated immunity, are produced by lymphocytes (B cells and T cells).

Humoral immunity

In this response, an invading antigen causes B cells to divide and differentiate into plasma cells. Each plasma cell, in turn, produces and secretes large amounts of antibodies (immunoglobulin molecules that interact with a specific antigen) into the bloodstream. Antibodies destroy bacteria and viruses, thereby preventing them from entering host cells. Five major classes of immunoglobulin exist:

- **Immunoglobulin (Ig) G** makes up 80% of plasma antibodies. It appears in all body fluids and is the major antibacterial and antiviral antibody.
- **IgM** is the first immunoglobulin produced during an immune response. It's too large to easily cross membrane barriers and is usually present only in the vascular system.
- **IgA** is found mainly in body secretions such as saliva, sweat, tears, mucus, bile, and colostrum. It defends against pathogens on body surfaces, especially those that enter the respiratory and GI tracts.
- **IgD** is present in plasma and is easily broken down. It's the predominant antibody on the surface of B cells and is mainly an antigen receptor.
- **IgE** is the antibody involved in immediate hypersensitivity reactions (or allergic reactions) that develop within minutes of exposure to an antigen. IgE stimulates the release of mast cell granules, which contain histamine and heparin.

Another part of humoral immunity, the **complement system,** is a major mediator of the inflammatory response. It consists of 20 proteins circulating as functionally inactive molecules. In most cases, an antigen-antibody reaction is necessary for the complement system to activate to destroy invading cells.

Cell-mediated immunity

In **cell-mediated immunity,** T cells respond directly to antigens (foreign substances such as bacteria or toxins that induce antibody formation). This response involves destruction of target cells — such as virus-infected cells and cancer cells — through the secretion of lymphokines (lymph proteins). Organ rejection is an example of cell-mediated immunity.

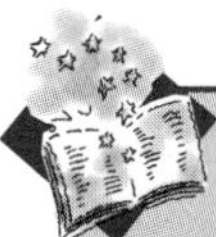

Beyond the dictionary

History of *spleen*

Since ancient times, the word **spleen** has been used to designate the largest lymphatic organ. The word probably first appeared in its modern form between 1250 and 1300, having been derived from the Latin word ***splen.*** The origins of the word go back even further, to the ancient Sanskrit ***plihan.***

Spleen: Cheerful or gloomy?

The spleen was considered to be the seat of various emotions or attributes. Some were positive, linking the spleen with cheerfulness, courage, and spirit. At other times, the spleen was thought to be the site of negative attributes, such as a bad temper and a spiteful or gloomy nature.

Acquired immunity

The body readily develops long-term immunity to specific antigens, including pollen, dust, mold, and invading organisms. There are four types of acquired immunity:

Natural, active immunity occurs when the immune system responds to a harmful agent and develops long-term immunity. For example, people develop immunity to measles after having the disease once.

Natural, passive immunity is the transfer of antibodies from a mother to her breast-fed infant, providing temporary, partial immunity.

Artificial, active immunity is obtained by vaccination with weakened or dead infectious agents introduced into the body to alert the immune system.

Artificial, passive immunity is provided by substances that provide immediate, but temporary immunity, such as antibiotics, gamma globulin, and interferon.

Physical examination terms

The following terms may be encountered when performing the physical examination:

- **Angioedema** is a subcutaneous and dermal eruption that produces deep, large, raised sections of skin (usually on the hands, feet, lips, genitals, and eyelids) and diffuse swelling of the subcutaneous tissue.
- **Butterfly rash** is a classic sign of **systemic lupus erythematosus (SLE).** Lesions appear on the cheeks and the bridge of the nose, creating a characteristic butterfly-shaped pattern.
- **Chills** (also called **rigors**) are extreme, involuntary muscle contractions with characteristic paroxysms of violent shivering and tooth chattering.
- **Lymphadenopathy** is enlarged lymph nodes.
- **Lymphangioma** is a benign tumor caused by congenital malformation of the lymphatic system.
- **Splenomegaly** is an enlarged spleen.
- **Urticaria** is more commonly known as **hives.**

Diagnostic tests

Most tests of the immune system use a combination of techniques to evaluate the body's immune response and break down the individual components.

Laboratory tests

Some common laboratory tests are:

- **ABO blood typing** classifies blood according to the presence of major antigens A and B on RBC surfaces and according to serum antibodies anti-A and anti-B. ABO blood typing is required before transfusion to prevent a lethal reaction.
- **Crossmatching** is an antibody detection test that establishes the compatibility of a donor's and recipient's blood.
- A **direct antiglobulin test (direct Coombs' test)** demonstrates the presence of antibodies (such as antibodies to the Rh factor) or complement on circulating red blood cells.
- **Enzyme-linked immunosorbent assay (ELISA)** identifies antibodies to bacteria, viruses, deoxyribonucleic acid, allergens, and substances such as immunoglobulins.
- **Erythrocyte sedimentation rate (ESR)** measures the degree of erythrocyte settling in a blood sample during a specified time period.
- **Human leukocyte antigen test (HLA)** identifies a group of antigens that are present on the surfaces of all nucleated cells but most easily detected on lymphocytes. These antigens are essential to immunity and determine the degree of histocompatibility between transplant recipients and donors.
- **Immunoelectrophoresis** identifies immunoglobulins in a serum sample. It evaluates the effectiveness of radiation therapy or chemotherapy and detects **hypogammaglobulinemias** (abnormally low levels of gamma globulins causing increased susceptibility to infection).
- The **platelet count** assesses the number of platelets in a microliter of blood.
- **RH typing** classifies blood by the presence or absence of the Rh_0(D) antigen on the surface of RBCs. In this test, a patient's RBCs are mixed with serum containing anti-

$Rh_0(D)$ antibodies and are observed for clamping together of antigen-bearing particles of similar size in a solution.

- **WBC count,** also called a leukocyte count, is part of a complete blood count. It indicates the number of WBCs in a microliter of whole blood.
- The **WBC differential** evaluates the type, number, and condition of WBCs present in the blood. WBCs are classified as one of five major types of leukocytes — neutrophils, eosinophils, basophils, lymphocytes, and monocytes — and the percentage of each type is determined in this test.
- **Western blot test** detects the presence of specific viral proteins.

Patch and scratch allergy tests

These skin tests evaluate the immune system's ability to respond to known allergens, which are applied to hairless areas of the patient's body.

Patch work

In **patch testing,** a dilute solution of each allergen is placed directly on the skin and covered with gauze. In 48 to 72 hours, the appearance of redness, vesicles, itching, or swelling shows a positive reaction.

Scratching the surface

Scratch tests introduce allergens into a scratched area on the patient's skin with a special tool or needle. Test sites are examined 30 to 40 minutes later and compared with a control site; redness, itching, or swelling are considered positive reactions.

Under your skin

Intradermal skin tests evaluate the patient's immune system by injecting **recall antigens** (antigens to which the patient may have been previously sensitized). Antigens are injected into the superficial skin layer with a needle and syringe or a sterile four-pronged lancet.

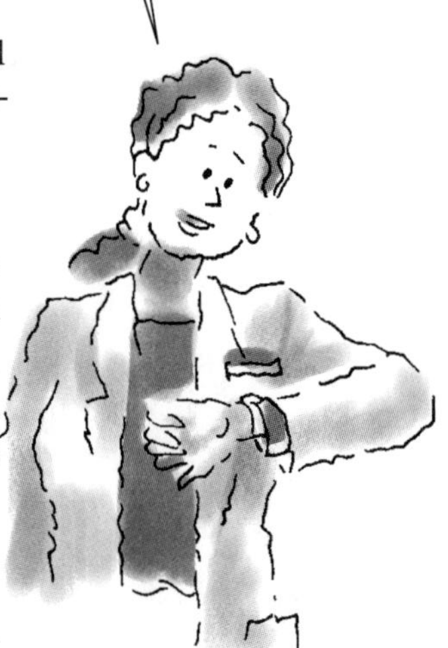
Patch tests show results in 2 to 3 days. Scratch tests work more quickly; results show in 30 to 40 minutes.

Lymphatic and immune disorders

Because of their complexity, the processes involved in host defense and immune response may malfunction. When the body's defenses are exaggerated, misdirected, or either absent or depressed, the result may be a hypersensitivity disorder, autoimmunity, or immunodeficiency, respectively. This section provides terminology associated with lymphatic and immune system disorders.

Hyperreactivity and **hypersensitivity** share a prefix. ***Hyper-*** comes from Greek and means *in excess of.* These are disorders that cause an excessive reaction or sensitivity in the immune system.

Hypersensitivity disorders

An exaggerated or inappropriate immune response may lead to various hypersensitivity disorders, such as asthma, allergic rhinitis, anaphylaxis, atopic dermatitis, latex allergy, and blood transfusion reactions.

Asthma

Asthma is a chronic, reactive airway disorder leading to episodes of airway obstruction with bronchospasms, increased mucus secretion, and mucosal swelling. (See *How do I (pant) say asthma?*)

Take a deep breath

Here are a few types of asthma:

- **Acute asthma** is an attack that can begin either dramatically with severe symptoms or slowly with gradual symptoms.
- **Extrinsic asthma** results from sensitivity to pollen, animal dander, mold, or other sensitizing substances.
- **Intrinsic asthma** is diagnosed when no extrinsic allergen can be identified.
- **Status asthmaticus** is a persistent, intractable asthma attack that can lead to acute respiratory failure.

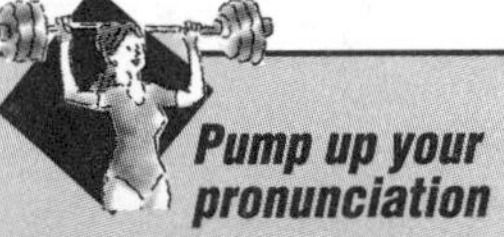
Pump up your pronunciation

How do I (pant) say asthma?

Asthma derives from the Greek and means *gasping* or *panting.* The grouping of consonants in its middle makes it look more difficult to pronounce than it actually is. The ***th*** is silent, leaving you with the easily pronounceable: AZ-MAH.

Allergic rhinitis

Allergic rhinitis is a reaction to airborne (inhaled) allergens. The resulting runny nose, itching, nasal obstruction, and congestion can be seasonal, **hay fever,** or year-round, **perennial allergic rhinitis.**

Anaphylaxis

Anaphylaxis is a dramatic, acute reaction marked by the sudden onset of rapidly progressive hives and respiratory distress.

Atopic dermatitis

Atopic dermatitis is a chronic skin disorder characterized by superficial skin inflammation and intense itching.

Latex allergy

Latex allergy is a hypersensitivity reaction to products that contain natural latex, which is derived from the sap of a rubber tree, not synthetic latex. These hypersensitivity reactions range from local dermatitis to a life-threatening anaphylactic reaction.

Blood transfusion reactions

Mediated by immune or nonimmune factors, a **transfusion reaction** happens during or after the administration of blood components. Symptoms can be mild (fever and chills) or severe (acute renal failure or complete vascular collapse and death), depending on the amount of blood transfused, the type of reaction, and the patient's general health.

Poorly made matches

Hemolytic reactions follow transfusion of mismatched blood. When this occurs, red blood cells clump together and break down, leading to kidney damage.

Less worrisome

Allergic reactions to transfused blood are fairly common and only occasionally serious. Patients may experience transient hives, itching, chills, and fever. Symptoms resolve quickly when the transfusion is stopped.

More common

Febrile nonhemolytic reactions, the most common type of reaction, apparently develop when antibodies in the patient's plasma attack antigens on lymphocytes, granulocytes, or plasma cells of the transfused blood.

Autoimmune disorders

Autoimmune disorders occur when a misdirected immune response causes the body's defenses to become self-destructive.

- **Ankylosing spondylitis** is a chronic, usually progressive, inflammatory disease that primarily affects the sacroiliac, apophyseal, and costovertebral joints and adjacent soft tissue.
- **Rheumatoid arthritis** is a chronic, systemic inflammatory disease that primarily attacks peripheral joints and surrounding muscles, tendons, ligaments, and blood vessels.
- **Scleroderma** is a diffuse connective tissue disease characterized by fibrotic, degenerative, and occasionally inflammatory changes in the skin, blood vessels, synovial membranes, skeletal muscles, and internal organs.
- **Sjögren's syndrome,** the second most common rheumatoid disorder, is marked by decreased secretions from the lacrimal and salivary glands.
- **Systemic lupus erythematosus (SLE)** is a chronic inflammatory disorder of the connective tissue. It affects multiple organ systems, is characterized by remissions and exacerbations, and can be fatal.
- **Vasculitis** includes a broad spectrum of disorders characterized by inflammation and necrosis of blood vessels.

Immunodeficiency disorders

In immunodeficiency, the immune system is absent or depressed, resulting in increased susceptibility to infection.

Opportunity knocks

Also known as **AIDS, acquired immunodeficiency syndrome** causes progressive damage to the body's immune response and gradual destruction of cells — including T cells. The retrovirus **human immunodeficiency virus (HIV)** causes AIDS.

Major immunity missing

DiGeorge syndrome, also called congenital thymic hypoplasia or aplasia, is a disorder characterized by the partial or total absence of cell-mediated immunity that results from a deficiency of T lymphocytes.

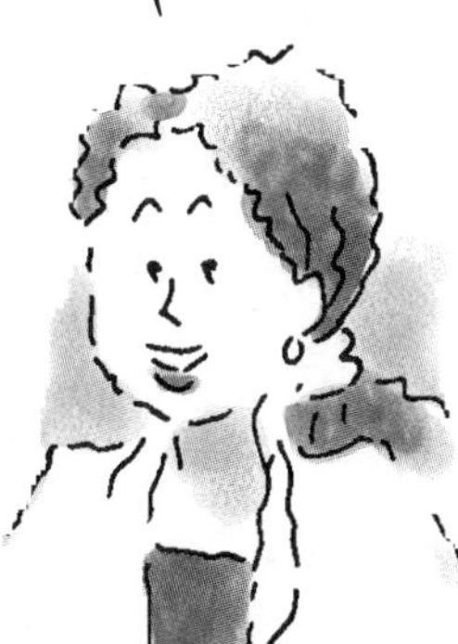
Lupus is Latin for wolf. It was first used as a medical term because disorders such as **systemic lupus erythematosus** were thought to devour the body like a hungry wolf.

Chemo complication

Iatrogenic immunodeficiency is a deficiency in the immune response that occurs as a complication of chemotherapy and other medical treatment.

Cancers

Several types of cancer can affect the lymphatic and immune system:

- **Hodgkin's disease** is a neoplastic disease characterized by painless, progressive enlargement of lymph nodes, spleen, and other lymphoid tissue.
- **Kaposi's sarcoma** is a cancer of the lymphatic cell wall. It involves the lymph nodes, viscera and, possibly, GI structures.
- **Malignant lymphoma** is a group of malignant diseases originating in lymph glands and other lymphoid tissue.

Treatments

A variety of methods are used to combat disorders to the lymphatic and immune system, including drug therapy, radiation, surgical removal of an infected organ, and bone marrow transplantation.

Drug therapy

Here is a list of drugs commonly used to treat immune and lymphatic disorders:

- **Antilymphocyte serum** or **antithymocyte globulin** is an anti-T-cell antibody that reduces the number and function of T cells. This suppresses cell-mediated immunity. The drug is used to prevent rejection of tissue grafts or transplants.
- **Corticosteroids** are adrenocortical hormones widely used to treat immune disorders because of their anti-inflammatory and immunosuppressant effects. These drugs stabilize the vascular membrane, blocking tissue infiltration by neutrophils and monocytes and thus inhibiting inflammation.
- **Cytotoxic drugs** kill immune cells while they're replicating. However, most cytotoxic drugs aren't selective

and interfere with all rapidly growing cells. As a result, they reduce the number of lymphocytes as well as phagocytes.

- **Cyclosporine** is an immunosuppressant drug that selectively suppresses T-helper cells, resulting in depressed immunity. It's used to prevent organ rejection in kidney, liver, bone marrow, and heart transplants.

Radiation therapy

Radiation therapy is the use of a radioactive substance to treat a disease. Radiation therapy of all major lymph node areas — known as **total nodal radiation** — is used to treat certain disorders, such as Hodgkin's disease.

Surgery

Surgeries include the removal of a lymph node, a lymph vessel, the spleen, or the thymus.

- **Lymphadenectomy** is surgical removal of a lymph node.
- **Lymphangiectomy** is surgical removal of a lymph vessel.
- **Splenectomy,** or removal of the spleen, causes increased risk of infection, especially from such bacteria as *Streptococcus pneumoniae.*
- **Thymectomy** is the surgical removal of the thymus.

Bone marrow transplantation

Bone marrow transplantation begins with the collection of marrow cells from a donor. The cells are then transferred to an immunosuppressed patient. There are three types of bone marrow transplant:

- **Allogeneic transplant** uses bone marrow from a compatible donor, usually a sibling.
- **Autologous transplant** uses marrow tissue that is harvested from the patient before he receives chemotherapy and radiation therapy, or while he's in remission, and frozen for later use.
- **Stem cell transplant** involves the transfusion of stem cells, which can develop into RBCs, WBCs, and platelets. Stem cells are typically donated by the patient before chemotherapy.
- **Syngeneic transplant** refers to the transplantation of marrow between identical twins.

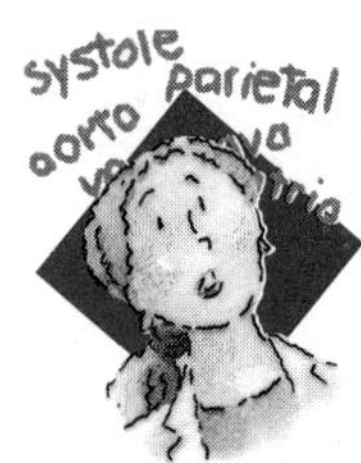

Vocabulary builders

At a crossroads

Completing this crossword puzzle will help you ward off an attack by incorrect lymphatic and immune system terms. Good luck!

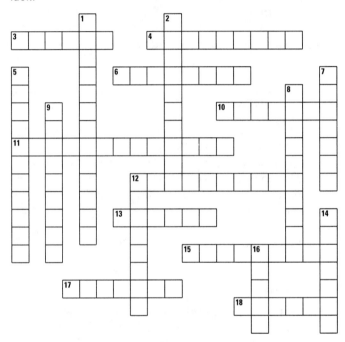

Across

3. The largest structure of the lymphatic system
4. Term indicating location behind the knee
6. Term used to refer to immune system organs and tissues
10. Eponym for the second most common autoimmune rheumatoid disorder
11. Process by which stem cells develop into blood cells or immune system cells
12. Immunodeficiency introduced by a medical treatment
13. Response activated by microorganisms
15. The type of transplant of marrow between identical twins
17. Tests that introduce allergens to the skin using a special tool, with results examined 30 to 40 minutes later
18. A chronic, reactive airway disorder

Down

1. The "S" in ESR
2. A group of 20 protein compounds that activate to destroy invading cells
5. Exaggerated systemic reaction of the immune system
7. Masses of lymphatic tissue located at the back of the mouth and throat
8. Bands of connective tissue
9. Reactions that follow transfusion of mismatched blood
12. The body's capacity to resist invading organisms and toxins
14. Lymphatic vessel located in the small intestine
16. Acronym for test that identifies antibodies to bacteria, among others

Answers are on page 316.

Match game

The long-term immunity the body develops to specific antigens is called acquired immunity. Match the following types of acquired immunity to their definitions.

Clues

1. Natural, passive ____
2. Artificial, active ____
3. Natural, active ____
4. Artificial, passive ____

Choices

A. When the immune system responds to a harmful agent and develops long-term resistance

B. The transfer of antibodies from a mother to her breast-fed infant, providing temporary, partial resistance

C. Obtained by vaccination with weakened or dead infectious agents

D. Provided by substances that give immediate, but temporary immunity, such as antibiotics, gamma globulin, and interferon

Scrambled or overeasy

Fill in the answers for the following questions, then unscramble the circled letters to find the answer to the puzzle.

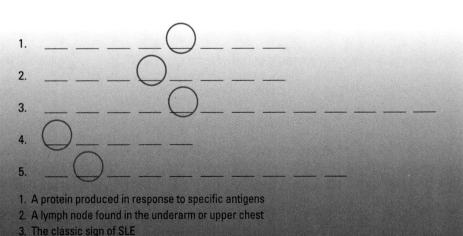

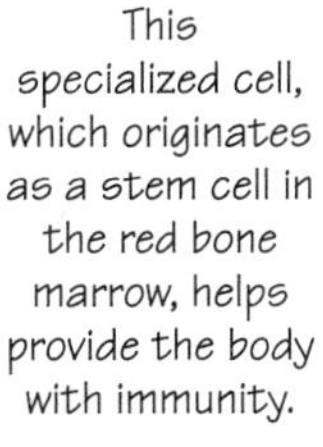

This specialized cell, which originates as a stem cell in the red bone marrow, helps provide the body with immunity.

1. ___ ___ ___ ___ ___ (___) ___ ___ ___
2. ___ ___ ___ (___) ___ ___ ___ ___
3. ___ ___ ___ ___ (___) ___ ___ ___ ___ ___ ___ ___ ___
4. (___) ___ ___ ___ ___
5. ___ (___) ___ ___ ___ ___ ___ ___ ___ ___

1. A protein produced in response to specific antigens
2. A lymph node found in the underarm or upper chest
3. The classic sign of SLE
4. A milky lymph fluid produced by lacteals
5. A type of transplant that uses bone marrow from a compatible donor

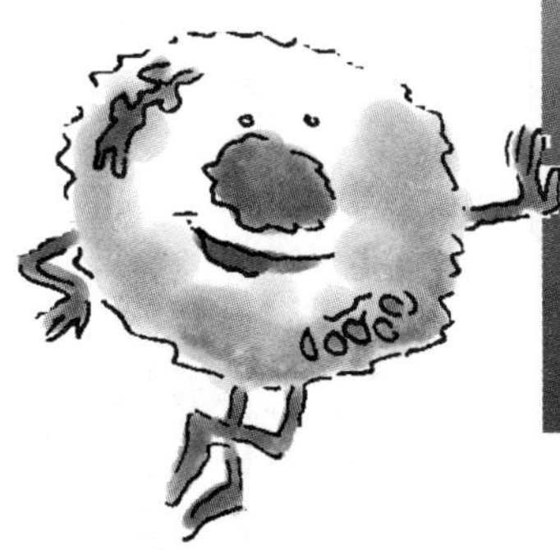

Answers are on page 316.

Answers

At a crossroads

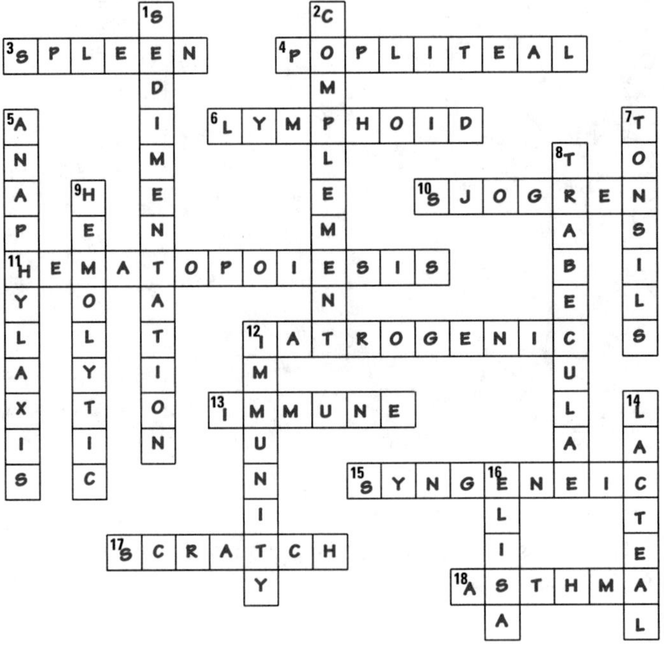

Match game

1. B; 2. C; 3. A; 4. D.

Scrambled or overeasy

1. Antibody; 2. Axillary; 3. Butterfly rash; 4. Chyle; 5. Allogeneic.
Solution to puzzle — B cell

Sensory system

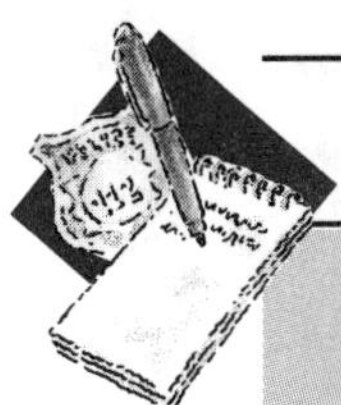

Just the facts

In this chapter you'll review:

- terminology related to the structure and function of the sensory system
- terminology needed for physical examination
- tests that help diagnose common sensory system disorders
- common sensory system disorders and their treatments.

Sensory structure and function

Sensory stimulation allows the body to interact with the environment. The brain receives stimulation from the sense organs — the eyes, the ears, and the **gustatory** (taste) and **olfactory** (smell) organs located in the nose and mouth. (See *Pronouncing key sensory system terms,* page 318.)

Vision

The **eye** is the sensory organ of sight and transmits visual images to the brain for interpretation. The eyeball occupies the **bony orbit,** a skull cavity formed by bones of the face. The term **optic,** as well as the prefixes ***oculo-*** and ***ophthalmo-,*** refers to the eye. (See *Eye terms,* page 318.)

The outer eye

Six cranial nerves serve the eye, the ocular muscles, and the **lacrimal apparatus.** The coordinated action of six

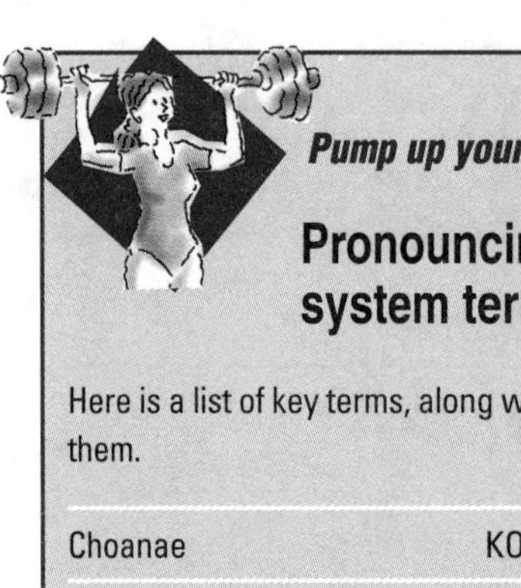

Pump up your pronunciation

Pronouncing key sensory system terms

Here is a list of key terms, along with the correct way to pronounce them.

Choanae	KOH-AH-NEE
Cilia	SILL-EE-AH
Eustachian	YOO-STAY-KEE-EHN
Osmesthesia	AWZ-MESS-THEE-ZEE-AH

muscles controls eye movement. Extraocular structures — the **eyelids, conjunctivae,** and lacrimal apparatus — protect and lubricate the eye.

Eye protectors

The **eyelids,** also called **palpebrae,** are loose folds of skin covering the front of the eye. They provide protection from foreign bodies, regulate the entrance of light, and distribute tears over the eye by blinking. The lid margins contain hair follicles, which in turn contain eyelashes **(cilia)** and sebaceous glands.

Conjunctivae are transparent mucous membranes that protect the eye from foreign bodies. The **palpebral conjunctiva** lines the eyelids and appears shiny and red. The **bulbar conjunctiva** joins the palpebral portion and covers the sclera up to the limbus. A small, fleshy elevation called the **caruncle** sits at the nasal aspect of the conjunctivae.

These crying eyes

The **lacrimal apparatus** lubricates and protects the eye with tears produced by **lacrimal glands.** After washing across the eyeball, tears drain through the **punctum,** a tiny opening at the junction of the upper and lower eyelids. From there, tears flow through **lacrimal canals** into the **lacrimal sac.** They then drain through the **nasolacrimal duct** and into the nose.

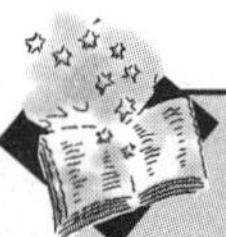

Beyond the dictionary

Eye terms

Common eye terms are often derived from Greek or Latin roots. Recognizing these roots will help you quickly understand many eye terms.

Eye know Greek

The term **optic** means *pertaining to the eye or sight,* and derives from the Greek word of the same meaning, ***optikos.*** The **optic disk,** therefore, is a round area within the eye. The ***opt-*** of optic is used as a prefix to form other terms pertaining to the eye, such as **optometry,** *the science of treating the human eye.*

Ophthalmo-, from the Greek word for eye, ***ophthalmos,*** forms "eye words," as well, such as **ophthalmoscope,** *an instrument used for examining the inner eye.*

Eye know Latin

The root ***oculo-,*** from the Latin word for eye, ***oculus,*** is also used to form many terms that refer to the eye; for example, **intraocular,** which means *within the eyeball* — as in **intraocular structures.**

The inner eye

The **sclera** is the white part of the eyeball, composed of fibrous tissue and fine elastic fibers. It's covered by the conjunctiva and bathed by tears from the lacrimal glands.

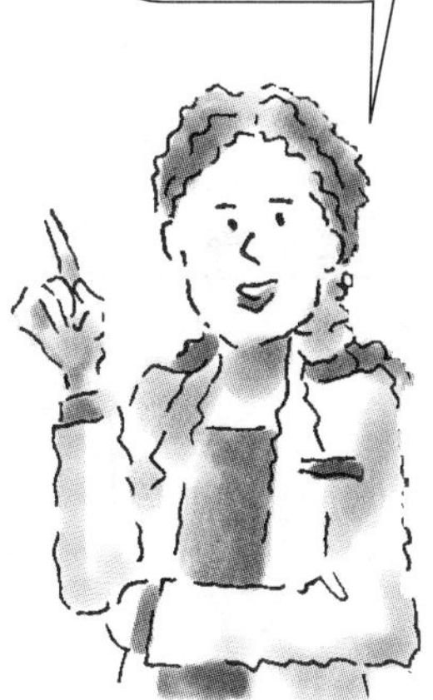

The light of the eye

The **cornea** is a smooth, transparent portion of the eyeball through which light enters the eye. It bulges slightly with a domelike protrusion and lacks blood vessels. The cornea is very sensitive to touch.

Looking straight in the eye

The **iris** is a circular disk in the center of the eye with the ability to contract. The **anterior** and **posterior chambers** of the iris are filled with a clear watery fluid called **aqueous humor.** This fluid drains through the trabecular meshwork into **Schlemm's canal** (a sinus at the junction of the cornea and the iris). **Intraocular pressure** is the balance of pressure between secretion and removal of fluid.

Focus on this

The **pupil,** or central opening of the iris, is black in color. By expanding and contracting, it regulates the amount of light admitted to the **lens,** enclosed in an elastic capsule directly behind the iris. The lens acts like a camera lens, refracting and focusing light onto the retina.

The reception area

The **retina** receives visual stimuli and sends them to the brain.

Optical equipment

The **optic disk** is a well-defined, round yellow to pink disk within the nasal portion of the retina. It allows the optic nerve to enter the retina at the **nerve head.**

Photoreceptors called **rods** and **cones**, named for their shape, are the visual receptors of the retina and are responsible for vision. The rods, located toward the outside of the retina, respond to low-intensity light and shades of gray. The cones are concentrated in the center and respond to bright light and color.

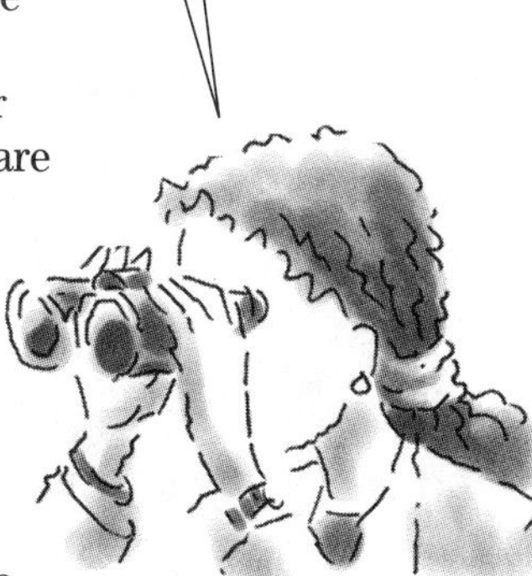

The lens of a camera or binocular, takes its name from the lens in our eyes. They perform the same function: refracting and focusing light.

It's all clear here

Located to the side of the optic disk is the **macula,** which is slightly darker than the rest of the retina. A region in the macula called the **fovea centralis** is the site of clearest vision, where cones are most concentrated and no rods are found. Because the fovea centralis contains the heaviest concentration of cones, it's a main receiver of vision and color.

Oh, say can you see

The process called **accommodation** allows the eyes to focus on light rays that are close or far away. The eyeballs are **converged** (move together) by muscles attached to the eyeball and the bones of the orbit.

Hearing

The **ear** is a sensory organ that enables hearing and maintains equilibrium. It's conveniently divided into the **external, middle,** and **inner ear.**

The external ear

The **auricle,** or **pinna** (pinna means *wing),* is the cartilage-based outer part of the ear. The **external auditory meatus** (opening) is the short passage leading into the ear. Earwax, called **cerumen,** lines this canal, which ends at the tympanic membrane.

Why is the **tympanic membrane** called the eardrum? For starters, the term comes from the Greek word for *kettle drum,* **tympanon,** and most importantly, it acts like a drum when struck by sound vibrations.

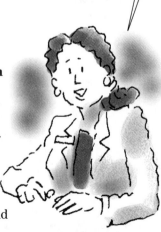

Drum roll, please...

The **tympanic membrane** separates the external ear from the middle ear. Also called the **eardrum,** it picks up sound waves and transmits them to the auditory nerve in the brain.

The middle ear

The **middle ear** is located in a small, air-filled cavity in the temporal bone called the **tympanic cavity.** It lies between the tympanic membrane and the inner ear and communicates with the throat by way of the **eustachian tube,** which keeps air pressure equal on both sides of the ear drum. The tympanic membrane is so sensitive to air pressure that rapid changes in altitude can produce pain, feelings of pressure, and ringing in the ears **(tinnitus).**

A hammer, anvil, and stirrup

The middle ear contains three small bones named for their shapes — the **malleus** (hammer), **incus** (anvil), and

stapes (stirrup). Connected by joints, their mechanical activity transmits sound waves to the inner ear. The three bones together are called the **auditory ossicles** (bones). The stapes sits in an opening called the **oval window (fenestra ovalis),** through which sound vibrations travel to the inner ear.

The inner ear

A bony and a membrane-covered labyrinth combine to form the inner ear. It consists of the **vestibule,** a small space at the beginning of a canal, and two systems of canals, the **cochlea** and the **semicircular.**

Ear-y canals

Sensory tissue in the semicircular canals maintains the body's sense of position and equilibrium. The **cochlea** (which means *spiral* or *shell-shaped)* contains three canals separated from each other by thin membranes:

- The **vestibular canal** connects with the oval window that leads to the middle ear.
- The **tympanic canal** is connected to the **round window,** which also leads to the middle ear. Both of these canals are bony and contain **perilymph fluid.**
- The **cochlear canal** is membranous and filled with **endolymph fluid.**

Located in the cochlear canal is the **organ of Corti,** a spiral-shaped membrane made up of cells with projecting hairs that transmit sound to the cochlear branch of the acoustic nerve.

Listen up

For hearing to occur, sound waves travel through the ear by two pathways:

1. **Air conduction** occurs when sound waves travel in the air through the external and middle ear to the inner ear.
2. **Bone conduction** occurs when sound waves travel through bone to the inner ear.

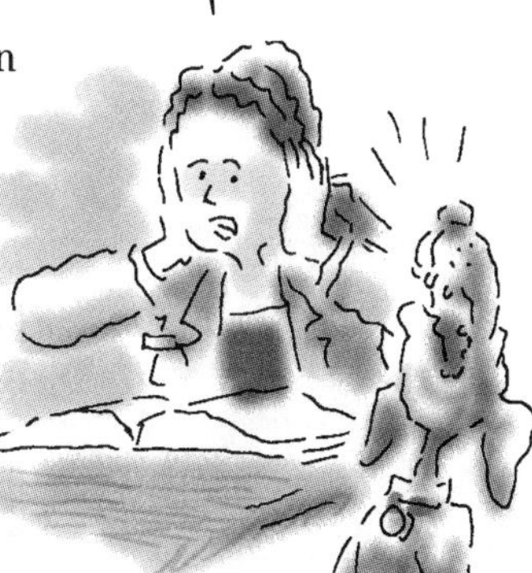

For me to hear this dog, the sound of his barking has to travel to my inner ear through **air conduction, bone conduction,** or both!

Smell

The sensory organ for smell, the **nose,** also warms, filters, and humidifies inhaled air. The word elements

naso- and ***rhino-*** and the term **olfactory** refer to the nose, including the external parts and internal cavities.

The nose knows

The **olfactory epithelium** within the nose is the actual organ of smell, perceiving odors when its cells are stimulated. **Olfactory receptors** are located in a narrow shelf formed by the **superior nasal concha,** the upper part of the **septum,** and bordering the **nostrils** on the lower part of each side — the winglike **alae.** Smells received by the olfactory epithelium are transmitted to the **olfactory bulb** and continue from there to olfactory centers in the brain. (See *Not that kind of factory.*)

> ***Beyond the dictionary***
>
> **Not that kind of factory**
>
> When studying the sense of smell and the nose, the term **olfactory** comes up often, as in **olfactory epithelium,** the actual organ of smell. Although the term olfactory suggests *a smell factory,* the term actually derives from the Latin word for *smell,* ***olfactus.***

Nosing around the inside of the nose

The upper third of the nose consists of bone and the lower two-thirds is made of cartilage. **Cilia,** tiny hairs that filter inhaled air, line the **vestibule,** the area inside the nostrils. The **nasal septum** separates the nostrils. Grooves called **meatuses** separate the three curved, bony structures called **turbinates (superior, middle,** and **inferior),** which aid breathing by warming, filtering, and humidifying inhaled air. Posterior air passages known as **choanae** lead to the oropharynx (throat).

And right out in front of your nose

The upper, narrow end of the nose is called the **root.** The **bridge** extends from the root to the **tip**. The **external nares** are the two outer openings, separated by the **nasal septum.** The **ala** flare out from either side of the nares.

Touch

The **skin** is the organ of touch, able to receive sensations of pressure, heat, cold, and pain. Touch, or light pressure perception, occurs when **dendrites** (free sensory nerve endings in the skin) are stimulated.

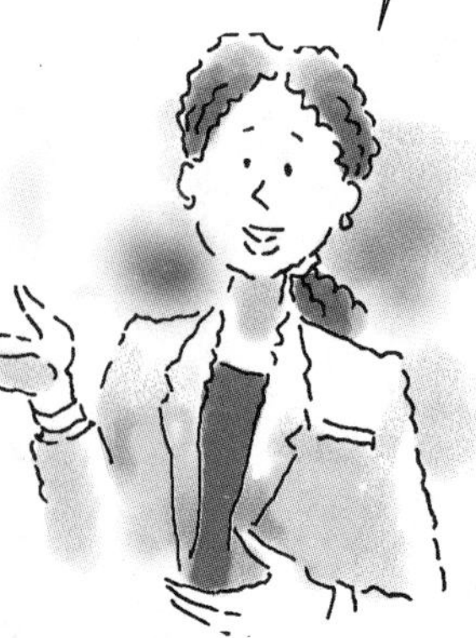

The nose can identify about 10,000 odors — but all result from combinations of the six basic odors: flowery, fruity, spicy, resinous, burned, and putrid.

A light touch

Merkel's disks are **tactile corpuscles** in the epidermis that relay light touch and superficial pressure. **Meissner's corpuscles** (in the corium below the epidermis), receive light pressure sensation. Heavy pressure is transmitted by **Pacini's corpuscles,** layered sensory nerve tissues in the skin's subcutaneous layer.

Touchy to temperature changes

The skin reacts to temperature changes of even a few degrees. Although the mechanism is unknown, skin capillaries, free nerve endings, and **Ruffini's corpuscles** (in the corium) help send temperature information to the brain.

Taste

The **taste buds** are the receptors for the taste nerve fibers located in the **papillae** (small projections on the tongue). A few taste buds are found in the mucous membranes of the soft palate, the opening from the mouth to the throat, and the epiglottis. (See *A tasteful history.*)

Beyond the dictionary

A tasteful history

The term **gustatory** pertains to the sense of taste and derives from the Latin word ***gustare,*** *to taste.* Another "tasteful" English word, or rather "distasteful," that is derived from that same Latin root is ***disgust,*** which literally means *to cause nausea.*

Physical examination terms

This section will provide terms you may need to know for a physical examination of the sensory system.

Examining vision

An **ophthalmoscope,** which contains a light, a mirror with a single hole, and several lenses, is used for examining the interior structures of the eye. This instrument is also called a funduscope. These terms are used in the physical examinations of the sense of vision:

- **anisopia** — unequal vision in the two eyes
- **blepharospasm** — spasms or constant blinking of eyelid
- **diplopia** — double vision
- **exophthalmos** — unilateral or bilateral bulging or protrusion of the eyeballs
- **floaters** — tiny clumps of vitreous gel appearing to float in the visual field (see *Keeping it simple*, page 324)
- **monochromatism** — total color blindness
- **myopia** — nearsightedness
- **nyctalopia** — night blindness
- **optic neuritis** — inflammation of the optic nerve
- **ptosis** — drooping of the eyelid
- **strabismus** — absence of coordinated eye movement, leading to misalignment of the eyes
- **uveitis** — inflammation of the uvea, including the iris, ciliary body, and choroid.

The term **ptosis** is from Greek and means *falling down.* It refers to the condition of a drooping eyelid. The *p-* is silent: TOH-sɪss.

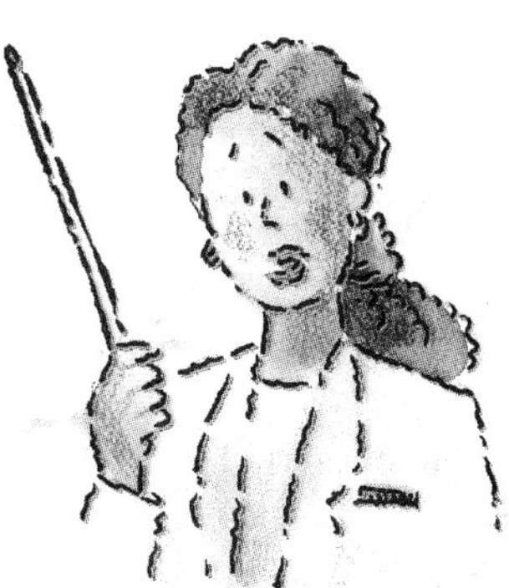

Examining hearing

An **otoscope** is a device for examining the ear, including the external ear, eardrum, and ossicles. This instrument includes a device for insufflation (blowing vapor or powder into a cavity), a light, and a magnifying glass. Here are terms involved with physical examination of the ear:

- **Otorrhagia** is bleeding from the ear.
- **Otorrhea** is a discharge from the ear.
- **Ototoxic** is a substance toxic to the eighth cranial nerve or the organs of balance and hearing.
- **Tinnitus** is a ringing in one or both ears.
- **Vertigo** is a sensation of movement in which the patient feels himself revolving in space or surroundings revolving about him; it may result from inner ear disease.

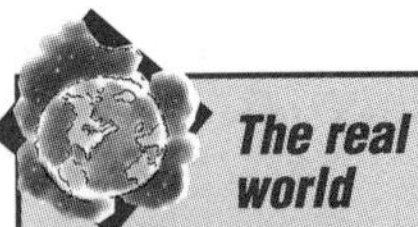

Keeping it simple

Not all medical terms are derived from Greek and Latin and contain many syllables. Sometimes a simple word best describes a medical phenomenon. Take, for example, the term **floaters**, a coined term for the tiny clumps of vitreous gel that appear to "float" in the eyes.

Examining the sense of smell

The following terms are used in the physical examination of the sense of smell:

- **anosmia,** absence of the sense of smell
- **dysosmia,** defect or impairment of the sense of smell
- **hyperosmia,** abnormal sensitivity to odors
- **osmesthesia,** inability to perceive and distinguish odors
- **osmodysphoria,** abnormal dislike of certain odors.

Examining the sense of taste

The following terms are used in the physical examination of the sense of taste:

- **ageusia,** an impaired or absent sense of taste
- **dysgeusia,** abnormal or perverted sense of taste
- **hypergeusia,** unusual acuteness of taste
- **hypogeusia,** impaired sense of taste.

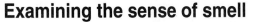

Diagnostic tests

Many methods are used to diagnose the origins of sensory diseases or conditions. Some tests measure an individual component's level of function in the sensory system, while others examine each component for injury. This section reviews diagnostic test terms for the sensory system.

Eye tests

Eye tests can be conducted either under direct evaluation or with radiologic and imaging equipment.

Direct evaluation

In direct evaluation, tests are applied directly to the eye by the examiner with the aid of various pieces of equipment.

Look into the light

Refraction is an examination to determine and correct refractive eye errors. The **ophthalmologist** usually performs a refraction with a **retinoscope.** In this test, the examiner uses the retinoscope to shine a light into the patient's eye. The examiner then notes the reflexive movements of the fundus.

In the spotlight

Slit-lamp examination gets its name from the piece of equipment used, an instrument equipped with a special lighting system and a binocular microscope that allows the examiner to view details of the eye, including the eyelids, eyelashes, conjunctiva, and cornea.

Eye know IOP

Tonometry permits indirect measurement of **intraocular pressure (IOP),** the pressure within the eyeball.

Radiologic and imaging studies

Radiologic and imaging equipment can make the inner eye visible for closer study.

Shutter bug

Fluorescein angiography records the appearance of blood vessels inside the eye through rapid-sequence photographs of the fundus. The photographs follow the I.V. injection of **sodium fluorescein,** a contrast medium.

Sounding it out

Ocular ultrasonography transmits high-frequency sound waves through the eye and measures their reflection from ocular structures.

Eye of the storm

Other eye examinations and terms include:

- **Orbital computed tomography (CT)** reveals abnormalities that can't be seen with standard X-rays. The orbital CT scan is a series of tomograms reconstructed by a computer and displayed as anatomic slices on a screen.
- **Orbital radiography** examines the orbit, the deep-set cavity housing the eye, lacrimal gland, blood vessels, nerves, muscles, and fat.
- A **scanning laser ophthalmoscope** is a laser device used to detect abnormal retinal secretions.

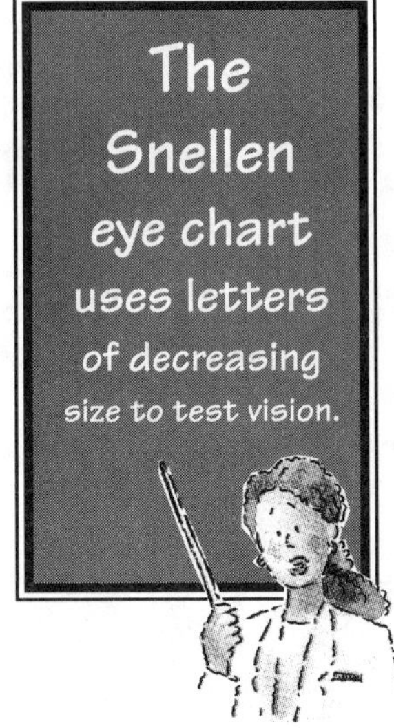

The Snellen eye chart uses letters of decreasing size to test vision.

Visual acuity tests

A **Snellen eye chart** is the standard chart used in eye examinations, containing block letters of decreasing size read by the patient from a distance.

Visual field tests determine the extent of the retinal area through which the patient can perceive visual stimuli.

Testing the ears

When performing diagnostic tests on the sense of hearing, the examiner generally needs the participation of the patient. After all, only the individual being tested can tell the examiner whether he heard something.

First look

Otoscopy is the direct visualization of the external auditory canal and the tympanic membrane through an instrument called an **otoscope.**

Tuning fork tests

Tuning fork tests such as the Weber's and Rinne tests are quick screening tools for detecting hearing loss.

Good vibrations

Weber's test evaluates bone conduction by placing a vibrating tuning fork on top of the patient's head at the midline or in the middle of the patient's forehead. The patient should perceive the sound equally in both ears.

The **Rinne test** compares bone conduction to air conduction in both ears by placing the base of a vibrating tuning fork on the mastoid process and noting how many seconds pass before the patient can no longer hear it.

Audiometric tests

Audiometric tests are performed by **audiologists** to confirm hearing loss. **Audiometry** is the evaluation of hearing using an **audiometer,** a device that measures perception of tones at various frequencies. (See *I hear.*)

Reaching the threshold

Pure-tone audiometry provides a record of the **thresholds** — the lowest intensity levels — at which a patient can hear a set of test tones through earphones or a bone conduction (sound) vibrator. The **test tones** are concentrated at certain frequencies labeled bone conduction thresholds and air conduction threshold. In **Békésy audiometry,** a patient pushes a button to indicate that a tone was heard.

Going with the flow

Acoustic admittance tests evaluate middle ear function by measuring sound energy's flow into the ear (admittance) and the opposition to that flow (impedance). Two tests are used to measure admittance:

- **Tympanometry** measures middle ear admittance in response to air pressure changes in the ear canal.
- The **acoustic reflex test** measures the change in admittance produced by contraction of the stapedius muscle as it responds to an intense sound.

Electrocochleography

Electrocochleography measures the electrical current generated in the inner ear after sound stimulation. The current is measured by an electrode in the external acoustic canal. (See *Isn't there an abbreviation?*)

Electronystagmography

In **electronystagmography,** eye movements in response to specific stimuli are recorded on graph paper and used to evaluate the interactions of the vestibular system and the muscles controlling eye movement in what is known as the vestibulo-ocular reflex.

Beyond the dictionary

I hear

You're probably familiar with the word **audio**. You own audio equipment (such as a radio) and maybe even consider yourself an **audiophile** *(one devoted to high-quality sound equipment)*. But did you know that ***audio*** is the Latin word for *I hear?* Therefore, it makes sense that tests that examine your ability to hear are called **audiometric.**

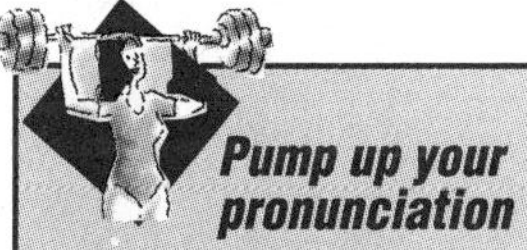

Pump up your pronunciation

Isn't there an abbreviation?

Generally, tests with long, hard-to-pronounce names like **electrocochleography** are referred to by an abbreviation. In this case, maybe ECG would be appropriate, but it's used for electrocardiogram. What do you do then? Take a deep breath and sound it out: EH-LECK-TROH-KAWK-LEE-AWG-RAH-FEE.

Tests for smell

The **Proetz test** measures the acuity of smell, using different concentrations of substances with recognizable odors.

Do you smell something?

The lowest concentration at which the patient recognizes an odor is called the **olfactory coefficient,** or **minimal identifiable odor.**

Sensory disorders

The sensory system is a complex system with even more complicated components. This section provides terminology related to disorders of the sensory system.

Eye disorders

Eye disorders can range from common irritation in and around the eyes to impaired vision.

Common inflammations and infections

- **Blepharitis** is a common inflammatory condition of the eyelids, lash follicles, and glands of the eyelids, characterized by swelling, redness, and crusts of dried mucus on the eyelids.
- **Conjunctivitis** is an inflammation of the conjunctiva, sometimes called **pinkeye.** (See *Is pinkeye pink?*)
- **Dacryocystitis** is a common infection of the lacrimal sac caused by an obstruction (**dacryostenosis**) of the nasolacrimal duct or by trauma.
- **Keratitis** is an inflammation of the cornea, usually confined to one eye, and it may be acute or chronic, superficial or deep.

Other eye disorders

One common cause of vision loss, a **cataract** is a gradually developing opacity of the lens or lens capsule of the eye.

Other eye disorders include:

- **Corneal abrasion,** a scratch on the surface epithelium of the cornea, is often caused by a foreign body.
- **Macular degeneration,** the atrophy or degeneration of the macular disk, is the most common cause of blindness in adults.
- **Nystagmus** is recurring, involuntary eyeball movement that produces blurred vision and difficulty in focusing. The movement may be horizontal, vertical, rotating, or mixed.

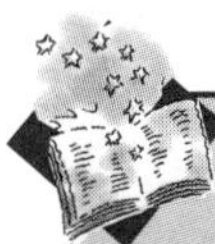

Beyond the dictionary

Is pinkeye pink?

The inflammation caused by **pinkeye** may strike some as pink in color and therefore explain the origin of its use, but the term probably derives from the Middle English word ***pinken,*** which means *to prick.*

Pinkeye originally was used to indicate *half-shut,* or what your eye would look like after it was pricked or poked, and what it may look like if you're suffering from pinkeye.

Too much pressure

Glaucoma is a group of disorders characterized by an abnormally high IOP, which can damage the optic nerve. Left untreated, it can cause blindness. Glaucoma occurs in several forms.

- **Chronic open-angle glaucoma** results from overproduction of aqueous humor.
- **Acute angle-closure glaucoma** results from obstruction to the outflow of aqueous humor.
- **Secondary glaucoma** can result from uveitis, trauma, or drugs such as steroids.

Looking to the retina

In **retinal detachment,** the retinal layers split and create a subretinal space, which fills with fluid (called **subretinal fluid**).

A genetically transmitted disorder, **retinitis pigmentosa** causes progressive destruction of the retinal rods and leads to eventual blindness.

Noninflammatory retinal disorders, called **vascular retinopathies,** result from disruption of the eye's blood supply. The two types of this condition are:

- **Hypertensive retinopathy** results from prolonged hypertensive disease, which produces retinal vasospasm and consequently damages and narrows the arteriolar opening.
- **Diabetic retinopathy** is retinopathy that results as a complication of diabetes.

Ear disorders

Ear disorders can range from common irritation to serious hearing loss.

Hearing loss

Hearing loss (deafness) results from a dysfunction in the mechanical or nervous system that disrupts transmission of sound waves. It's classified as:

- **conductive loss** — interrupted transmission of sound impulses from the external ear to the junction of the stapes and oval window
- **mixed hearing loss** — combined conductive and sensorineural dysfunctions
- **otosclerosis** — slow growth of a spongy bone in the otic capsule, particularly at the oval window (the most common cause of progressive conductive hearing loss)
- **sensorineural loss** — impaired cochlear or acoustic nerve function that prevents transmission of sound impulses within the inner ear or brain.

The older we get

Presbycusis, an effect of aging, results from the loss of hair cells in the organ of Corti. This disorder causes sensorineural hearing loss, usually of high-frequency tones.

Ear disorders without chronic hearing loss

Here are some common disorders of the ear that generally have no long-term affect on hearing:

- **Infectious myringitis** is characterized by inflammation, hemorrhage, and effusion of fluid into the tissue and at the end of the external ear canal and tympanic membrane.
- **Labyrinthitis,** an inflammation of the labyrinth of the inner ear, frequently causes severe vertigo.
- **Mastoiditis** is a bacterial infection and inflammation of the mastoid antrum air cells and is often a complication of chronic or acute otitis media.
- **Ménière's disease,** also called **endolymphatic hydrops,** is a labyrinthine dysfunction known to cause violent attacks of severe vertigo lasting from 10 minutes to several hours.
- **Otitis externa** is an inflammation of the external ear canal, which may be acute or chronic.
- **Otitis media** is an inflammation of the middle ear.

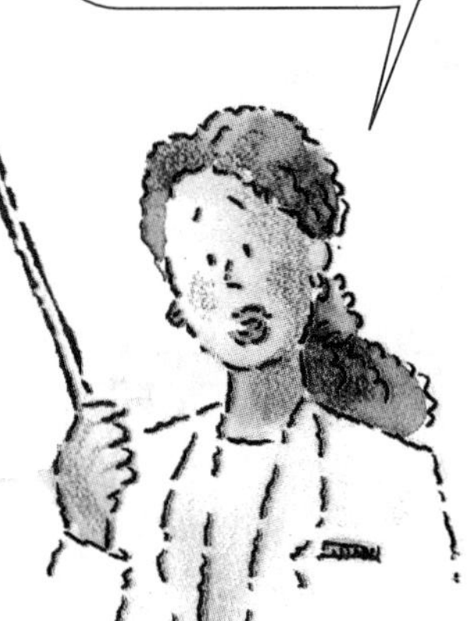
Mastoiditis is an infection and inflammation of the **mastoid antrum** cells. The mastoid antrum takes its name from the Greek word for *breasts*, ***mastos,*** because it is breast-shaped.

Treatments

Treatment options for sensory system disorders include drug therapy, surgical intervention and, in some cases, a transplant replacing a damaged component.

Eye treatments

Drug therapy is a common treatment for eye disorders.

Drug therapy

The most frequently used drugs include:
- **Anti-infectives,** such as bacitracin and erythromycin, are used to treat infection.
- **Anti-inflammatory agents,** such a dexamethasone, are used to treat inflammatory conditions of the eye.
- **Artificial tears** provide moisture for the eyes when insufficient tear production is a problem.
- A **miotic** is an agent that causes constriction of the pupil.
- **Mydriatics** are agents that dilate the pupil of the eye.
- **Ophthalmic anesthetics** prepare the eye for procedures, such as tonometry, suture removal from the cornea, or removal of foreign bodies.

Eye surgery

Surgery may involve the repairing, removal, or transplant of a failing component of the eye. Surgeons often employ **laser surgery,** using a laser that generates focused, or monochromatic, light waves; it then magnifies their power by deflecting them off a series of mirrors. The result: a finely focused, high-energy beam.
- **Cataracts** are removed by one of two methods. In **intracapsular cataract extraction,** the entire lens is removed, most often with a **cryoprobe,** a surgical instrument that freezes and adheres to the lens, making the lens easier to remove. **Extracapsular cataract extraction** removes the patient's anterior capsule, cortex, and nucleus, leaving the posterior capsule intact. This technique uses irrigation and aspiration or **phacoemulsification.** Phacoemulsification uses an ultrasonic probe to break the lens into minute particles and aspirate them. (See *How do I say phacoemulsification?*)

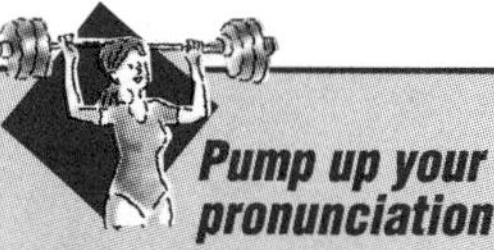
Pump up your pronunciation

How do I say phacoemulsification?

Phacoemulsification is the process by which an ultrasonic device disintegrates a cataract. ***Phakos*** is Greek for *lens* and ***emulsification*** is the process by which something is *emulsified* or *broken down.* It becomes easier to pronounce when you break it down phonetically — FACK-OH-EE-MULL-SIH-FIH-KAY-SHUN.

• Performed by laser or standard surgery, an **iridectomy** reduces IOP by improving the drainage of aqueous humor. The procedure makes a hole in the iris, creating an opening though which the aqueous humor can flow to bypass the pupil.
• A **radial keratotomy** is a treatment for myopia (nearsightedness) that involves the creation of small radial incisions in the cornea. These incisions flatten the cornea and help properly focus light on the retina.
• **Sclerectomy** is excision of part of the sclera.
• **Scleral buckling** is surgical repair of a detached retina, in which indentations of the sclera are made over the retinal tears to promote retinal adherence to the choroid.
• **Trabeculectomy** is a surgical filtering procedure that removes part of the trabecular meshwork, allowing aqueous humor to bypass blocked channels. This procedure creates a filtering bleb or opening under the conjunctiva.
• A microsurgical procedure, **vitrectomy** removes part or all of the vitreous humor — the transparent gelatinous substance that fills the cavity behind the lens. It's also used for removal of foreign bodies and infection within the eye.

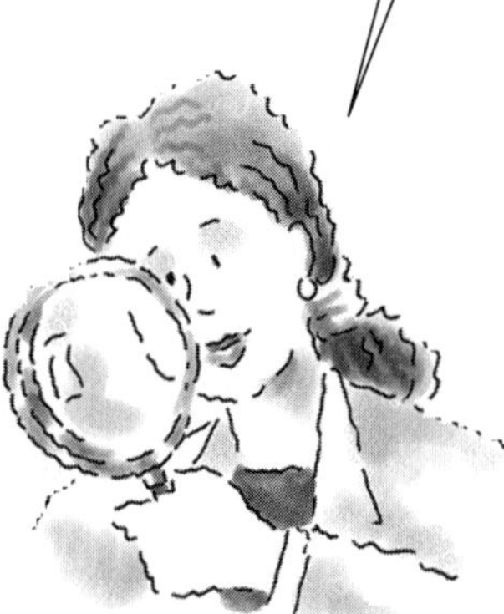
A corneal transplant uses corneal tissue from a human donor to replace a damaged part of the cornea.

Restoring clarity

In a **corneal transplant,** healthy corneal tissue from a human donor replaces a damaged part of the cornea. The transplant can take one of two forms:

1. **Full-thickness penetrating keratoplasty** involves excision and replacement of the entire cornea.

2. **Lamellar keratoplasty** removes and replaces a superficial layer of corneal tissue.

Ear treatments

Treatments for ear disorders range from drug therapy to surgical intervention.

Drug therapy

The following drugs are used to treat otic disorders:
• **Acetic acid,** or **Domeboro's Solution,** treats ear canal infections (and prevents "swimmer's ear").
• **Anesthetics** treat pain from otitis media and assist with removal of cerumen.

- **Antibiotics** treat external ear canal infection.
- **Cerumeolytics** help remove impacted cerumen.
- **Corticosteroids,** such as hydrocortisone, treat inflammation of the external ear canal.

Ear surgery

Surgical procedures can either repair or remove a failing component.

Drum repair

Myringotomy is a surgical incision into the tympanic membrane to relieve pain and drain pus or fluid from the middle ear. **Myringoplasty** is performed to repair a ruptured tympanic membrane. The surgeon approximates the edges of the membrane or applies a graft taken from the temporalis muscle.

Taking off the stirrups

Stapedectomy removes all or part of the stapes. A **total stapedectomy** involves removal of the entire bone, followed by insertion of a graft and prosthesis to bridge the gap between the incus and the inner ear.

In a **partial stapedectomy,** the surgeon removes part of the bone and rebuilds what is left with a prosthesis. **Laser stapedectomy,** a relatively new technique, is easier to perform but carries a risk of the laser beam penetrating the bone.

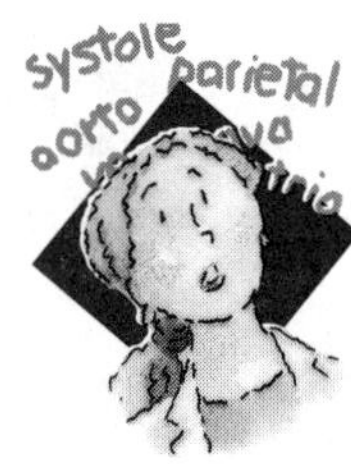

Vocabulary builders

At a crossroads

Completing this crossword puzzle will help you come to your senses about correct sensory system terms. Good luck!

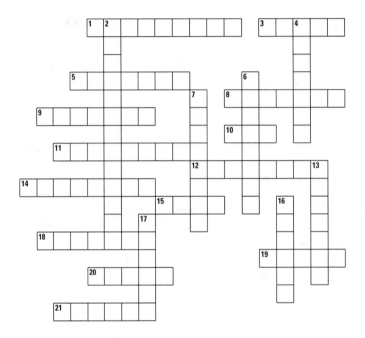

Across

1. Another name for eyelids
3. Eponym for the spiral-shaped membrane that transmits sound to the cochlear branch
5. Absence of the sense of smell
8. Latin term for *teardrop*
9. Term for earwax
10. Number of basic odors
11. Free sensory nerve endings
12. Particles of calcium carbonate in the small sacs of the vestibule
14. Ringing in the ears
15. Organ of touch
18. Air passages from the nose that lead to the throat
19. This test evaluates bone conduction
20. The eyeball occupies the bony ___
21. The white part of the eyeball

Down

2. Process that allows eyes to focus on light rays that are close or far away
4. Eponym for corpuscles that are involved in sending temperature information to the brain
6. Location of taste buds
7. Unequal vision in the two eyes
13. Name that lends itself to the standard eye chart
16. This test measures the acuity of smell
17. Part of the eye that receives visual stimuli

Answers are on page 336.

Finish line

Tears protect and lubricate the eye. **Lacrimal** pertains to tears and comes from the Latin ***lacrima***, which means tear. Fill in the blanks for the eye structures involved in tear production.

1. The **lacrimal** _____ lubricates and protects the eye with tears.
2. The **lacrimal** _____ produce tears.
3. The **lacrimal** _____ are where tears flow after draining through the punctum.
4. The **lacrimal** _____ is where the tears then collect.
5. The ___-**lacrimal** ___ is where tears drain through into the nose.

Scrambled or overeasy

Fill in the answers for the following questions, then unscramble the circled letters to find the answer to the puzzle.

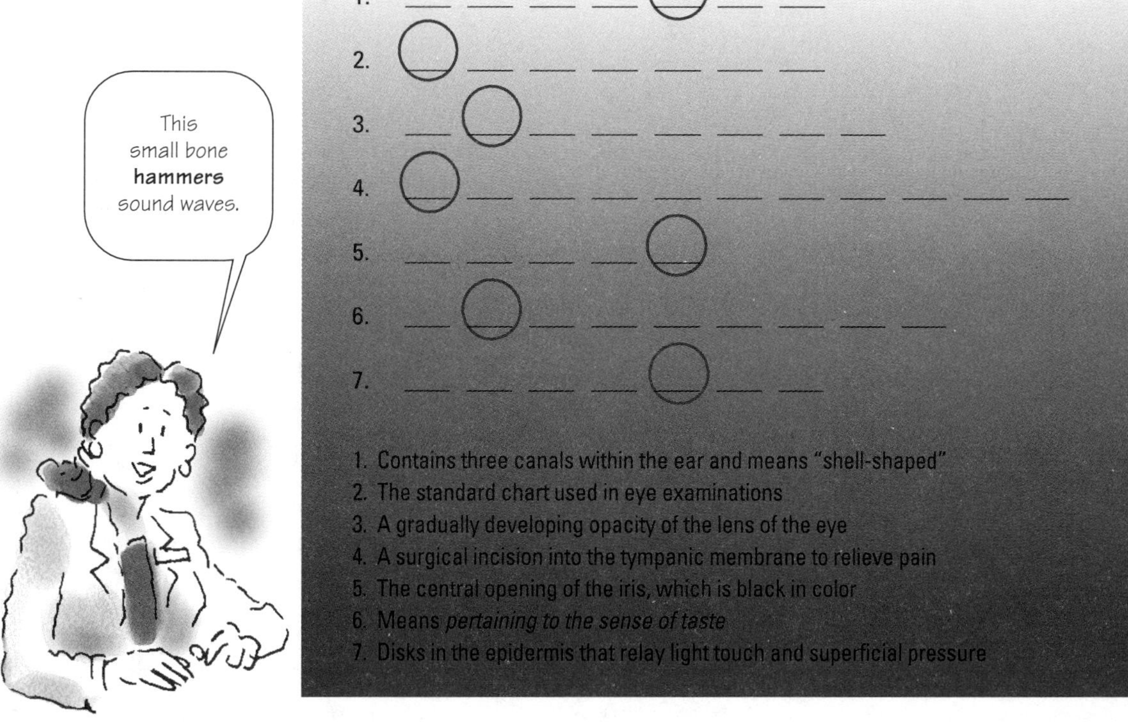
This small bone **hammers** sound waves.

1. Contains three canals within the ear and means "shell-shaped"
2. The standard chart used in eye examinations
3. A gradually developing opacity of the lens of the eye
4. A surgical incision into the tympanic membrane to relieve pain
5. The central opening of the iris, which is black in color
6. Means *pertaining to the sense of taste*
7. Disks in the epidermis that relay light touch and superficial pressure

Answers are on page 336.

Answers

At a crossroads

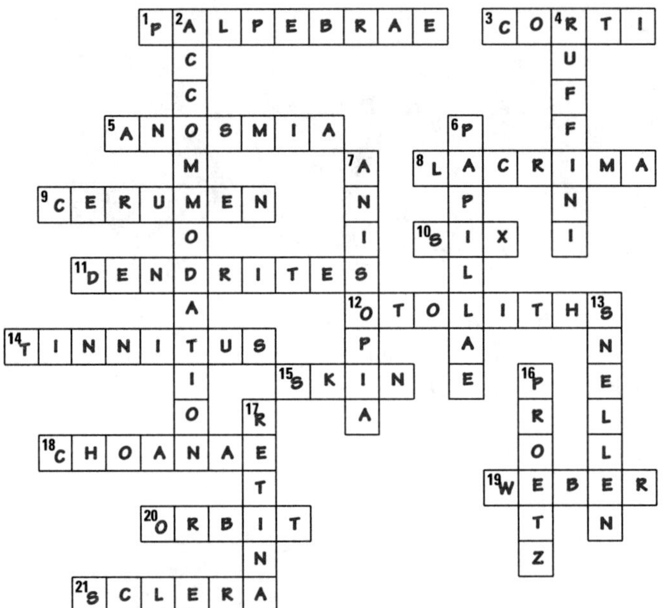

Finish line

1. Apparatus; 2. Glands; 3. Canals; 4. Sac; 5. Naso-, Duct.

Scrambled or over easy?

1. Cochlea; 2. Snellen; 3. Cataract; 4. Myringotomy; 5. Pupil; 6. Gustatory; 7. Merkel's.
Solution to puzzle — Malleus

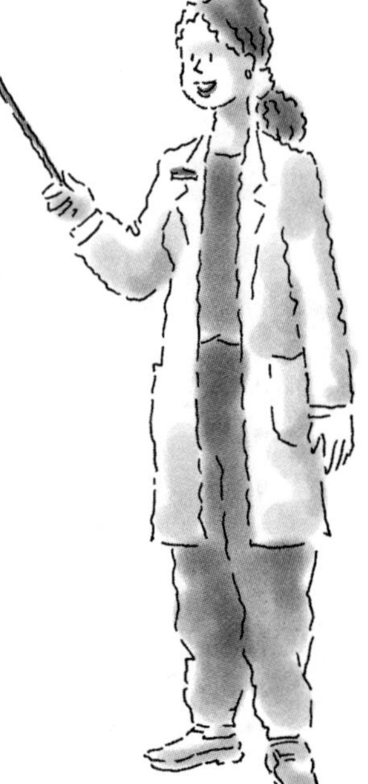

Appendices and index

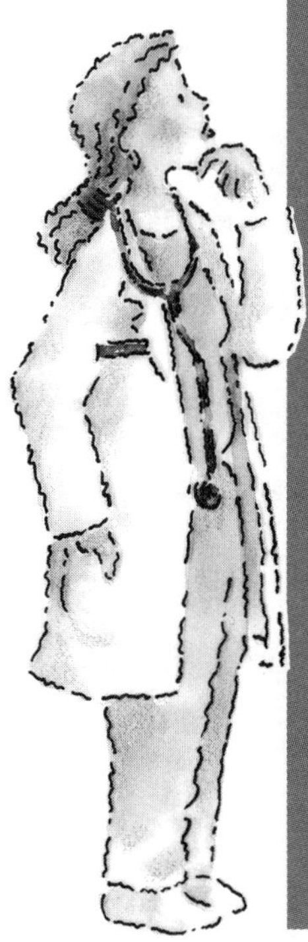

Appendix A

Cancer terminology

Cancer begins when a group of cells grow and multiply uncontrollably, eventually forming a mass of tissue called a **tumor.** This chart presents important medical terms associated with cancer care.

A note on names

Cancer is generally named for its location in the body. For example, **colorectal cancer** is cancer involving the colon and rectum. Cancer can also have a more technical name that refers to its location, such as **hepatic carcinoma** (liver cancer). Or, a cancer may be named after an individual, such as **Hodgkin's disease,** a lymphatic cancer. Certain cancers, such as brain cancer, also have specific tumor types. These tumor types are discussed in the chart below.

Terms	Definitions
Cancer diagnosis terms	
Metastasis	Growth of cancer cells away from the site of primary involvement
TMN staging system	System for tumor description, with **T** as **t**umor size, **M** as **m**etastatic progress, and **N** as **n**odal involvement
Blood and other sample tests	
Bone marrow analysis	Examination of aspirated bone marrow for diagnosis of leukemia and myeloma
Carcinoembryonic antigen (CEA) test	Measurement of CEA levels by immunoassay; useful for staging and monitoring treatments of different cancers
Cell washing	Rinsing of bronchial tree, esophagus, stomach, or uterine cavity with solution, loosening exfoliated cancer cells; solution is then aspirated and cells collected for analysis
Cytologic tests	Study of body cells to detect cancer; can determine presence of cancer but not location or size of malignancy
Fecal occult blood test	Study of paper slide prepared with guaiac (resin from certain Caribbean trees) to detect blood in a stool smear; used for early detection of colorectal cancer
Papanicolaou test	Commonly known as Pap test or Pap smear; analysis of secretions from a patient's cervix to detect cervical cancer
Prostate-specific antigen (PSA) test	Measurement of serum levels of PSA, a substance secreted by the prostate gland; tests for benign prostatic hyperplasia and prostate cancer
Radioimmunoassay (RIA)	Measurement of antigens or antibodies by tagging them with radioactive isotopes; used to measure hormones secreted by malignant tumors

Terms	Definitions
Imaging and scanning tests	
Mammography	Radiographic technique used to detect breast cysts or tumors
Radionuclide imaging	Use of a special gamma scintillation camera or scanner to provide images of an organ after patient receives an I.V. radionuclide (contrast medium); specific tests include brain scan, bone scan, and renal scan
Tumor types	
Brain tumors	
• Acoustic neuroma	• Originates from eighth cranial (acoustic) nerve
• Astrocytoma	• Arises from astrocytes
• Ependymoma	• Derives from the ependymal cells of the lining of the ventricles and aqueducts of the brain
• Glioblastoma	• Originates from undifferentiated glial cells
• Glioma	• Originates in the neuroglial tissue
• Hemangioma	• Derives from the blood vessel wall
• Medulloblastoma	• Derives from undifferentiated glial cells
• Oligodendroglioma	• Arises from oligodendrocytes
Leukemia	
• Acute lymphoblastic leukemia	• Abnormal growth of immature lymphocytes
• Acute myeloblastic leukemia	• Rapid accumulation of myeloblasts
• Chronic lymphoblastic leukemia	• Uncontrollable spread of abnormal, small lymphocytes in lymphoid tissue, blood, and bone marrow
• Chronic myeloblastic leukemia	• Overgrowth of immature granulocytes in bone marrow, peripheral blood, and body tissues
Lung cancer	
• Adenocarcinoma	• Originates in glandular tissue
• Large-cell carcinoma	• Originates in large, undifferentiated cells
• Small-cell carcinoma	• Originates in small, oval, undifferentiated cells; also known as oat cell carcinoma
• Squamous cell carcinoma	• Originates from squamous epithelial tissue
Skin cancer	
• Basal cell carcinoma	• Slow-growing, destructive tumor that usually occurs on sun-exposed skin, especially the face
• Malignant melanoma	• Arises from melanocytes (cells that produce pigment)
• Squamous cell carcinoma	• Arises in the epidermal cells and usually appears on sun-damaged areas of skin; invasive tumor with metastatic potential

Terms	Definitions
Treatments	
Chemotherapy	Use of one or more drugs to destroy cancer cells or halt their growth
• Alkylating agents	• Inhibit cell division at any point in the cell's life cycle
• Antimetabolites	• Interfere with deoxyribonucleic acid (DNA) synthesis
• Antibiotic antineoplastics	• Bind with DNA to inhibit the functioning of both normal and malignant cells
• Hormonal antineoplastics	• Inhibit tumor growth in specific tissues without directly damaging cells; mechanism of action not completely known
External radiation	Radiation delivered by a standard X-ray machine to shrink tumors before surgery or destroy remaining cancer cells after tumor removal
Internal radiation	Radioactive device implanted in the patient's body; can be interstitial (within a tumor) or intracavitary (within a cavity)
Surgery	Removal of the tumor and a margin of normal tissue (if possible)

Appendix B

Commonly used medical abbreviations

ā	before
āā	of each
AAA	abdominal aortic aneurysm
ABG	arterial blood gas
a.c.	before meals
ACE	angiotensin-converting enzyme
ACLS	advanced cardiac life support
ACTH	adrenocorticotropic hormone
a.d.	right ear
ADH	antidiuretic hormone
ADL	activity of daily living
AED	automated external defibrillator
AFIB	atrial fibrillation
AIDS	acquired immunodeficiency syndrome
AKA	above-knee amputation
ALL	acute lymphocytic leukemia
ALS	amyotrophic lateral sclerosis
AMA	against medical advice
AP	anteroposterior; apical pulse
ARDS	adult respiratory distress syndrome
ARF	acute renal failure; acute respiratory failure
AROM	active range of motion; artificial rupture of membranes
a.s.	left ear
ASA	acetylsalicylic acid (aspirin)
ASD	atrial septal defect
a.u.	both ears
AV	atrioventricular; arteriovenous
AVM	arteriovenous malformation
BBB	bundle-branch block
BCP	birth control pill
BE	barium enema
b.i.d.	two times per day
BKA	below-knee amputation
BM	bowel movement
BMR	basal metabolic rate
BP	blood pressure
BPH	benign prostatic hyperplasia
BRP	bathroom privileges
BSA	body surface area
BUN	blood urea nitrogen
BW	birth weight
bx	biopsy
C	centigrade; Celsius
c̄	with
CA	cancer
Ca	calcium
CABG	coronary artery bypass graft
CAD	coronary artery disease
CAPD	continuous ambulatory peritoneal dialysis
CAVH	continuous arteriovenous hemofiltration
CBC	complete blood count
CC	chief complaint
cc	cubic centimeter
CCU	coronary care unit
CDC	Centers for Disease Control and Prevention
CEA	carcinoembryonic antigen
CF	cystic fibrosis
CK	creatine kinase

CMV	cytomegalovirus; continuous mandatory ventilation
CNS	central nervous system
CO_2	carbon dioxide
C/O	complains of
COPD	chronic obstructive pulmonary disease
CP	cerebral palsy
CPAP	continuous positive airway pressure
CPP	cerebral perfusion pressure
CPR	cardiopulmonary resuscitation
CS	cesarean section
C&S	culture and sensitivity
CSF	cerebrospinal fluid
CT	computed tomography
CV	cardiovascular
CVA	cerebrovascular accident
CVP	central venous pressure
CXR	chest X-ray
DC	direct current
D/C	discontinue; discharge
D&C	dilatation and curettage
D&E	dilatation and evacuation
DIC	disseminated intravascular coagulation
DJD	degenerative joint disease
DKA	diabetic ketoacidosis
DM	diabetes mellitus
DNR	do not resuscitate
DOA	date of admission; dead on arrival
DOB	date of birth
DPT	diphtheria, pertussis, and tetanus
DSM-IV	*Diagnostic and Statistical Manual of Mental Disorders,* 4th ed.
DVT	deep vein thrombosis
D_5W	dextrose 5% in water
Dx	diagnosis
ECF	extended care facility; extracellular fluid
ECG	electrocardiogram
ECHO	echocardiography
ECMO	extracorporeal membrane oxygenator
ECT	electroconvulsive therapy
ED	emergency department
EDC	estimated date of confinement
EDD	estimated date of delivery
EEG	electroencephalogram
EENT	eyes, ears, nose, and throat
EF	ejection fraction
ELISA	enzyme-linked immunosorbent assay
EMG	electromyogram
EMS	emergency medical services
ENT	ear, nose, and throat
ER	emergency room; expiratory reserve
ERCP	endoscopic retrograde cholangiopancreatography
ERV	expiratory reserve volume
ESR	erythrocyte sedimentation rate
ETOH	ethanol (ethyl alcohol)
F	Fahrenheit
FBS	fasting blood sugar
FDA	Food and Drug Administration
FEF	forced expiratory flow
FEV	forced expiratory volume
FFP	fresh frozen plasma
FH	family history
FHR	fetal heart rate
FRC	functional residual capacity
FSH	follicle-stimulating hormone
FUO	fever of unknown origin
FVC	forced vital capacity
Fx	fracture

G	gravida
g	gram
GB	gallbladder
GBS	gallbladder series
GFR	glomerular filtration rate
GI	gastrointestinal
GP	general practitioner
gr	grain
GTT	glucose tolerance test
gtt	drops
GU	genitourinary
GVHD	graft-versus-host disease
GYN	gynecology
Hb	hemoglobin
HBIG	hepatitis B immunoglobulin
HBsAg	hepatitis B surface antigen
HCG	human chorionic gonadotropin
HCT	hematocrit
Hg	mercury
H&H	hemoglobin and hematocrit
HHA	home health aide
HHNS	hyperosmolar hyperglycemic nonketotic syndrome
HIV	human immunodeficiency virus
HLA	human leukocyte antigen
HMO	health maintenance organization
H_2O	water
H_2O_2	hydrogen peroxide
H&P	history and physical
HPI	history of present illness
h.s.	hour of sleep
HSV	herpes simplex virus
HTN	hypertension
HX	history

IABP	intra-aortic balloon pump
ICD	implantable cardioverter defibrillator
ICP	intracranial pressure
ICU	intensive care unit
I&D	incision and drainage
I.M.	intramuscular
I&O	intake and output
IOP	intraocular pressure
IPPB	intermittent positive-pressure breathing
IU	international unit
IUD	intrauterine device
I.V.	intravenous
K	potassium
KCl	potassium chloride
kg	kilogram
KUB	kidneys, ureters, and bladder (X-ray)
KVO	keep vein open
L	left, liter
LDL	low-density lipoprotein
LE	lower extremity
LH	luteinizing hormone
LLL	left lower lobe
LLQ	left lower quadrant
LMP	last menstrual period
LP	lumbar puncture
LUE	left upper extremity
LUL	left upper lobe
LUQ	left upper quadrant
LVEDP	left ventricular end-diastolic pressure
LVH	left ventricular hypertrophy
MAO	monoamine oxidase
MAP	mean arterial pressure
mcg	microgram
MCL	midclavicular line

mEq	milliequivalent
Mg	magnesium
mg	milligram
MI	myocardial infarction
ml	milliliter
MRI	magnetic resonance imaging
MS	multiple sclerosis; mitral stenosis
Na	sodium
N/A	not applicable
NaCl	sodium chloride
NAD	no acute distress
NAS	no added salt
NB	newborn
neg.	negative
NG	nasogastric
NICU	neonatal intensive care unit
NKA	no known allergies
NMR	nuclear magnetic resonance
NPO	nothing by mouth
NSAID	nonsteroidal anti-inflammatory drug
NSR	normal sinus rhythm
N&V	nausea and vomiting
NWB	non-weight bearing
O_2	oxygen
OB	obstetrics
OD	right eye
o.d.	daily
OL	left eye
OOB	out of bed
OPV	oral polio vaccine
OR	operating room
ORIF	open reduction internal fixation
OT	occupational therapy
OU	both eyes
P	pulse
$\bar{p}$	after
PAP	Papanicolaou (test); pulmonary artery pressure
PAT	paroxysmal atrial tachycardia
PAWP	pulmonary artery wedge pressure
p.c.	after meals
PCA	patient-controlled analgesia
PDA	patent ductus arteriosus
PE	physical examination
PERRLA	pupils equal, round, react to light and accommodation
PET	positron-emission tomography
PICC	peripherally inserted central catheter
PID	pelvic inflammatory disease
PIH	pregnancy-induced hypertension
PKU	phenylketonuria
PMH	past medical history
PMI	point of maximal impulse
PMS	premenstrual syndrome
P.O.	by mouth
pr	per rectum
PRBC	packed red blood cells
p.r.n.	as needed
PROM	passive range of motion
PT	prothrombin time, physical therapy
PTCA	percutaneous transluminal coronary angioplasty
PTT	partial thromboplastin time
PVC	premature ventricular contraction
PVD	peripheral vascular disease
q	every
q.d.	every day
q.h.	every hour
q.o.d.	every other day
q.s.	quantity sufficient

RA	rheumatoid arthritis; right atrium; right arm; renal artery
RAI	radioactive iodine
RAP	right atrial pressure
RBBB	right bundle-branch block
RBC	red blood cell
REM	rapid eye movement
Rh	Rhesus factor
RLE	right lower extremity
RLL	right lower lobe
RLQ	right lower quadrant
RML	right middle lobe
R/O	rule out
ROM	range of motion
RR	respiratory rate
R/T	related to
RUL	right upper lobe
RUQ	right upper quadrant
Rx	prescription, treatment, or therapy
$\bar{s}$	without
S.C.	subcutaneous
SG	specific gravity
SIDS	sudden infant death syndrome
S.L.	sublingual
SLE	systemic lupus erythematosus
SNF	skilled nursing facility
SOB	shortness of breath
SSE	soapsuds enema
stat	immediately
STD	sexually transmitted disease
STS	serologic test for syphilis
SVD	spontaneous vaginal delivery
$S\bar{v}o_2$	venous oxygen saturation
Sx	symptoms
T	tablespoon; temperature
T&A	tonsillectomy and adenoidectomy
TAH	total abdominal hysterectomy
TB	tuberculosis
TENS	transcutaneous electrical nerve stimulation
TIA	transient ischemic attack
t.i.d.	three times per day
T.O.	telephone order
TPN	total parenteral nutrition
TPR	temperature, pulse, and respirations
TUR	transurethral resection
TURP	transurethral resection of the prostate
U	unit
UA	urinalysis
UE	upper extremity
URI	upper respiratory infection
USP	United States Pharmacopeia
UTI	urinary tract infection
UV	ultraviolet
VAD	vascular access device; ventricular assist device
VC	vital capacity
VD	venereal disease
VDRL	Venereal Disease Research Laboratory (test)
VF	ventricular fibrillation
V.O.	verbal order
VSD	ventricular septal defect
VT	ventricular tachycardia
V_T	tidal volume
WBC	white blood cell
WNL	within normal limits
WPW	Wolff-Parkinson-White (syndrome)

Index

A

B

i refers to an illustration; t refers to a table.

E

i refers to an illustration; t refers to a table.

F

G

H

i refers to an illustration; t refers to a table.

M

N

O

i refers to an illustration; t refers to a table.

i refers to an illustration; t refers to a table.

T

i refers to an illustration; t refers to a table.

i refers to an illustration; t refers to a table.